Living in the Shadows of China HIV/AIDS Epidemics

Identifying the existing challenges and shortfalls of China's current HIV/AIDS programming, this book provides an understanding of the history of HIV/AIDS in China, comparing government responses to global best practice in prevention and treatment.

Considering three key populations in China, namely, female sex workers, people who inject drugs and floating migrants, *Living in the Shadows of China's HIV/AIDS Epidemics* highlights the effects of high mobility and marginalisation on the spread of HIV in China. It is argued that these groups often suffer from stigmatisation and a lack of human security, resulting in sub-optimal outcomes for HIV/AIDS intervention and prevention efforts and the reinforcement of high-risk behaviours, further contributing to the transmission of the virus to the general population. In adding to the emerging body of literature, this book further elucidates the myriad of challenges posed by HIV/AIDS epidemics, allowing sustained engagement and a fresh insight into how governments might respond to the needs of individuals living with HIV/AIDS, both in China and globally.

Including case studies which give voice to research participants in a rich and engaging way, this book will appeal to students and scholars of Chinese Studies, Asian Studies, International Relations and Political Science, as well as those engaged in epidemiological studies in the Health Sciences.

Shelley Torcetti received her PhD from Bond University, Australia, with a research focus on human security, people migration, trafficking, sex work, drug use and HIV/AIDS in China and South-East Asia.

Routledge Contemporary China Series

For more information about this series, please visit: www.routledge.com/ Routledge-Contemporary-China-Series/book-series/SE0768

Living in the Shadows of China's HIV/AIDS Epidemics

Sex, Drugs and Bad Blood

Shelley Torcetti

Routledge
Taylor & Francis Group

LONDON AND NEW YORK

First published 2020
by Routledge
2 Park Square, Milton Park, Abingdon, Oxon OX14 4RN

and by Routledge
52 Vanderbilt Avenue, New York, NY 10017

Routledge is an imprint of the Taylor & Francis Group, an informa business

First issued in paperback 2021

British Library Cataloguing-in-Publication Data
A catalogue record for this book is available from the British Library

Library of Congress Cataloging-in-Publication Data
A catalog record has been requested for this book

ISBN: 978-0-367-21116-5 (hbk)
ISBN: 978-1-03-209132-7 (pbk)
ISBN: 978-0-429-26548-8 (ebk)

Typeset in Times New Roman
by Wearset Ltd, Boldon, Tyne and Wear

For Lachlan and Tahlya

Contents

Illustrations

Acknowledgements

This book would not have been possible without the assistance and encouragement of a vast number of people. I would particularly like to thank the individuals from organisations in China who were willing to talk with me about the HIV/AIDS situation. Additionally, the many people living with HIV/AIDS, sex workers and people who inject drugs I met while undertaking research in China and Australia. Dr Anna Hayes, you are an absolute rock star. Dr Jonathan Ping, you told me I could do it.

Finally, because they mean the most, I would sincerely like to thank my wonderful friends and family (particularly my amazing children, Lachlan and Tahlya and Colin, who is the best kind of Superman) for their encouragement and support; endless cups of coffee; and willingness to forgive my distraction, many absences and general air of madness.

Abbreviations

AIDS	Acquired Immunodeficiency Syndrome
ART	antiretroviral therapy
ARV	antiretroviral drugs
AUSAID	Australian Government Overseas Aid Program
CBO	community-based organisation
CDC	Chinese Centre for Disease Control
CDC	Centers for Disease Control
CMOH	China's Ministry of Health
CRF	circulating recombinant form
COPRI	Copenhagen Peace Research Institute
CSW	commercial sex worker
FPD	former plasma donor
FSW	female sex worker
GALT	gut-associated lymphoid tissues
GBP	global best practice
GONGO	government-operated non-governmental organisation
GRD	Gay Related Immunodeficiency Deficiency
HAARP	HIV/AIDS Asia Regional Program
HIV	human immunodeficiency virus
HIV+	HIV-positive
HPV	human papilloma virus
IDU	intravenous drug use
IDU	injection drug user
ILO	International Labour Organisation
INGO	international non-governmental organisation
MDG	Millennium Development Goal
MMT	methadone maintenance treatment
MSM	men who have sex with men
MTCT	mother-to-child transmission
NEP	needle exchange programme
NGO	non-governmental organisation
NSP	needle-syringe programme
OI	opportunistic infection

PEP	post-exposure prophylaxis
PLWHA	people living with HIV/AIDS
PMTCT	prevention of mother-to-child-transmission
PRC	People's Republic of China
PrEP	pre-exposure prophylaxis
PWID	people who inject drugs
SARS	severe acute respiratory syndrome
SIV	simian immunodeficiency virus
SIVcpz	simian immunodeficiency virus chimpanzee
SIVsm	simian immunodeficiency virus sooty mangabeys
STI	sexually transmitted infection
TasP	treatment as prevention
TG	transgender
UN	United Nations
UNAIDS	Joint United Nations Programme on HIV/AIDS
UNDP	United Nations Development Programme
UNICEF	United Nations Children's Emergency Fund
UNODC	United Nations Office on Drugs and Crime
URFs	unique recombinant forms
VCT	voluntary counselling and testing
WHO	World Health Organization

1 Living in the shadows

A mountain cannot turn, but a road can.

山不转路转

China's ghost people

In China, there are groups of people living on the fringes of society. They are difficult to reach and often live in fear, not only of arrest but also of the inimical reactions of those with whom they come in contact. They are commercial sex workers (CSWs) (*xing gongzuozhe*), people who inject drugs (PWID) (*zhushe xidu zhe*), and China's 'floating' or undocumented internal labour migrants passing between provinces within China (*liudong renkou*), and they constitute key populations in the spread of human immunodeficiency virus/acquired immunodeficiency syndrome (HIV/AIDS) and other communicable diseases in China.

These groups operate as separate entities but are paradoxically interconnected with each other and the population as a whole. They live in the shadows both as a part of and distinct from the lives of everyday Chinese citizens. Although generally used within China to refer to transgender individuals, the term 'ghost people' (*ren yao*) also seems a fitting representation of many of the individuals from other key populations. The high mobility and marginalisation of these groups pose significant challenges to the implementation of HIV/AIDS programmes and, as such, they not only suffer from a lack of security but also constitute a non-traditional security threat to China and its proximate nation-states. This book identifies HIV/AIDS as a non-traditional security threat, and in particular a threat to human security, within these groups in China's Yunnan Province.

Yunnan is located in South-western China and borders Myanmar, Laos and Vietnam (Map 1.1). Yunnan has been selected as the site for this analysis due to its high percentages of HIV/AIDS infection; and its geographic propinquity to other states and the drug production and trafficking areas of the 'Golden Triangle'. The Golden Triangle is a major opium/heroin production area spanning the mountainous areas of Myanmar, Thailand, Laos and Vietnam (the black triangle in Map 1.1) It is close to the borders of Southern China and maintains major drug trafficking routes throughout China's Southern provinces, including

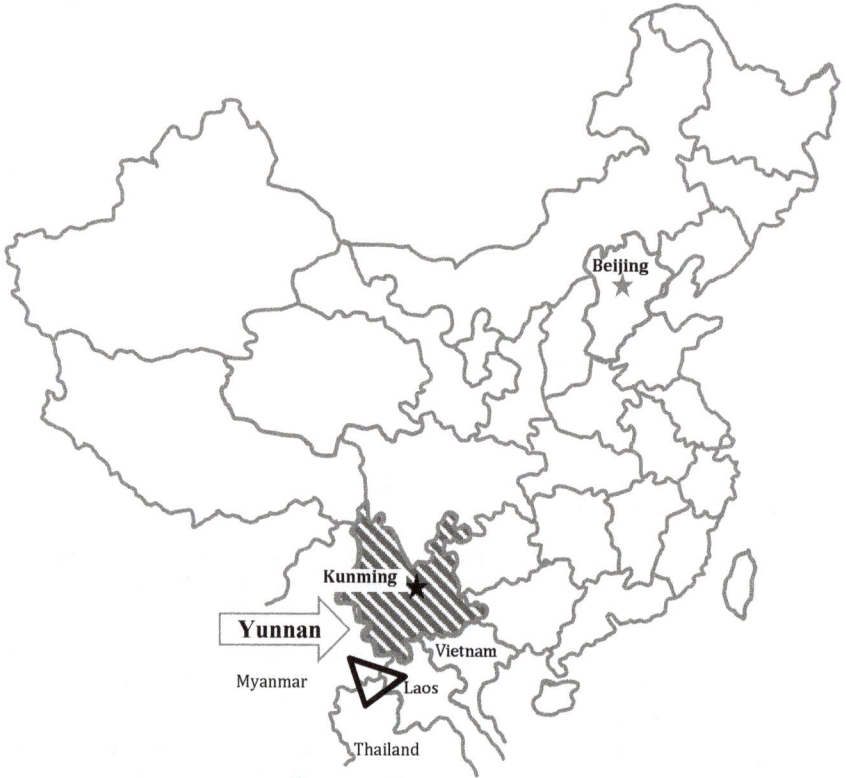

Map 1.1 Location of Yunnan Province in China.

Yunnan. These factors contribute to high rates of intravenous drug use (IDU), commercial sex work and labour migration in this site.

Within Yunnan, cross-border trade and travel between the ethnic minorities in China and bordering countries are common (Lu et al., 2008). Unfortunately, while there is cross-border trade in legitimate goods and services, there is also an illegal trade in drugs and women for both the sex industry and to be sold into coerced marriages with Chinese men (Duong, Bélanger & Hong, 2005; Qian, Schumacher, Chen & Ruan, 2006; Zhao, 2003). Significantly, Yunnan's close vicinity to its neighbours and the movement of ethnic groups straddling porous political borders allow the diffusion of HIV in and out of China, as disease crosses borders along with the migration flows of people from one locality to another (Map 1.2). Infectious disease, in this case, HIV/AIDS, threatens states not only due to a reduction in the labour force owing to illness or death but also because of the high costs associated with the treatment, prevention and education programmes targeted at reducing the impact of the disease on communities.

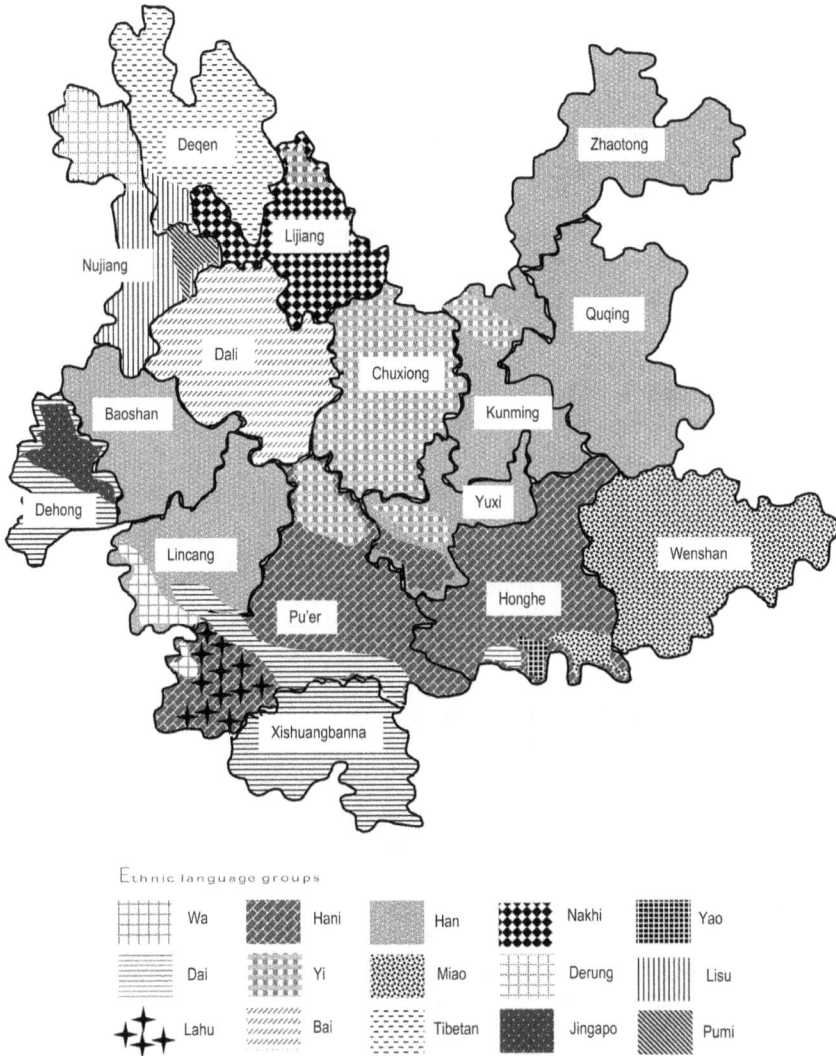

Map 1.2 Approximate distribution of ethnic minority groups in Yunnan prefectures.

Additionally, China's floating population is significant because of its large numbers (over 250 million) and the complexities of China's internal registration system. Unlike international migrants, who cross borders between countries, the floating population moves in search of work opportunities within China. This is particularly the case for rural residents who migrate into urban areas. They often do not change their provincial registration details and, as such, are considered undocumented, and therefore unable to access government services in their new location.

Additionally, these migrants are likely to return to their place of birth at significant Chinese holidays, and in particular the Chinese New Year, which may enable the transmission of communicable diseases, such as HIV. This is particularly serious for several reasons:

- an inadequate response to the escalating epidemic in the Yunnan region;
- the transnational importance of this epidemic to both China and its regional neighbours;
- the implication of these migrants in the changing transmission routes of HIV away from transmission via intravenous drug use (IDU) into a sexually driven epidemic among key populations and the wider general population.

These three cohorts share a symbiotic relationship and are generally mobile because of the demands of the labour market or fear of arrest and incarceration due to the illegal nature of their activities (Pirkle, Soundardjee & Stella, 2007; Yi, Mantell, Wu, Lu, Zeng & Wan, 2010). Not only does the HIV/AIDS epidemic disproportionally affect these marginalised groups in both concentrated and generalised epidemics but also they are often left out of AIDS programmes and face legal and structural barriers in accessing existing services (UNAIDS, 2011, p. vii). Health and prevention programmes are thus difficult to deliver and implement in mobile populations due to their constant mobility and often illegal status.

In addition to the preceding rationales for locating the research in Yunnan, China's first HIV/AIDS outbreak among people who inject drugs (PWID) was identified in 1989 in the border town of Ruili (Jia, Wang, Dye, Bao, Liu & Lu, 2010). Yunnan was not only the first to report an outbreak of HIV; it also has China's highest percentage of people living with HIV/AIDS (PLWHA) in the groups being researched (Qian, Schumacher, Chen & Ruan, 2006). These factors make it an appropriate region for this research. In the field of epidemiology 'patient zero' is of paramount importance in discerning the spread and treatment of a disease. Likewise, Yunnan is 'ground zero' for China's HIV/AIDS epidemics and therefore invaluable for clearly understanding the spread of the virus throughout the nation-state.

Consequently, the ever-changing health environment resulting from the high mobility of these groups negatively impacts the efficacy and delivery of the HIV programmes currently being offered. Therefore, this book will examine current education and prevention programmes by government, non-governmental organisations (NGOs) and international non-governmental organisations (INGOs), aimed at reducing the transmission of HIV/AIDS in these highly mobile populations. In addition to identifying the challenges of current HIV/AIDS practices in PLWHA populations, some of the shortfalls of current Chinese policies and their connection to Beijing's lack of perception of HIV/AIDS as a human security threat will be highlighted.

HIV/AIDS as a non-traditional threat to security

Traditional concerns with security have focused on realism and state-centric Westphalian notions of sovereignty and the threats from external sources faced by nation-states because of military engagements. These realist ideas of security can be observed in Cold War-type security dilemmas that use the threat of armed force, or non-military coercion in the form of political and economic sanctions, and consider nation-states to be the most important actors (Alkire 2003; Dahl-Eriksen, 2007; Newman, 2010; Selgelid & Enemark, 2008).

In International Relations, realism posits that people are basically egotistical and selfish. In addition, the international system is viewed as anarchic and, within this setting, war is not only probable but acceptable. Finally, as proposed by realist thinker Hans Morgenthau, international relations are thereby a struggle for power, and, as a result, ethical considerations cannot govern the actions of a state (Donnelly, 2005). Although traditional security issues are still a dominant concern for states, there has been a shift in thinking in the post-Cold War period. While traditional concerns with security previously concentrated on external threats to the state, this has altered somewhat due to the impacts of globalisation.

The forces of globalisation and the rapid growth in technology have redefined the space of security dialogue since the Cold War. With the advent of globalisation has come disempowerment for weaker communities and social inequalities that have created an environment for unprecedented types of security threats (Annan, 2000a; Bowsher, Milner & Sullivan, 2016). Additionally, what happens within nation-state borders can now significantly influence international spaces (Alkire 2003; Dahl-Eriksen, 2007; Newman, 2010). As such, it is no longer just states but people and the pervasive threats they face, such as poverty and infectious disease, which have increasingly become a major focus of security dialogues and, in particular, of those addressing issues of human security or the lack of human security (also termed insecurity).

Human security shares conceptual space and complements human development and human rights but differs slightly from both these concepts. Human development is broader and more holistic than human security and of concern to all states, whether rich or poor (Alkire, 2003, p. 7). Unlike human rights, human security is focused on feasibility and only addresses particular rights and freedoms directed at protecting individuals from 'freedom from fear' and 'freedom from want' (Annan, 2000b). When applied in an HIV/AIDS context, it is a useful tool for establishing those fears and wants that hamper the efforts of governments and PLWHA to halt and potentially reverse HIV/AIDS epidemics.

Thus, the following United Nations (UN) broad definition of human security, as articulated by then UN Secretary-General Kofi Annan, has been adopted as the best platform for understanding the position of PLWHA in mobile and marginalised communities in China. He stated:

> Human security, in its broadest sense, embraces far more than the absence of violent conflict. It encompasses human rights, good governance, access to

education and health care and ensuring that each individual has opportunities and choices to fulfil his or her potential. Every step in this direction is also a step towards reducing poverty, achieving economic growth and preventing conflict. Freedom from want, freedom from fear, and the freedom of future generations to inherit a healthy natural environment – these are the interrelated building blocks of human – and therefore national – security.

(Annan, 2000b, para 3)

This definition clearly articulates human security as protective and perpetrating the rights of individuals to be free from threats pertaining to their economic, food, health, environmental, personal, community and political security (Alkire, 2003; UNDP, 1994, pp. 24–25).

Within human security frameworks, these seven essentials are interlinked and affect each other. For example, economic security impacts food security; personal, political and community security can have direct impacts on an individual's ability to access health security; and food security impacts on an individual's ability to attain economic and health security; environmental security can also affect economic, community and political security (Figure 1.1). When

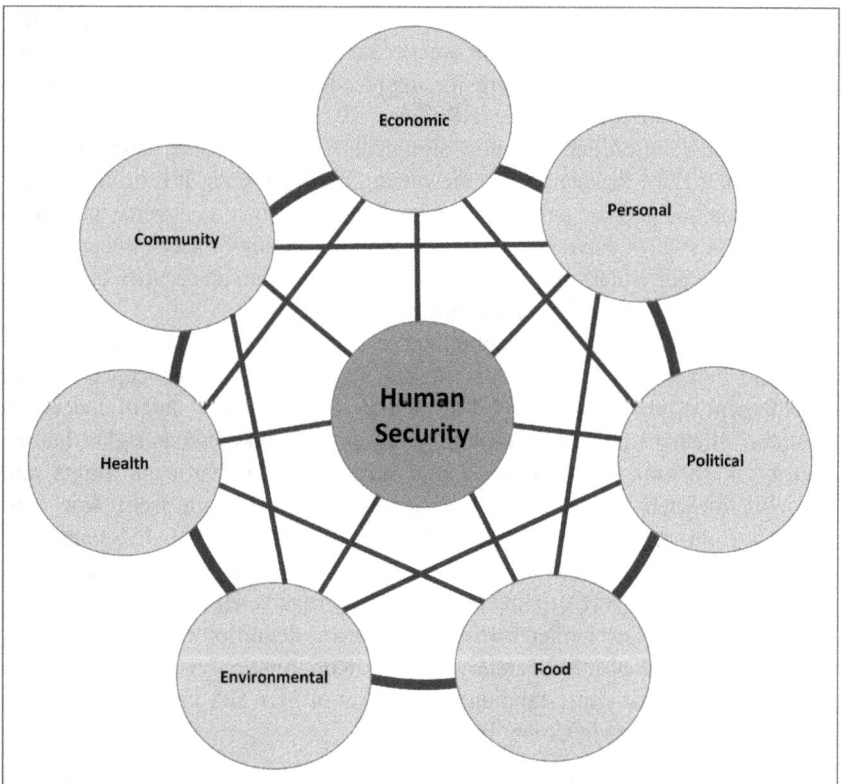

Figure 1.1 Human security.

considering these same elements ensuring security from the standpoint of insec-urity it is also accurate to state that insecurity in any one of these areas can cause insecurity in another.

Food insecurity is of particular concern within HIV/AIDS epidemics, as not only does it hinder the biological impacts and sustainability of antiretroviral therapy (ART), it also leads to high-risk behavioural pathways within HIV/AIDS epidemics (Figure 1.2). Structural drivers at a community level, such as poverty, stigmatisation and ecological (or environmental) factors, have a direct correl-ation to food insecurity. This impacts households through behaviour, poor mental health and poor nutrition. Ultimately, these make the individual more vulnerable to contracting HIV.

Thus, on an individual level, food insecurity generates three main pathways to HIV acquisition (Weiser et al., 2011). Nutritional pathways leading to

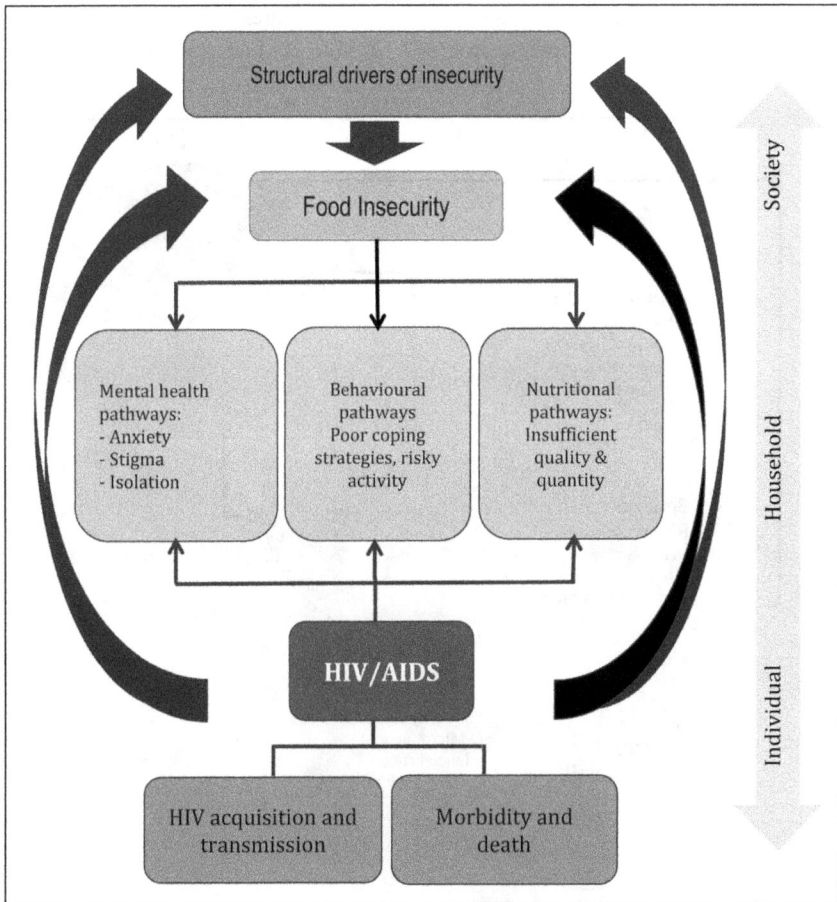

Figure 1.2 Conceptual framework for food insecurity and HIV/AIDS links.

compromised mucosal and gut integrity and micronutrient deficiencies have an effect on the PLWHA individual's abilities to maintain ART and the suppression of HIV within the body. Mental health pathways may lead to high-risk behaviours, such as alcohol abuse and drug-taking in an attempt to deal with depression and anxiety. The resulting behavioural pathways are well documented as having direct influences on HIV infectious spread and include: needle-sharing, sex in exchange for drugs, food or money, unprotected sex and increased labour migration (Figure 1.3).

Therefore, bolstering human security and addressing the areas of insecurity of PLWHA are mandatory when considering that HIV/AIDS can only be spread through the sharing of bodily fluids: (1) mucus and/or blood during sexual intercourse; (2) through the exchange of blood (e.g. sharing used injection equipment); or (3) through ingesting breast milk. It is essential therefore that treatment and prevention programmes targeting key populations approach the problem from the bottom-up. The virus is most often shared or disseminated in the intimate spaces, between individuals. This is not to suggest that sharing is always consensual. It might be forced, coerced, or due to peer pressure, gendered

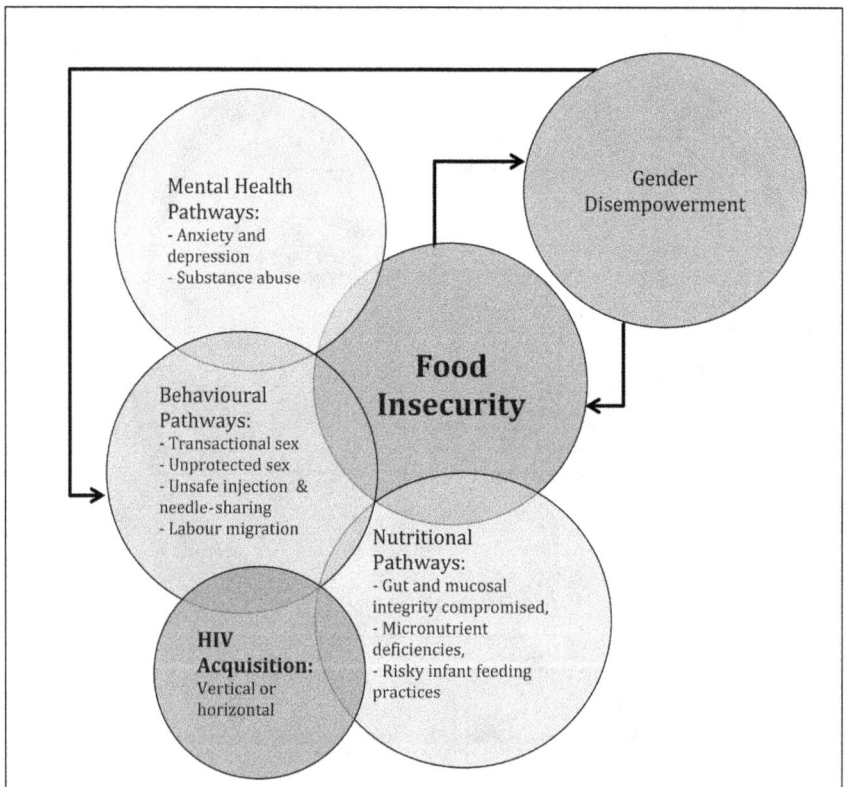

Figure 1.3 Food insecurity and HIV acquisition.

stereotypes, and so forth. However, the space where that event generally takes place is still intimate – person-to-person.

The virus cannot be contracted through contact with a residue or breathed through the air. Two (or more) people must make contact and share an event that leads to the virus transmission from one to the other. This is particularly so since iatrogenic transmission through blood transfusion, while still occurring occasionally, is now considered unacceptable due to regulated blood collection practices. If the disease spreads in the intimate spaces, the solutions must also be implemented in the intimate spaces. Thus, the risk-taking behaviours, and the human insecurity instigating those behaviours, must be addressed before sustainable change can occur on the macro-level of the nation-state and the global community.

This is certainly the case in China simply due to the size of the population, and the potential that the current HIV/AIDS epidemic could rapidly spread if not well managed. For example:

> If a pandemic of HIV/AIDS occurs in Mainland China, which has over 1/5 of the world's population, it will not only damage the national economy of China but also it can be an economic disaster for the rest of the world.
>
> (Qin et al., 2005, p. 1480)

Undoubtedly, the HIV/AIDS epidemic in China is a human security threat, not only to the economic growth and poverty reduction of the state but also to the health and well-being of individuals, particularly those who are hard to reach due to stigmatisation and marginalisation.

The extent of China's epidemic

The most recent China AIDS Response Progress Report of the Joint United Nations Programme on HIV/AIDS (UNAIDS, 2015, p. 15) announced figures, generated by 1,881 sentinel surveillance sites in China, revealing 103,501 newly reported cases of HIV in China. The overall number of reported cases of PLWHA in China was stated to be 501,000 at the conclusion of 2014 (UNAIDS, 2015, p. 7). Interestingly, the previous 2014 report states that 437,000 PLWHA were reported to be living in China at the end of 2013 (UNAIDS, 2014a). This shows an increase of 64,000 PLWHA over the course of one year. The discrepancy in the two figures presented in 2014 and 2015 does not seem to correlate to a decreasing epidemic. Additionally, there were a number of deaths from AIDS; which were recorded as 159,000 (UNAIDS, 2015, p. 7).

Figures are fluid and problematic to verify concerning HIV/AIDS in China. As an example of this, in contrast to the lower 2015 figures (501,000), the 2012 AIDS response progress report estimated the epidemic in China at 780,000 PLWHA (UNAIDS & CMOH, 2012, p. 6). The 2017 figures were once again reported as 758,610 with 134,512 newly diagnosed infections (NCAIDS, NCSTD, China CDC, 2017; Su et al., 2018). It is possible that the divergent nature of the 2012, 2017 and 2015 figures is due to one being an estimate and the others being actual reported cases, but if that is so, then the 2015 figure needs to be revised upwards to account for PLWHA who remain ignorant of their HIV+ status. Apart from the undiagnosed status of some PLWHA, there is also evidence to suggest that figures are impacted by under-reporting of HIV/AIDS in China (Saich, 2006). Additionally, China's surveillance coverage is reliant on key populations accessing health services, but disadvantaged subgroups are likely to be under-represented (L. Zhang et al., 2013). As a result of the difficulties in determining the veracity of China's HIV/AIDS figures, caution needs to be exercised in representing those figures.

What the reports do agree on is that China's HIV/AIDS epidemics are being expanded by a number of newly diagnosed PLWHA every year. Overall, in the Asian region, responses to the epidemic are being outpaced and there are nearly two newly diagnosed HIV infections for every HIV+ individual commencing antiretroviral therapy (ART) (UNAIDS, 2011, p. 20). In light of the infection rates globally, and in China specifically, preventative measures need to be escalated and effects of human insecurity mitigated in order to halt the continued spread of HIV.

UNAIDS, and the HIV/AIDS community at large, currently support the 'know your epidemic, know your response' message. This message advocates that HIV/AIDS data collection efforts should be fine-tuned to understand the dimensions of local epidemics in drafting effective national responses (Kurth, Celum, Baeten, Vermund & Wasserheit, 2011; Mishra et al., 2012; Sgaier et al., 2012; UNAIDS, 2011). From the start of the epidemic in China HIV/AIDS has predominantly affected people who inject drugs (PWID) but, in 2007, the Joint Assessment on AIDS in China identified that the main route for transmission of HIV in China had changed from PWID to heterosexual transmission with female sex workers (FSWs) (*jinü* or more recently *Xiaojie*) acting as bridging populations to the general community (Figure 1.4).

Historically, in China, drug abuse and prostitution have been considered social evils, as they operate outside the acceptable moral practices espoused by Chinese Confucian philosophy (Ding, Li & Ji, 2011; Qian et al., 2006; Yang & Kleinman, 2008). As a result, commercial sex workers (CSWs) and PWID are often stigmatised and marginalised. While Confucianism is only one of many reasons for this stigmatisation, it does play a part in the overall situation for PWID and FSWs and particularly those who are PLWHA. Although, stigmatisation is a problem for PLWHA globally, and in situations where Confucianism is not followed, it is driven by cultural beliefs unique to each particular society. Confucianism remains an underpinning belief system in China and it is therefore appropriate to comment on the effect that it has within a China HIV/AIDS context.

People live within a variety of social contexts and these contexts provide the frameworks used to ascertain whether someone is a good or bad person (Hwang, 1999). Additionally, the concept of filial piety informs Chinese patterns of socialisation, creating a hierarchical social structure and a ubiquitous propensity

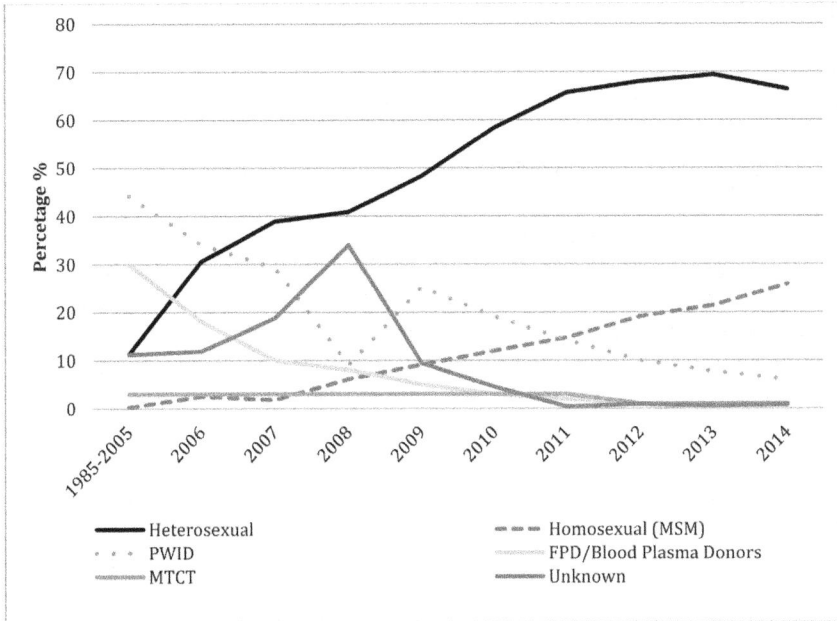

Figure 1.4 Transmission modes of newly diagnosed cases of HIV/AIDS by year, 1995–2014.

to judge individuals against moral standards and precepts (Hwang, 1999). Individuals operating within these filial attitudes are found to be more likely to subscribe to fatalistic, superstitious and stereotypical beliefs and have personal characteristics such as dogmatism, authoritarianism and high conformity (Hwang, 1999, p. 178). Thus, when the moral standards, attitudes and modes of behaviour operating within Confucian culture judge drug use and sex work to be social evils and those practising them to be bad, individuals within a society follow this stereotypical belief, which results in stigmatisation.

When the issue of living with HIV/AIDS is added to the mix, these groups are pushed even further back to the periphery of society, making them not only difficult to interact with, but to all intents and purposes shadow populations within their own country. Thus, highly mobile PLWHA might be seen as a new type of minority group beyond the interest and care of Beijing and conservative Han society (Hood, 2005). The stigmatisation and marginalisation of this new shadow minority have been exacerbated by state-sanctioned media portrayals reflective of Beijing's general attitude towards PLWHA. PLWHA are often portrayed as being unsafe, and only belonging to a certain class, occupation or ethnicity.

This has led to individuals believing themselves to be immune to HIV and therefore engaging in high-risk behaviours. They may also be afraid to be tested due to concerns that a HIV+ diagnosis will lead to stigmatisation and discrimination (Burki, 2011; Hood, 2012; Li, Wu, Wu, Sun, Cui & Jia, 2006). One of the outcomes of an individual's disinclination to be tested for HIV/AIDS is the potential skewing of HIV/AIDS sentinel surveillance figures leading to underestimation of HIV/AIDS statistics. Stigma and marginalisation also greatly contribute to the likelihood that PLWHA will suffer from human insecurity, and be unable to procure ART medications, access health services or prevention initiatives.

Therefore, this potential community rejection of PLWHA has consequences not only for the spread of HIV but also for the management of HIV health programmes and ART maintenance (Lin, Li, Wu, Wu & Jia, 2008; L. Li, et al., 2010). Those working in health care settings that offer services to PLWHA may also perpetuate and suffer from the same issues of stigmatisation and are therefore reluctant to treat PLWHA (L. Li et al., 2007; Lin, Wu, Wu, Rotheram-Borus, Detels & Jia, 2007; Lin et al., 2008). This has obvious implications for the expansion of HIV in China as a non-traditional security threat to China and the world. If those who are tasked with providing their medical assistance are reluctant to engage with PLWHA, this patient group cannot receive efficient, or sufficient, assistance to manage their disease or understand prevention initiatives.

Since HIV first became recognised as an epidemic in Yunnan, it has spread throughout all of China's provinces, with two other distinct outbreaks in PWID in Xinjiang and former plasma donors (FPD) in Henan. Blood selling to unregulated blood collectors (known as blood-heads), clinics and other pharmaceutical concerns became popular as way to raise revenue for impoverished farmers in Henan during the 1990s. However, unsafe collection practices, including reinjection of pooled blood donations, led to high numbers of donors, in particular, majority Han Chinese, becoming infected with HIV (Hayes, 2005). This group of PLWHA was significant as the virus was impacting the ethnic majority and could no longer be considered a disease exclusive to ethnic minorities and morally corrupt people.

When HIV was believed to be confined to foreigners, ethnic minorities and injecting drug users, Beijing and China's general population seemed to have little sympathy for those living with the virus. Even as late as the end of the 1990s, most urban Chinese were unaware of PLWHA in the Han ethnic majority. There was no politically sanctioned media discourse of the rising epidemic, and the government, while making some preparations, largely ignored the problem (Hayes, 2005; Hood, 2012). Two events occurred to change the situation in the very late 1990s and early 2000s: (1) the Chinese government were forced to acknowledge the problem after UNAIDS released their 2002 *HIV/AIDS: China's Titanic Peril* report, predicting that, without action, China could have 10–20 million HIV+ people by 2010; and (2) several doctors began diagnosing HIV and reporting their findings to the authorities and the media (Hood, 2012).

Significantly, it was not until the public were made aware of HIV in the Henan blood plasma donors, a disaster made public despite reporters being told to 'tread carefully' due to state media prohibitions (Stern & O'Brien, 2011, p. 8), that both community and government support began to be mobilised. One reason for this was that the Henan plasma donors (while still enduring stigma) were deemed to be innocent sufferers; and as they had not violated the values esteemed by society, they were afforded some sympathy. Even so, Beijing still expended little effort to address the burgeoning problem of HIV/AIDS in China.

The pivotal health care nexus inducing Beijing to seriously consider the ramifications of HIV/AIDS epidemics within the country occurred due to the events surrounding the severe acute respiratory syndrome (SARS) outbreak.[1] Beijing was finally pushed to contemplate HIV as a non-traditional security threat requiring serious discourse. The cover-ups and deceptions that had proliferated during the SARS crisis were greeted unfavourably by the international community and Beijing was motivated to address the issue as a threat to all nations; therefore, as a follow-on from this, China began to seriously examine the issue of HIV within its borders (Knutsen, 2012; Wishnick, 2010). Thus, with these external and internal push-pull factors placing Beijing under international scrutiny and increasing public pressure, the state began implementing health policies specifically dealing with HIV/AIDS (Knutsen, 2012).

This resulted in harm reduction programmes for injecting drug users and a national HIV health care programme labelled the 'Four Free and One Care'. This policy states:

> Free ARV drugs will be given to all rural AIDS patients and urban AIDS patients facing financial difficulties; free voluntary counseling and testing (VCT) will be provided in high prevalence areas; free VCT and prevention of mother-to-child transmission (PMCT) services will be provided for pregnant women; free education will be available for children orphaned by HIV/ AIDS; and care will be given to all AIDS patients facing financial difficulties.
>
> (Zhang et al., 2006, p. 98)

Regardless of the implied intent of the Four Free and One Care policy to make HIV/AIDS care available to everyone, there is still a lack of adequate care for PLWHA in China. Additionally, there is a lack of equity in the distribution of services under this programme.

Continuing concerns regarding the expansion of HIV/AIDS in China include

- the epidemics' concentration in rural areas;
- chronic under-funding of rural health services, resulting in low capacity to deal with a burgeoning HIV epidemic;
- high costs of services which place them out of reach of many patients;
- under-reporting of cases and misdiagnosis;
- poor levels of training and lack of personnel to conduct laboratory testing;
- the refusal of some hospitals to accept HIV patients (Saich, 2006; Yip, 2006; Zhang et al., 2006).

Added to which, there have been new concerns about China's blood collection practices, with blood supplies reportedly found to be contaminated with HIV as recently as February 2019 (Needham, 2019).

Although costs of health care for PLWHA are high, they will only continue to increase unless a solution is found. At the present moment ,there is a narrow window of opportunity to obviate an epidemic that will be even costlier with regards to human suffering and increased medical system costs from treating high numbers of patients (Saich, 2006, pp. 93–94). With rates of HIV increasing in China, there were a reported 103,501 new infections in 2014 (UNAIDS, 2015, p. 15), thus, it is essential that Beijing should address the shortfalls in current HIV policies. An essential component in addressing the current shortfalls is mitigating the threats to the human security of PLWHA, particularly in key populations, who are generally very vulnerable and most in need of holistic interventions to tackle the disease and associated essentials, such as poverty alleviation, stigma and community engagement.

In summary, while in part working within a non-traditional security threat context as a result of SARS, to date, Beijing seems to have no intention of embracing a human security framework in shaping an effective response to the HIV/AIDS epidemic. Their responses have been inadequate, particularly in mobile populations. Although there are many vectors[2] or modes of transmission for HIV in China, such as men who have sex with men (MSM), former plasma donors (FPD), mother-to-child transmission (MTCT), CSWs, PWID and some migrant populations, rates of infection differ across these cohorts. Therefore, CSWs (specifically FSWs due to their higher numbers and increased vulnerability based on unfavourable gendered norms), PWID and the undocumented floating migrant population will be the focus of this book, as the groups with the highest rates of infection found in China's Yunnan Province.

In order to effectively prevent the transmission of HIV among these highly mobile and marginalised populations, it is important to examine the factors that increase HIV vulnerability. There is also a lack of human security encountered within a state and society that stigmatises, marginalises, and thereby places key populations at the threshold of the conventional assistance offered by Beijing. As such, there needs to be a more complete understanding of the characteristic value of human security frameworks in dealing with the existing HIV/AIDS epidemic in China.

Methodology

The interviews that inform the analysis were undertaken from October to December 2013 and June 2014 in Beijing and Yunnan Province in Southern China. All interviews were conducted with members of NGOs and community-based organisations (CBOs) operating in an HIV/AIDS context in China. Additionally, all participants held posts of authority within their organisations or operated as leaders or peers in HIV/AIDS outreaches and are thus sufficiently knowledgeable in their areas of operation. The expert nature of these individuals and the peer workers operating within key populations allows a comprehensive understanding of the underpinning issues faced by the majority of individuals in these contexts. Moreover, there was consensus among all interview participants. The issues, or challenges and shortfalls, identified within China's HIV/AIDS contexts (as negotiated by these experts in the field) were similar in Beijing, and the areas in and around Kunming and Ruili where most interviews and observations were conducted.

Due to the highly sensitive nature of the research, the anonymity of all participants was assured and, as such, any information allowing the identification of any person has been removed. This includes names of participants, the names of the organisations, and the names of some townships where observations were carried out. Rather, participants will be identified in this chapter by replacing their real names with some of the most common surnames in China. This was necessary to ensure that people had the confidence to provide comprehensive information regarding the situation. Without these assurances of strict confidentiality, it would have been virtually impossible to find any willing participants, due to fear of reprisals.

The main reason for this emphasis on anonymity is that in China there is still a culture of reluctance to be seen to be criticising the government. Members of some other NGOs who were approached declined to participate, regardless of assurances of anonymity, as they felt that there was still some risk implicit in speaking on the subject at all. Some commented that meeting a HIV/AIDS researcher in even the most casual of encounters might shine a spotlight on them or possibly get them into trouble. In email conversations where interviews were declined, stated reasons included, As there is a stigma when dealing with HIV etc, [*sic*] these projects might be a bit sensitive to interview' (pers. comm., 10 March, 2013) and, 'I have spoken to our leaders and we all agree that due to the sensitivity of these projects, we can't have any interventions at this stage' (pers. comm., 3 July, 2013).

This reluctance to talk did cause some limitations on the number of participants who were willing to be interviewed, and it speaks volumes about the operational climate for NGOs involved in this area. It appears that HIV/AIDS is still a sensitive subject for Beijing. This obviously has implications for those who are working on the ground but it appears that some NGOs are prepared to work in a restrictive environment if it means that they can deliver HIV/AIDS programmes. When their safety was assured, there were a number of people keen to identify areas where current programmes and policy might be improved. They were able to provide valuable insights into the current HIV/AIDS situation in China and identify emerging trends for the spread of infection in Yunnan specifically and China in general.

While undertaking the research, there was opportunity to observe several programmes in action and gain an understanding of the restrictions as well as the accessibility that NGO workers face on the ground. This ethnographic approach allowed the observation of interactions between NGO staff and recipients. It also permitted an insight into the living situation and daily issues facing HIV+ individuals in

Yunnan. It is one thing to understand the literature but quite another to gain an understanding of the issue in situ (some of these examples are presented in the case studies concluding each chapter). This was particularly the case when the opportunity arose to spend time visiting HIV+ PWID and FSWs in their township environments where they live. All recipients of the NGOs' resources were living in poverty, were unemployed (unless engaged in sex work) and highly stigmatised by the rest of the township.

While the names of some smaller townships have been omitted and the interview participants may have travelled from other areas, it is possible to say that interviews took place in Beijing, Kunming and Ruili. The interview participants were all employed in both paid and/or volunteer positions with organisations currently active in the delivery and preparation of HIV/AIDS programmes in highly mobile population groups in China. Some of the individuals spoken to (via an NGO interpreter) were employed by NGOs in peer roles and were themselves PWID, FSWs or migrants (or a combination of two or more of the three cohorts), all of whom were HIV+. Although there was an opportunity to ask questions, these interactions are not considered as interviews and rather come under the umbrella of incidental conversations and their value lies solely in their contribution to a general understanding of the HIV/AIDS situation in China. In saying that, they have also featured in a number of the case studies.

According to the data gathered during interviews, incidental conversations and observations, improvements must be made before China effectively deals with its still expanding HIV epidemic. While there have been enormous strides forward over the past two decades, there are a number of areas where effective interventions appear to be lacking in scope and number. Some of the reasons for this may stem from the basic premise with which the epidemic is viewed in China. Stigma and discrimination of PLWHA are continuing problems that may stem directly from the lack of basic human security.

Study limitations

Doing research in China can prove problematic. Chinese authorities are often reluctant to grant foreign scholars entry into areas that it deems to be sensitive and which may possibly cause the government to 'lose face' (Yang & Le, 2008, p. 117). Significantly, this reluctance to lose face in the international community can cause Beijing to 'brush aside concerns' and avoid accepting blame for sensitive issues (Bate, 2012, pp. 178–179).

The key populations being examined are highly mobile and operate on the fringes of society. This is in part, due to their illegal status and the covert nature of their practices (Ding et al., 2005). This results in members of the communities being suspicious of strangers and fearful of drawing attention to themselves. This mistrust may well extend to include health workers and organisations that interact with the populations being researched. For politically sensitive issues such as HIV, there is a lot of mistrust of researchers because of concerns that they will not correctly interpret the facts, which may potentially result in damage to the country as a whole (Yang & Le, 2008, p. 122).

China has many vectors for the spread of HIV but the focus of this book is PWID, CSWs and the floating migrant populations. While there are reasonably high rates of infection in MTCT, MSM, and FPDs, they constitute a smaller number of the overall epidemic. Conversely, there are still high numbers of new infections in PWID populations. However, this is changing with China's highest rates of new infection occurring through sexual interactions, including those in MSM populations. Migrant populations are implicated in the spread of HIV, both due to an adoption of high-risk behaviours away from their home communities, and the potential for introducing HIV into a number of new areas as they move from one location to another. Additionally, FSWs, PWID and the floating populations are currently those with the highest rates of HIV and include the initial cohort for the spread of HIV in China and the primary sources of emergent infections.

In summary, due to the difficulties involved in researching sensitive issues in China, the reluctance of Chinese authorities to grant foreign researchers access to target sites and populations and, given the nature of cross-cultural research, there are several limitations on this study. Even so, these limitations have not precluded the gathering of valuable and pertinent information that highlight China's current policies on HIV/AIDS in mobile populations and their recognition or lack thereof of HIV as a non-traditional (human security) threat.

Issues of human security

The fact that China approaches the epidemic almost solely from a public health model means that their concern lies with the general public and halting the spread of HIV into the general population. While it is essential to deal with the spread of HIV into the general population, this should not be done in a manner that deprives those who are already HIV+ from having their basic human security needs addressed. Perfunctorily, it seems reasonable to disregard the human security of PLWHA in the pursuit of the greater good. However, if their right to human security for all is upheld, it will make a positive contribution to the prevalent non-traditional threat to security that the epidemic poses to China as well as contributing to halting the spread of the disease.

The human security of the individual should become paramount in the midst of HIV/AIDS epidemics (McIntosh & Hunter, 2010). The UN has contextualised the situation within a human security framework (UN, 2000). In protecting the human security of the individual, both PLWHA and those in the general population, the dilemma of whether to consider the rights of the individual or the population as a whole becomes a moot point. They are complementary goals (Ogata & Sen, 2003). When PLWHA are enabled and free from fear and want, then they can become productive members of society; less of a burden on the financial agendas of the government; and they will suffer less under the burden of marginalisation and stigma (Fukuda-Parr, 2003; Nishikawa, 2009).

When introducing the subject of human security during research interviews, most participants felt that Beijing was too little concerned. Two participants conceded that the rights of PLWHA and high-risk individuals were important as long as they did not interfere with the overarching goal of assuring public health (Chen, pers. comm., October 2013; Wang, pers. comm., November 2013). Therefore, all concerns with the individual are circumvented when they are perceived to impinge upon public rights and concerns with safety. Moreover, there was no consensus concerning the point where the rights of the individual no longer mattered. Rather, there was just a general idea that the public good mattered more. This seems particularly concerning, given that these populations are already highly vulnerable, marginalised and stigmatised.

Therefore, what if it were deemed best for public health if PLWHA were hidden from interaction with the public at all? China already has mandatory re-education and treatment centres for FSWs and PWID. It may seem a trifle extreme to consider the option of mandatory treatment centres for HIV/AIDS in China, but where the human security of the individual is disregarded when juxtaposed with that of the general public, then it becomes a possibility. No one who was interviewed or observed implementing HIV/AIDS programmes was of the opinion that PLWHA should be detained. One person actually pointed out that the PLWHA they were assisting were fathers and mothers who worked to support family units and positively contributed to the economy (Liu, pers. comm., October 2013).

However, in incidental conversations with some members of the general public, they expressed the belief that they would feel safer if detention became a reality. It seems that, in some quarters at least, there is still a sense of fear concerning the potential metastasising of HIV/AIDS among the general population. One person who held this view was university educated. Thus, it is not just a lack of education per se at the root of this disquieting opinion but rather a lack of effective education on the topic of HIV/AIDS. This is even more concerning when coupled with the understanding that school children and university students do receive some education on HIV/AIDS. Consequently, the question arises whether they fully understand the educational materials and information provided or whether the materials and methods are effective.

World AIDS Day activities

In China, World AIDS Day is traditionally the day for the dissemination of HIV/AIDS-related material. It is seen as an opportunity to educate students and the general public concerning issues of stigma; the vectors for the spread of HIV; and steps that can be taken to reduce the risk of contracting the disease. During the research in Kunming, the press and web pages (such as *GoKunming*) were scanned regularly, television programmes were watched, and, in particular, any events that were being hosted on World AIDS Day were attended. While there was one television advertisement dealing with the issue of HIV, there were no specific newspaper articles and only the *China Daily*, (as the paramount broadsheet newspaper) was scrutinised.

The *China Daily*, Kunming television programming and *GoKunming*, an English-language website detailing what is on in Kunming, were specifically chosen for scrutiny as these information platforms are the most popular sources of news and community information for the majority of Kunming residents. Thus, any attempts to disseminate information with the intention of reaching the highest volume of audience when advertising World AIDS Day activities would certainly have appeared in the *China Daily*, Kunming television programmes or on *GoKunming*. What was concerning was the lack of any obvious mention, in any of the sources perused, of any events to attend in Kunming on World AIDS Day.

When one interview participant was asked why this was the case, they commented that in China World Aids Day events had been very 'low key' for that year (2013) (Chen, pers. comm., October 2013). They volunteered the information that all major international non-governmental organisations (INGOs) had recently withdrawn or were in the process of withdrawing from China (with the exception of the Gates Foundation, which is still currently supporting at least one NGO employing one of the interview participants). As a result of this withdrawal and the handing over of the financial burden to Beijing, a funding freeze had been instigated while extensive research was done on the best allocation of funds. As such, it is possible that the withdrawal of major HIV/AIDS INGOs from China and Beijing's subsequent freeze on funds may have contributed to the lack of HIV/AIDS education and awareness events in Kunming.

While the majority of this research took place from October 2013 to December 2013, a follow-up visit to China took place in July 2014 and one of the interview respondents, Chen (none of the other respondents indicated a willingness for further contact) was re-interviewed. Chen revealed that the 2014/2015 funding year, budget figures for HIV/AIDs expenditure for the entire Yunnan Province had been released the day before the interview. It totalled 5 million yuan or, as he stressed, 1 million Australian dollars. When asked if he thought this was sufficient, Chen replied, 'Of course not. But in China we can do a lot with a little bit of money' (pers. comm., July 2014). Chen stated that the allocation of these funds was for the entirety of HIV/AIDS services and that of the amount allocated, 35 per cent of that amount would be used for NGO wages and other running costs. In real terms then, only 65 per cent of the fund were available for programming activities.

Chen went on to state that in the entire province of Yunnan, there were only a handful, less than six, full-time HIV/AIDS NGOs in operation. In practice, NGOs formed or disbanded as funding became available. Since there is no ongoing funding, they must apply for funding grants for specific HIV/AIDS initiatives and when the money runs out, they are forced to close their doors. Even though Chen worked in one of the full-time HIV/AIDS NGOs in China, he stated that it was still necessary to apply for further funding from INGOs and other donors to maintain existing projects. He ended the interview on a positive note stating that although there had been some challenges, including a lack of funding, a lot of good work had been done in the six months between interviews.

This included working to set up a permanent camp for homeless PWID, several initiatives with Myanmar cross-border PLWHA and support for programmes in refugee camps along the China/Myanmar border.

In order to test the veracity of the information provided by Chen (pers. comm., July 2014), information was sought from members of the China Centre for Disease Control (CDC). This took place at the AIDS 2014 conference in Melbourne, where there were several members of China's CDC in attendance. When questioned about the 5 million yuan figure, they were unwilling to make a comment except to say that it seemed low and therefore could not be correct. However, they did confirm Chen's statement that NGOs were seeking extra funding from sources other than Beijing. Additionally, although they declined to produce any data in support of their argument against the information provided by Chen, they were particularly concerned that the figure of 5 million yuan should not be made public, directly requesting that it not be presented in this book. They were also keen to find out the name of my source and seemed to be unimpressed and slightly agitated when that information was not forthcoming. Thus. it is apparent that Beijing is still reluctant to be open and forthcoming concerning the exact nature of the HIV/AIDS operational environment in China.

Literature review

Over the past 30 years, the global HIV/AIDS pandemic has been of persistent concern to governments, researchers and individuals. In 2014, UNAIDS set a new target for the end of the AIDS epidemic by 2030. The 90–90–90 cascade care targets for HIV state that, by 2020, 90 per cent of PLWHA will be diagnosed; 90 per cent of those diagnosed will be on ART; and 90 per cent of the people on treatment will achieve viral suppression (UNAIDS, 2014b). These initiatives rely on HIV testing, ART scale-up and viral suppression (Marukutira et al., 2018). As a result, by 2020, 73 per cent (86 per cent by 2030) of all PLWHA should be virally suppressed and on ART (Granich, Williams, Montaner & Zuniga, 2017). These targets were expanded in 2016 to include a rapid scale-up of prevention and treatment services, such as

- the eradication of new infections for children;
- access to combination HIV prevention options;
- pre-exposure prophylaxis (PrEP);
- male circumcision;
- elimination of gender inequity and violence;
- the adoption of a zero discrimination policy (Marukutira et al., 2018).

Although UNAIDS data suggest that in recent years the incidence of infection has stabilised, and even began to wane in some countries with generalised epidemics, there are still an alarming number of people becoming infected every year. UNAIDS (2011, p. 1) estimates that 2.7 million people, equating to almost 7,500 people per day, were newly affected with HIV in 2010.

Country-specific figures suggest China's current estimated HIV/AIDS burden to be 780,000 PLWHA with some 103,501 new infections for 2014 (UNAIDS, 2015, p. 15; UNAIDS & CMOH, 2012, p. 6). Much research has been done on the HIV/AIDS pandemic globally (particularly in Sub-Saharan Africa) and in China, and, therefore, it is possible to gain a comprehensive understanding of the general trajectory of China's site-specific HIV/AIDS epidemics. When considering the high numbers of new infections, and the continuing financial and social burden of the disease on states and their populace, it is apparent that HIV/AIDS persists as a significant non-traditional security threat.

HIV/AIDS first became securitised by the UN in the year 2000 with the drafting of Resolution 1308, and since that time there has been vigorous debate about how best to contextualise the issue as a human security threat or, indeed, whether it should be done at all (Elbe, 2006; Kettemann, 2006). The literature on International Relations theory, concerning the conceptual shift in the previously state-centric viewpoint of security since globalisation, is well represented by Alkire (2003), Fukuda-Parr (2003), Dahl-Eriksen (2007) and Newman (2010). They suggest that while traditional concerns with security are still prominent, issues faced by individuals and their rights to live in 'freedom from fear' and 'freedom from want' are becoming more important to policy-makers. Conceptualised by human security theories, issues such as poverty, environmental devastation, hunger, gender inequity and infectious disease are now on the international agenda.

In presenting HIV/AIDS as a non-traditional security threat at the UN Security Council, Gore (2000) used traditional concerns with security as a scaffold by conceptualising the struggle against the HIV epidemic as a war, stating: 'The United Nations was created to stop wars. Now, we must wage and win a great and peaceful war of our time – the war against AIDS' (para. 25). In July 2000, UN Resolution 1308 was passed, raising concerns with HIV/AIDS in a human security context to appear on the UN agenda. This was the first time that HIV/AIDS had been considered in the context of a non-traditional threat to security. While it was the USA who first presented HIV as a non-traditional threat to security, they were not alone in situating HIV as a threat. Due to the scale and impact of HIV/AIDS globally, there was a distinct desire internationally to securitise HIV, and understandings of its risk to security have continued to develop since this time (Hindmarch, 2016).

Since that time the UN has continued to develop a common understanding of human security. In September 2012, at the 66th UN General Assembly, the UN adopted a consensus text on human security as proposed in paragraph 143 of the 2005 World Summit Outcome stating:

[A] common understanding on the notion of human security would include the right of people to live in freedom and dignity; a call for people-centred, comprehensive, context-specific and prevention-oriented responses that strengthened the protection and empowerment of all people and all

communities; and recognition of the interlinkages between peace, development and human rights, and equally considered civil, political, economic,
social and cultural rights.

(para. 20)

However, there is continuing conceptual debate about human security and
whether infectious diseases such as HIV/AIDS should be securitised. Some
debates on human security focus on the lack of clarity and the range of current
definitions and question their workability in international arenas (Aldis, 2008;
Kettemann, 2006; Newman, 2010).

Newman (2010, p. 78) submits that human security is normative and involves
reshaping security around the individual according to international standards of
human rights and governance. He suggests that '[it] seeks to challenge attitudes
and institutions that privilege so-called 'high politics' above individual experiences of deprivation and insecurity' (2010, p. 79). A report by the Commission
on Human Security states:

> Human security complements state security, enhances human rights and
> strengthens human development. It seeks to protect people against a broad
> range of threats to individuals and communities and, further, to empower
> them to act on their own behalf. And it seeks to forge a global alliance to
> strengthen the institutional policies that link individuals and the state – and
> the state with a global world.
>
> (Ogata & Sen, 2003, pp. 2, 4)

In other words, the ultimate purpose of human security is to establish safeguards
for the vital core of human life by protecting individuals from pervasive threats
and thereby enable long-term human fulfilment (Alkire, 2003, p. 2). Hayes
(2007, 2012) touches on some similar issues and introduces the concept of
human security as it applies to the HIV situation in China. Therefore, a human
security framework is essential in shaping responses to the ubiquitous non-
traditional security threats, including HIV/AIDS, faced by states and individuals
in the current globalised environment.

However, human security is not as firmly entrenched in international security
dialogues as many people believe. Rushton (2010) suggests that the UN has not
really accepted HIV/AIDS as a human security threat. Rushton's stance is reiterated in a corroborative article with McInnes, suggesting that securitisation of
HIV/AIDS was only partially successful (McInnes & Rushton, 2010, p. 234). To
the contrary, these arguments are questionable in light of the 2012 resolution by
the UN to seek common understandings of human security (UN, 2012). Clearly,
human security is still on the UN agenda and as yet there has been no repeal of
the existing broader definitions such as those submitted by Annan (2000a) and
Gore (2000), which includes infectious disease and HIV/AIDs specifically.
Despite this, there is no consensus on whether infectious disease should be conceptualised as a human security threat.

Scholars such as Aldis (2008), Wishnick (2010) and Selgelid and Enemark (2008) suggest that the securitisation of infectious disease can be problematic due to associated stigma and suspicion related to definitions pertaining to health security. Wishnick (2010, p. 463) uses the HIV pandemic and the SARS outbreak in China as case studies and suggests that securitisation can lead to certain groups having their civil liberties restricted or being stigmatised, resulting in refusals to share data and in excessive penalties. Other theorists question the effectiveness or benefit of securitising diseases such as HIV/AIDS (Rushton, 2010). Additionally, some proponents of the Copenhagen School suggest securitisation of infectious disease can create some situations where resources and political will are disproportionate to the problem, resulting in fear and loss of freedoms and human rights for individuals (Newman, 2010).

In contradiction with these scholars, De Waal, Klot, Mahajan, Huber, Frerks and M'Boup (2010, p. 25) confirm that HIV/AIDS does pose diverse threats to international, national and human security. There are many positive outcomes for the securitisation of HIV, including attracting attention and proportionate resources to the problem and mobilising political will (Wishnick, 2010). Human security in a health setting is also beneficial in that it focuses on the risks of rapid change that have led to better surveillance mechanisms and added focus on early warning and prevention efforts (Fukuda-Parr, 2003). Regardless of the debates concerning human security frameworks, scholars do agree that there is a greater acceptance of the concept of health security in the literature and public policy (Aldis, 2008; Davies, 2008; Newman, 2010).

Nevertheless, Aldis (2008) argues that the definitions of health security are too broad in scope and not clearly understood by stakeholders; which can lead to a breakdown in global cooperation. Newman (2010), in agreement with Aldis, suggests that definitions should be more delineated and less opaque. Newman concedes that there is no uncontested definition or approach to human security. However, he suggests that a broad approach, such as that adopted by the UN, attracts the most critics who argue:

> the broad approach is so inclusive – in considering potentially any threat to human safety – that as a concept it becomes meaningless. It does not allow scholars or policy makers to prioritise different types of threats, it confuses sources and consequences of insecurity, and it is too amorphous to allow analysis with any degree of precision.
>
> (Newman, 2010, p. 82)

Newman accepts that human security can be considered analytically weak (while normatively attractive); but counters that for many stakeholders interested in promoting human security, the real issue is the improvement of lives that are dangerously insecure (pp. 82–83). Shaw, MacLean and Black (2006) advocate something similar and suggest that 'freedom from want' has been displaced by 'freedom from fear' as it is definitionally narrower and more compatible with state-centric frameworks (p. 4). The debate and analytical coherence are incidental and non-essential as many interested in promoting human security are simply interested in its impact on policy.

This policy-driven approach to human security and its concerns with assisting those that are least empowered and most insecure is useful for analysis. However, human security dialogues do need to confront the internal contradictions and analytical confusion surrounding the scope and application of human security in order to get past the debates about definition. In doing so, human security can be academically viable, positively contribute to security studies and remain policy-relevant (Newman, 2010, p. 92). Therefore, even while lacking in the area of definition, human security frameworks are still useful and worthy of increased adoption and adaptation. During the recent sixty-seventh UN General Assembly, Member States committed to further dialogue concerning human security and internationally agreed goals (UN, 2012).

China, however, has a sceptical approach to human security. In the Sixty-Fourth UN General Assembly, China's representative, La Yifan, presented their concept of human security, identifying that:

> [It] pertained to many different fields, and his delegation considered that it was still a broad and abstract idea that did not enjoy international consensus. Member States needed to engage in further discussion on the matter to arrive at a clearer definition of the concept and mechanisms through which it would be applied. In all that, China believed that Governments retained the primary responsibility of ensuring the security of their citizens.
>
> (UN, 2010, para. 58)

While La Yifan does indicate China's willingness to engage in further discussion concerning the concepts and mechanisms of human security, the above statement clearly indicates that China presently has a limited engagement in issues of human security and that traditional forms of security are still predominant in the PRC security discourses.

Much earlier, Chu (2002) provided an informative background on China's reluctance to embrace the term 'human security',[3] identifying their strong bias towards traditional forms of security, inviolable sovereignty and reluctance to allow humanitarian intervention or interference in their internal affairs as a key part of Beijing's reluctance to embrace such an approach to security. He suggested that China is rather concerned with 'people's safety' somewhat fashioned on UN concepts of human security. Chu cautioned that while Beijing is open to embracing its citizens' right to 'safety', it does not accept that individual human rights rank higher than state sovereignty (p. 5). Therefore, when contemplating La Yifan's announcement and Chu's article in the light of global ramifications of HIV/AIDS and the agreed necessity for collaboration, PLWHA in China may still presently face a lack of effective infrastructure in addressing the HIV epidemic.

That is not to suggest that Beijing has made no attempts to deal with the HIV/AIDS epidemic in China. However, several scholars have questioned the effectiveness and affordability of HIV/AIDS programmes, including ART (Yu, Souteyrand, Banda, Kaufman & Perriëns, 2008; Zhou et al., 2011), prevention education programmes and harm reduction and methadone maintenance programmes for PWID in China (Hood, 2011; Li, Ha, Zhang & Liu, 2010; Pirkle, Soundardjee & Stella, 2007; Qian et al., 2006; Tsai, Morisky & Chen 2010, p. 546; Tucker et al., 2011). Knutsen (2012) suggests that Beijing's conventional approach has led to human rights violations through mandatory detention and mass screenings but believes that Beijing has adopted a more human rights approach in recent years and, as such, has more effectively addressed the epidemic.

However, some researchers, such as Philbin and Zhang (2010) and Sun et al. (2010), argue that even though Beijing has made inroads into providing universal access to HIV/AIDS prevention and treatment programmes in China, there are still important gaps. This is exacerbated by China's decentralised health structure (Gill, 2006; Hood, 2011; Liu & Kaufman, 2006; Saich, 2006; Sun et al., 2010). Additionally, much of the literature negatively comments on the stigmatisation, risk of arrest and lack of access to services that arise from current laws criminalising sex work and drug use in China and how they increase the spread of HIV (Hammett et al., 2007; Li et al., 2010; Philbin & Zhang, 2010; Qian et al., 2006). In considering the shortfalls and challenges faced by Beijing in dealing with the HIV epidemic, a human security lens is useful to focus on the current gaps in policy and provision of services, in particular, those for highly mobile populations.

Many researchers agree that successful control of HIV in China's health care sector requires strong international collaboration, as well as the development of grassroots organisations to deliver efficacious HIV/AIDS programmes and ongoing ART maintenance (Sun et al., 2010; Wu, Wang, Detels & Rotheram-Borus, 2010). Liu and Kaufman (2006), submit that it is essential that there should be a 'comprehensive intersector response' and 'collaboration between different stakeholders' (p. 93). This is reinforced by Zhang, Hsu, Yu, Wen and Pan (2006), who examine the ART programme in China and suggest that a patient's social environment plays a vital role in the success of ongoing adherence to ART regimes.

Even so, scholars recognise that while government-organised NGOs are involved with HIV programmes in China, there are still a lack of independent INGOs and NGOs (Qian et al., 2006; Tucker et al., 2011). Tuñón (2006) and Stern and O'Brien (2011) all remark on the independent organisations in China but disagree somewhat as to their effectiveness and acceptability in the Chinese context. Tuñón praises the organisations and their effectiveness while Stern and O'Brien believe them to be troubled by blurred operational boundaries and PRC 'crackdowns' (2011, p. 14). Du Guerny, Hsu and Hong (2003) suggest that formal intervention programmes are ineffective and suggest a more situation-specific approach is needed. This would particularly apply in scenarios involving highly mobile people groups who may not access conventional programmes.

Independent organisations play an important role in mobile and marginalised populations as they cater to people who are unlikely to access state-run HIV/AIDS outreach programmes due to fear of stigmatisation and arrest. A number of scholars state that conventional HIV outreach programmes are not generally successful in accessing these mobile populations and that intervention programmes need to be tailored for their needs (Chu & Liu, 2011; Du Guerny et al., 2003; Li et al., 2010; Sun et al., 2010). Fortunately, in recent years, there have been a number of different studies concentrating on the HIV vulnerabilities faced by mobile people groups and the health care initiatives supporting them (Knutsen, 2012; Tucker et al., 2011; Wang et al., 2007).

Tuñón (2006) provides particularly helpful information concerning the *hukou* system of registration and the lack of health care for workers who have an undocumented status. However, his research is concerned with all aspects of labour mobility rather than HIV specifically. Nonetheless, he does discuss the interconnectedness of these groups and their vulnerability to HIV. In HIV/AIDS settings, migrant populations, FSWs and PWID are often interconnected and individuals may be classified as belonging to one or all of the groups mentioned. Mao et al. (2010) state, 'Effective responses to infectious disease epidemics depend on timely information' (p. ii80). This is particularly so considering HIV/AIDS epidemics are concentrated in these highly mobile high-risk groups and the epidemic can change substantially depending on site-specific circumstances.

UNAIDS confirms that the overwhelming burden of the disease rests with CSWs, PWID, migrants, MSM, transgender (TG) people and prisoners. Significantly, although there have been commitments made to respect the human rights of these high-risk populations, they still 'continue to face violence, social stigma and poor access to HIV services in many settings, a situation compounded by laws that criminalise homosexuality, drug use and sex work' (UNAIDS, 2011, p. 4). Researchers such as Zhang et al. (2006) confirm that in China this global trend of stigmatisation and marginalisation is evident among PLWHA. Other researchers have noted that stigma and discrimination have resulted in gaps in HIV policy and that high-risk groups are not receiving the assistance they need (Hood, 2012; Kaufman & Meyers, 2006; Li et al., 2006; Lin et al., 2007; Sun et al., 2010). Naiqun (2006, p. 194) suggests that the spread of HIV in China implies specific political and economic inequalities.

Philbin and Zhang (2010, p. 626) advise that this high rate of discrimination has resulted in PWID avoiding harm reduction programmes due to fear of arrest and stigmatisation once their HIV status becomes known. Pirkle et al. (2007) submit that FSWs are 'doubly marginalised, as they are both at high STI/HIV risk and subject to government sanctioned prosecution' (p. 696). In reality, this is a trend which is apparent not only in China's marginalised populations but also in the segments of the general population affected by HIV/AIDS.

Sandra Hyde (2007) has written an excellent work on the cultural politics of AIDS in South-West China that covers some similar issues to those being proposed for this research. She considers the mobility and multiplication patterns of disease as it passes through different locations and its impact on the culture and politics of individuals and groups, concluding that belonging to an ethnic minority, engaging in sex work and involved in people movement creates a nexus exacerbating HIV transmission.

In many ways, her work is similar to that of Hood (2005). Hood (2005) submits that people with HIV-positive (HIV+) status have become a separate type of minority group with a reconceptualised identity as an 'AIDS minority' (*Aizu*) (p. 24). Hayes (2012) proposes that this new minority status supplants other ethnic identifications and that although one might be born in the Han Chinese majority, being publicly known to be HIV+ simply makes one identifiable as a person with HIV, therefore, stripping away any of the privileges Han ethnicity may provide to the individual, compared to their non-Han counterparts. Kaufman and Meyers (2006) suggest that stigma related to group identification contributes to HIV vulnerability through impacts of marginalisation and limitations in accessing the employment and services.

Hood's (2012) more recent research considers HIV/AIDS in the context of media portrayals of PLWHA and the impact that this has on issues of stigma and resulting lack of access to medical interventions. Therefore, without financial resources and access to services, these groups cannot connect with prevention initiatives, treatment or education programmes on the risk factors contributing to the metastasising of HIV throughout the state. This is particularly so in the case of China, where stigmatisation and marginalisation of 'morally corrupt individuals' are condoned by the Chinese Confucian philosophy (Li et al., 2006; Lin et al., 2010; Tang & Hao, 2007).

This is reflective of Dikötter (1998) who proposes that a eugenic discourse, which elevates the gene pool above the rights and needs of the individual, is operating in China and that medical and economic explanations are used to control marginalised people who are considered not fit to live in society. He indicates that, in addition to focusing on genetic disease, information about genetics can be used against virtually anyone considered to be socially undesirable or economically burdensome. Whether deliberate eugenic discourses are operating within China or not, these scholars are in agreement that PLWHA in China are stigmatised and generally considered undesirable.

An article by Burki (2011) confirms that stigmatisation is still a major problem for PLWHA in China. Burki refers to a report co-issued by the International Labour Organisation (ILO) and China's Centre for Disease Control (CDC), which stated that the national policy for recruiting civil servants and sanitation employees working in public places excluded those suffering from sexually transmitted infections (STIs) and HIV from employment. This is in spite of policies and laws prohibiting discrimination against these groups of people. Burki suggests that this is in part due to common misperceptions and prejudices[4] concerning HIV/AIDS and a clause in the 2007 Employment Promotion Law forbidding infected individuals doing any jobs where they may expose someone to the disease (Burki, 2011, p. 286). There were also troubling reports of health care workers violating the privacy of clients and revealing their HIV status to employers. Stigmatisation clearly has a substantial impact on the human security of PLWHA in China.

Cai et al. (2007) and Cao et al. (2006) suggest that discrimination and stigmatisation result in weak HIV/AIDS programmes and that PLWHA are afraid to assert their rights. They submit that effective HIV outreach needs the participation of PLWHA and thus that they need to feel safe enough to contribute. In attempting to ascertain general attitudes towards PLWHA, Li, Liang et al. (2010) undertook research that suggests that stigma reduction programmes can change attitudes towards PLWHA and thereby can have positive effects on participation in HIV programmes. The researchers propose that this may be assisted by the integration of HIV prevention and stigma reduction frameworks. While there are some significant gaps in this research – for example, this study did not approach PLWHA concerning the ways in which they perceive stigma – it does confirm a link between stigma and the efficacy of HIV programmes. Stigma, and the resulting marginalisation of individuals, obviously play an important role in the expansion of HIV in China.

This is significant in places such as Yunnan, where there are high numbers of FSWs, PWID and migrant workers who already suffer from marginalisation even without the added stigma of HIV (Xiao, Kristensen, Sun, Lu & Vermund, 2007). Yunnan Province is a rural area populated by a large number of ethnic minorities and bordered by several states. Researchers such as Beyrer et al. (2006) and Philbin and Zhang (2010) identify how Yunnan's proximity to trafficking routes and the drug production areas of the Golden Triangle have contributed to high rates of IDU and subsequent HIV infection. Yunnan has the highest rates of infection for HIV/AIDS in China (UNAIDS, 2011, Jia et al., 2008; Jia et al., 2010).

Scholars researching the epidemic in China suggest that the highest concentrations (estimated at 80 per cent) of PLWHA are residents of rural areas (Gill, 2006; Jia et al., 2010; Xiao et al., 2007; Yip 2006; Zhang et al., 2006). Saich (2006) and Yi et al. (2010) agree that there is a lack in rural health care spending and desultory health care access for poor rural inhabitants. Gill (2006) concurs and comments on the asymmetrical nature of rural HIV/AIDS policy in comparison to that of urban centres. Considering that much of the floating population originates from rural communities, this is an area of urgent concern as these highly mobile, high-risk population groups are residing in and passing through these communities.

Many scholars agree that the HIV/AIDS epidemic in China still bears further scrutiny particularly in the previously mentioned mobile and marginalised communities (Kaufman, Kleinman & Saich, 2006; Yi et al., 2010; Zhao et al., 2005). In considering the literature it becomes clear that in order to deal with the epidemic in China, it is essential to gain a comprehensive understanding of how these groups have been affected by the disease, and the impact they have on communities. While there have been many studies on the HIV/AIDS situation faced by PWID due to their status as the HIV ground zero population in China, there is less information available on FSWs and limited information on floating migrants (Knutsen, 2012; Li et al., 2009; Tucker et al., 2011; Wang et al., 2007; Yang, Latkin, Luan & Nelson, 2010; Yi et al., 2010).

The HIV/AIDS epidemic in China was first identified in PWID in Yunnan Province and as a cohort they have the highest rates of PLWHA in China. The existing literature on PWID in China, particularly in Yunnan and Xinjiang Provinces in China, reveal globally established trends for the transmission of HIV, both within IDU communities and the expansion into the general population. Studies have found that illicit drug networks, needle-sharing and other high-risk behaviours, such as trading sex for drugs or money to buy drugs, were implicated in the spread of HIV (Beyrer et al., 2006; Che et al., 2011; Hammett et al., 2006; Hu et al., 2011; Li, He, Wang & Williams, 2009; Qian et al., 2006). Much of the literature indicates that PWID are closely connected to other high-risk groups.

One cross-sectional research study of FSWs by Wang et al. (2009, p. 162) found that injection drug use was the single largest factor for HIV infection in these groups. They collected blood and questioned participants to obtain information about drug habits, condom usage, and a range of other social interactions. However, their study was limited, and results possibly misclassified, due to its reliance on self-reporting from participants. Their outcomes were consistent with other studies concerning FSWs in China (Hu et al., 2011; Yao et al., 2009). Additionally, Wang et al. were unable to discover whether infection was initially caused through sex or drug networks. As a result, they advocate further research into the associations of drug and sex work in China (2009, p. 167).

Huda (2006) and Skeldon (2000) provide data on the ways that migration and sex trafficking impact on the expansion of HIV. Migrants are considered high-risk groups as they are far from their usual support networks; young and often single; and open to risk behaviours, such as drug use and sexual promiscuity (Knutsen, 2012; Liu, 2011; Merli & Hertog, 2010; Thiesmeyer, 2005; C. Yang et al., 2010). In a study by Wang, Li, Stanton, Fang, Lin et al. (2007, p. 2), it was found that migrants had significantly higher rates of HIV. This was confirmed by Jun et al. (2008, p. 558) with the authors referring to studies done in Shandong and Shanxi, which found that almost 70 per cent of all PLWHA were migrants.

However, Jun et al. (2008) also discussed the results of another study that found low or no HIV prevalence in migrants, leading them to caution that other factors might contribute to HIV in migrant cohorts. Contrary to this, Yang, Derlega and Luo (2007) suggest that they might be pivotal to the expansion of HIV in China. Piot, Greener and Russel (2007, p. 1571) confirm this, stating that infection patterns are influenced by the increase of men and women looking for work within and across borders and that mobility correlates to higher rates of infection. When considering this in the light of migrants' limited access to PMTCT health services (Liao et al., 2011), lack of health insurance and undocumented status (Tuñón, 2006), it is essential to gain an expanded understanding of the human security threats faced by floating migrants.

This has become even more important with recent studies confirming that transmission of HIV in China has changed from being driven by IDUs to being driven by sexual contact (Merli & Hertog, 2010; UNAIDS, 2011; C. Yang et al., 2010; Yi et al., 2010). This is significant considering the overall numbers of sex workers in China, with some scholarly estimates of between 4–6 million in 2000

(Pirkle et al., 2007). Elaine Jeffreys in her work, *Sex in China,* draws upon a number of different sources providing estimates between 4–20 million sex workers, including those who occasionally accept gifts, money or rent in exchange for sexual services (Jeffreys, 2015, p. 92). As with HIV/AIDS estimates, it is impossible to ascertain an absolute number of CSWs in China. Therefore, while they are interconnected with other mobile groups, it is essential to focus on the challenges faced by this specific group and their escalating role as a potential bridging population for the spread of HIV.

Contemporary studies have been undertaken concerning the impact of sex workers as bridging populations between high-risk groups and the general population in China (Jin et al., 2010). This is confirmed by Huang, Henderson, Pan and Cohen (2004) and Yi et al. (2010), who have carried out noteworthy research on the structural hierarchies of sex workers. However, they comment that the HIV risk and lack of ability to negotiate safer sex are increased in the lower level of sex work, such as streetwalkers.

There are many different types of sex worker and variations in sexual practice and risk (Parish & Pan, 2006; UNAIDS, 2011, p. 20; C. Yang et al., 2010, p. 293). This is also established by Burger (2012) who presents seven tiers of sex work, in a hierarchy, depending on the services they offer, namely:

- Tier one: *Ernai.*
- Tier two: *Baopo.*
- Tier three: *Santing.*
- Tier four, *Dingdong* girls.
- Tier five, *Falangmei.*
- Tier six, *Jienu* sex workers.
- Tier seven, *Xiagongpeng.*

Overall, the numbers and different hierarchies or tiers of CSWs present a formidable challenge to HIV/AIDS outreach programmes, treatment, prevention and education efforts.

These challenges are highly prevalent when examining issues surrounding condom use, as highlighted in much of the literature. It has been well documented that CSWs' multiplicity of sexual interactions with both commercial clients and non-commercial partners can lead to sub-optimal condom use (Hu et al., 2011; Jun et al., 2008; Knutsen, 2012; Merli & Hertog, 2010; Wang et al., 2009; C. Yang et al., 2010; Yi et al., 2010). Disinclined to use condoms with non-commercial partners, CSWs are also often the least powerful in negotiating condom use with clients, therefore researchers recommend that they cannot be held solely responsible for prevention methods (Huang et al., 2004; C. Yang, 2010; Yi et al., 2010). Therefore, these clients need to become more of a focus in prevention programmes and more research in this area is essential.

In conclusion, it is clear from a review of the existing literature that there are still significant gaps in the present understandings of HIV/AIDS as a non-traditional (human security) threat. This is particularly so in the mobile and marginalised populations in China. China's representatives in UN General Assemblies have indicated that they do not fully adopt human security frameworks. Additionally, the literature reveals a need for more research into the ways in which Beijing is currently addressing the needs of PLWHA and whether they are achieving success in populations who are highly mobile, marginalised and stigmatised. IDUs, FSWs and floating labour migrants face unique challenges in accessing health initiatives that need to be more clearly understood in order to successfully address the expansion of HIV in China.

Structure of the book

This introductory chapter provides an overview of the book's topic: the theoretical frameworks and study limitations. Additionally, it includes a review of the relevant literature discussing the ramifications of HIV/AIDS as a non-traditional security threat to China and its proximate states. It also reviews the literature on China's HIV/AIDS epidemics, particularly those most applicable to the book's research cohorts (FSWs, PWID and floating migrants).

At the end of each chapter there is a case study. These case studies are short renderings of the real encounters I had with people living in Yunnan. Not all of them were living with HIV/AIDS (although most were) but the disease in one way or another had affected all of them. They are written in a narrative style and in the first person as a deliberate (potentially jarring) juxtaposition to the academic writing style and theory in each chapter. Each of the case studies focuses on an aspect of human insecurity for PLWHA living in communities that often do not understand, and fear, HIV/AIDS and those living with the disease. The case studies serve as a catapult to throw the reader from theory to reality. These are real stories about the lives of real individuals, living with the daily ramifications of HIV/AIDS.

Sometimes, as researchers, it can be difficult to divorce ourselves from the statistics and realise that we are viewing the situation from a position of safety. While this is essential, it can be meaningful to remember that each of those statistics represents a person just trying to live their lives in the best way possible. My hope is that by introducing you to each one of them, they will no longer just be individuals within key populations but identified as sisters, mothers, fathers and friends affected but not defined by a disease. Also, it provides the opportunity to understand how human insecurity has very tangible effects on people's lives.

This chapter lays the foundation for the topic and provides basic information on Yunnan Province and the challenges faced by PLWHA due to porous borders, multiple minority groups and a diversity of languages. It also introduces the reader to the three main cohorts being considered. It includes a section on methodology; recounts information gathered in interviews during field research and the operation situation in Yunnan; considers the limitations inherent in obtaining data from China on sensitive topics, such as HIV/AIDS; and introduces the reader to the concept of human security as an overview.

Chapter 2 provides the theoretical foundation for considering HIV/AIDS as a non-traditional security threat. It ascertains the implications of securitising the disease and discusses HIV/AIDS impacts on the human security of PLWHA and whether current insecurities are contributing to the expansion of HIV/AIDS in China. Additionally, it considers the ongoing debate by scholars of International Relations concerning the definitions of human security and their applicability to the HIV/AIDS pandemic. China's disinclination to adopt the concept of human security and the ramifications of their current frameworks are also considered. The chapter queries whether there is any gap between international human security practice and China's official state practices in perceiving HIV/AIDS as a non-traditional human security threat. Additionally, Beijing's current policies concerning non-traditional security and in particular human security threats are examined.

Case study 1.1 Lily's story

Lily is a Myanmar sex worker who has worked in brothels on both sides of the Chinese border. She explained that the borders are so porous that girls travel and set up operations from one country to another with great ease. She also described the current work practices for sex workers and the prevailing drug culture. The majority of the towns and villages along Yunnan's border regions are also transit points for drug trafficking from the Golden Triangle production areas.

Chapter 3 provides an overview of the pathogenesis and epidemiology of HIV, highlighting the problematic nature of the virus. The virus poses significant challenges for PLWHA. Understanding how the virus is introduced into the body and the ways that it overcomes the immune functions of the host provides readers with the necessary framework for comprehending the difficulties faced by researchers attempting to create vaccines and efficient antiretroviral medications. The chapter then discusses the various strains of the virus, how they form recombinants and the specific strains found in the provinces in China. The role of STIs and the manner in which they are inextricably linked to, and exacerbate, the ongoing spread of HIV are described. Finally, the chapter provides a rendering of the history of HIV/AIDS globally.

Case study 1.2 Daiyu's story

Diayu is an injection drug user who lives in a village within a day's drive from Kunming. She inherited her family home after the death of her parents. It is a large sprawling building that used to operate as a boarding house run by Daiyu and her sister. However, after the death of her sister from an AIDS-related illness and Daiyu's own HIV+ status, no one will rent rooms from her any more. As a result, she has had to turn to sex work to support her drug habit and give her enough money to survive. Daiyu lives on ¥5 a day which allows her to buy one meal. She said she is just waiting to die.

Chapter 4 introduces the concept of global best practice (GBP) for dealing with HIV/AIDS epidemics. These practices have generally proven to be successful over a range of scenarios and are readily adaptable to country-specific epidemics. GBP specifically deals with the three most current practices: (1) treatment as prevention; (2) 'know your epidemic, know your response'; and (3) the cascade of care. It also comments on more long-term strategies including stigma reduction programmes, condom distribution, and methadone maintenance treatment (MMT) and syringe programmes. It then examines Beijing's adoption, or lack thereof, of HIV/AIDS GBP in China. It also considers China's current policies and practices concerning NGOs, in particular, INGOs, and how their efforts are aided or otherwise by Beijing.

Case study 1.3 Guoliang's story

Guoliang is an injection drug use peer worker in a city in Yunnan Province. He is HIV+ and is currently on a methadone maintenance programme; he also runs a drop-in centre for PWID. He describes the situation faced by PWID in Yunnan and the challenges that they face in providing services. Once or twice a week, he and his fellow workers travel to the border areas and help those who are homeless and living in ad hoc shelters. He said that many of them are HIV/AIDS-affected and have infected sores at injection sites. They have no access to health care and little access to food.

Chapter 5 presents a historical overview of HIV/AIDS in China. There are four distinct stages in China's handling of HIV/AIDS from the first encounter until the present time:

- Phase one, the introduction phase, provides information of how HIV/AIDS was first discovered in China.
- Phase two concerns China's classification of HIV/AIDS as a western disease, resulting in delayed action.
- Phase three is the diffusion period in China's epidemics where HIV was spreading rapidly throughout key populations.
- Phase four is the current stage where rampant prevalence has seen the virus become sexually driven and generalised in certain populations.

Additionally, this chapter examines the current situation of HIV/AIDS in China's Yunnan Province and whether the cultural diversity within Yunnan adds to the difficulties of delivering HV/AIDS programmes.

Case study 1.4 Ming-Hua's story

Ming-Hua took me to her small home, which she shared with her son. Everything that they owned was shoved into the space. It had no running water and they used a bucket tucked into a corner for their latrine. She said she used to run a noodle shop but that no one would buy noodles from her any more because they were scared. She was now a widow and had become HIV+ after her husband had acquired the virus as an injection drug user. She recounted that although people didn't blame her for her problems, they were scared that if they ate her noodles, then they too would catch HIV. She had a child to care for and was afraid of what would happen to him when she died.

Chapter 6, 'HIV/AIDS-affected populations', considers key populations in HIV/AIDS epidemics. The chapter gives a brief overview of the various pathways for the spread of the virus throughout key populations and among the general population. A population is considered key in HIV/AIDS epidemics due to generally high infection rates and the role that they can play in spreading HIV. They are also considered key populations due to the vulnerability they face whether through systematic violence, risk behaviours or mobility. These key populations include CSWs, PWID, HIV+ pregnant women, FPD and MSM. The impact of PRC laws regarding the criminalisation or illegality of FSWs, IDUs, and undocumented workers will be considered in light of the spread of HIV/AIDS in Yunnan and nearby areas.

Case study 1.5 Yong's story

Yong lived in a makeshift dwelling in Yunnan Province. He was sharing a dwelling the size of a small tent with two other people. Yong is an injection drug user who had just been released from a mandatory detention centre where he was supposed to be rehabilitated. He said that the first thing that he did when he was released was find a heroin supplier. He knew that he was better off not taking drugs but said that he now had no choice because his body needed it. He said that he and the other two people he lived with all did whatever they needed to in order to survive.

Chapter 7 examines the specific cohorts of this book (FSWs, PWID and floating migrants) in some depth and in the Chinese context. The chapter also reveals the shortfalls and challenges in HIV/AIDS prevention and treatment programmes in China. Discussions took place with NGOs and CBO dealing with the specific cohorts in China and many of their observations and experiences are examined in this chapter. Some of the programmes currently underway in China were also discussed, as were the current funding shortages.

Case study 1.6 Chen's story

Chen is an NGO worker, whom I was able to connect with in Yunnan. He was very forthcoming when discussing the HIV/AIDS situation in China. He expressed the opinion that there is never enough money. They do what they can but it really doesn't make much impact on the overall situation. He discussed the official HIV/AIDS figures and said that he didn't think it could be possible that they were correct. Yunnan Province alone diagnoses more than 10,000 new cases of HIV every year. He expressed his frustrations at the lack of support for HIV/AIDS initiatives and feared that the situation would continue to grow worse.

Chapter 8 considers the burden that HIV epidemics place on populations and the threat they pose to China and its neighbouring states. This chapter highlights the seven pillars of human insecurity: economic, food, health, environmental, personal, community and political security as the elements of human security most threatened in HIV/AIDS situations. Understanding the impacts of human insecurity in HIV/AIDS epidemics provides a scaffold for the book's contention that human security is a legitimate and useful framework for understanding China's HIV/AIDS epidemics. Moreover, it suggests that using such a framework will assist in addressing both the challenges and shortfalls of existing programmes.

Case study 1.7 Lijuan's story

Lijuan lives in a small house in a village near Kunming. Her home is a dark small room with a small antechamber. She has no running water and no electricity. She is in her eighties and told me that she often has no food to eat. She once had three sons but all of them had become drug users and contracted HIV, two of them had died from AIDS-related causes. She told me that she received no help from anyone although sometimes her neighbours would give her a meal or some work. At the time of my visit she had not eaten for several days and was destitute.

The book's concluding chapter contextualises the HIV/AIDS situation in China and considers both the ramifications of HIV/AIDS on China's state security, and the human security threats faced by PLWHA. In doing so, it identifies the shortfalls in existing programmes and highlights the challenges inherent in managing HIV/AIDS epidemics within China. Ultimately the conclusion makes the case for HIV/AIDS prevention and treatment programmes to operate from the bottom up in accordance with human security frameworks, placing the individual as the referent object.

Notes

1 SARS, a part of the coronavirus family, is a serious and highly infectious form of pneumonia that first appeared in Guangdong Province in southern China in November 2002, then spread to 28 countries, infecting 8,096 people and resulting in 774 deaths (Wishnick, 2010, p. 457).
2 Vector is a medical/epidemiological term for agents (people, animals or other organisms) that carry and transmit infectious disease (such as HIV) from one host to another.

3 Beijing considers that the term '*security* should be reserved for issues of national importance, whereas the term *safety* better reflects individual concerns' (Chu, 2002, p. 2).
4 He comments on statistics that suggest 51 per cent of people would not shake hands with a HIV+ person and 80 per cent would not buy a product from them.

References

Aldis, W. (2008). Health security as a public health concept: A critical analysis. *Health Policy and Planning, 23*(6), 369–375. doi:10.1093/heapol/czn030.

Alkire, S. (2003). A conceptual framework for human security. Working Paper no. 2. Centre for Research on Inequality, Human Security and Ethnicity (CRISE). Oxford University.

Annan, K. (2000a). *We the people: The role of the United Nations in the 21st century.* New York, NY: United Nations Department of Public Information.

Annan, K. (2000b). Secretary-General salutes international workshop on Human Security in Mongolia. Ulaanbaatar, 8–10 May. Press Release SG/SM/7382. Retrieved from www.un.org/News/Press/docs/2000/20000508.sgsm7382.doc.html

Bate, R. (2012). *Phake: The deadly world of falsified and substandard medicines.* Washington, DC: AEI Press.

Beyrer, C., Suwanvanichkij, V., Mullany, L. C., Richards, A. K., Franck, N., Samuels, A. & Lee, T. J. (2006). Responding to AIDS, tuberculosis, malaria, and emerging infectious diseases in Burma: Dilemmas of policy and practice. *PLoS Medicine, 3*(10), e393.

Bowsher, G., Milner, C. & Sullivan, R. (2016). Medical intelligence, security and global health: The foundations of a new health agenda. *Journal of the Royal Society of Medicine, 109*(7), 269–273.

Burger, R. (2012). *Behind the red door: Sex in China.* Hong Kong, China: Earnshaw Books.

Burki, T. K. (2011). Discrimination against people with HIV persists in China. *The Lancet, 377*(9762), 286–287.

Cai, G., Moji, K., Honda, S., Wu, X. & Zhang, K. (2007). Inequality and unwillingness to care for people living with HIV/AIDS: A survey of medical professionals in southeast China. *AIDS Patient Care & STDs, 21*(8), 593–601. doi:10.1089/apc.2006.0162.

Cao, X., Sullivan, S. G., Xu, J., Wu, Z. & China CIPRA Project 2 Team. (2006). Understanding HIV-related stigma and discrimination in a "blameless" population. *AIDS Education & Prevention, 18*(6), 518–528.

Che, Y., Assanangkornchai, S., McNeil, E., Li, J., You, J. & Chongsuvivatwong, V. (2011). Patterns of attendance in methadone maintenance treatment program in Yunnan Province, China. *The American Journal of Drug and Alcohol Abuse, 37*(3), 148–154.

Chu, S. (2002). China and human security. North Pacific policy papers No. 8. Northeast Asia Cooperation Project. Institute of Asian Research. Vancouver, Canada: University of British Columbia.

Chu, Y. & Liu, H. (2011). Advances of research on anti-HIV agents from traditional Chinese herbs. *Advances in Dental Research, 23*(1), 67–75.

Dahl-Eriksen, T. (2007). Human security: A new concept which adds new dimensions to human rights discussions? *Human Security Journal, 5*, Winter, 16–27.

Davies, S. E. (2008). Securitizing infectious disease. *International Affairs, 84*(2), 295–313. doi:10.1111/j.1468-2346.2008.00704.x.

De Waal, A., Klot, J. F., Mahajan, M., Huber, D., Frerks, G. & M'Boup, S. (2010). *HIV/ AIDS, security and conflict: New realities, new responses AIDS, security and conflict initiative.* New York, NY: Social Science Research Network.

Dikötter, F. (1998). Race culture: Recent perspectives on the history of eugenics. *The American Historical Review, 103*(2), 467–478.

Ding, Y., Detels, R., Zhao, Z., Zhu, Y., Zhu, G., Zhang, B., … & Xue, X. (2005). HIV infection and sexually transmitted diseases in female commercial sex workers in China. *Journal of Acquired Immune Deficiency Syndromes, 38*(3), 314–319.

Ding, Y., Li, L. & Ji, G. (2011). HIV disclosure in rural China: Predictors and relationship to access to care. *AIDS Care, 23*(9), 1059–1066. doi:10.1080/09540121.2011.554524.

Donnelly, J. (2005). Realism. In S. Burchill (Ed.), *Theories of international relations,* (pp. 29–54). New York, NY: Palgrave Macmillan.

Du Guerny, J., Hsu, L. N. & Hong, C. (2003). *Population movement and HIV/AIDS: The case of Ruili, Yunnan, China.* UNDP South East Asia HIV and Development Programme. Retrieved from www.hivdevelopment.org/Publications_english/The%20 case%20of%20Ruili.htm

Duong, L. E. B., Bélanger, D. & Hong, K. T. (2005). Transnational migration, marriage and trafficking at the China-Vietnam border. In I. Attané & C. Z. Guilmotow (Eds.), *Watering the neighbour's garden: The growing demographic female deficit in Asia* (pp. 393–425). Paris, France: Committee for International Cooperation in National Research in Demography.

Elbe, S. (2006). Should HIV/AIDS be securitized? The ethical dilemmas of linking HIV/ AIDS and security. *International Studies Quarterly, 50,* 119–144.

Fukuda-Parr, S. (2003). New threats to human security in the era of globalization. *Journal of Human Development, 4*(2), 167–179. doi:10.1080/146498803200008752.

Gill, B. (2006). China's health care and pension challenges. Testimony before the US-China Security and Economic Review Commission hearing on major internal challenges facing the Chinese Leadership, February, 2. Washington, DC. Retrieved from www.uscc.gov/hearings/2006hearings/written_testimonies/06_02_02_bates.pdf

Gore, A. (2000). Remarks prepared for delivery by Vice President Al Gore in U.N. Security Council session on AIDS in Africa. Washington, DC: The White House. Retrieved from http://clinton4.nara.gov/WH/EOP/OVP/speeches/unaid_health.html

Granich, R., Williams, B., Montaner, J. & Zuniga, J. M. (2017). 90–90–90 and ending AIDS: Necessary and feasible. *The Lancet, 390*(10092), 341–343.

Hammett, T. M., Kling, R., Johnston, P., Liu, W., Ngu, D., Friedmann, P., … & Des Jarlais, D. C. (2006). Patterns of HIV prevalence and HIV risk behaviors among injection drug users prior to and 24 months following implementation of cross-border HIV prevention interventions in northern Vietnam and southern China. *AIDS Education & Prevention, 18*(2), 97–115.

Hammett, T. M., Wu, Z., Tran, T. D., Stephens, D., Sullivan, S., Liu, W., … & Des Jarlais, D. C. (2007). 'Social evils' and harm reduction: The evolving policy environment for human immunodeficiency virus prevention among injection drug users in China and Vietnam. *Addiction, 103*(1), 137–145. doi:10.1111/j.1360-0443.2007.02053.x.

Hayes, A. (2005). AIDS, bloodheads & cover-ups: The "ABC" of Henan's aids epidemic. *AQ: Australian Quarterly, 77*(3), 12–40.

Hayes, A. (2007). Women's vulnerability to HIV/AIDS in China: A case study for the engendering of human security discourse. Unpublished doctoral thesis, University of Southern Queensland, Australia.

Hayes, A. (2012). HIV/AIDS in Xinjiang: A serious "ill" in an "autonomous" region. *IJAPS, 8*(1), January, 77–102.

Hindmarch, S. (2016). *Securing health: HIV and the limits of securitization.* London, UK: Routledge.

Hood, J. (2005). *Narrating HIV/AIDS in the PRC media: Imagined immunity, distracting others, and the configuration of race, place and disease.* Canberra, Australia: Australian National University.

Hood, J. (2011). *HIV/AIDS, health and the media in China.* London, UK: Routledge.

Hood, J. (2012). HIV/AIDS and shifting urban China's socio-moral landscape: Engendering bio-activism and resistance through stories of suffering. *IJAPS, 8*(1), 125–144.

Hu, Y., Liang, S., Zhu, J., Qin, G., Liu, Q., Song, B., ... & Qian, H. (2011). Factors associated with recent risky drug use and sexual behaviors among drug users in southwestern China. *Journal of AIDS Clinical Research, 2*(120), 3. Retrieved from www.omicsonline.org/2155-6113/2155-6113-2-120.php

Huang, Y., Henderson, G. E., Pan, S. & Cohen, M. S. (2004). HIV/AIDS risk among brothel-based female sex workers in China: Assessing the terms, content, and knowledge of sex work. *Sexually Transmitted Diseases, 31*(11), 695–700.

Huda, S. (2006). Sex trafficking in south Asia. *International Journal of Gynecology & Obstetrics, 94*(3), 374–381.

Hwang, K. K. (1999). Filial piety and loyalty: Two types of social identification in Confucianism. *Asian Journal of Social Psychology, 2*(1), 163–183.

Hyde, S. T. (2007). *Eating spring rice: The cultural politics of AIDS in southwest China.* Berkeley, CA: University of California Press.

Jeffreys, E. (2015). *Sex in China.* Chichester, UK: John Wiley & Sons.

Jia, Y., Sun, J., Fan, L., Song, D., Tian, S., Yang, Y., ... & Zhang, S. (2008). Estimates of HIV prevalence in a highly endemic area of China: Dehong prefecture, Yunnan province. *International Journal of Epidemiology, 37*(6), 1287–1296.

Jia, Z., Wang, W., Dye, C., Bao, Y., Liu, Z. & Lu, L. (2010). Exploratory analysis of the association between new-type drug use and sexual transmission of HIV in China. *American Journal of Drug & Alcohol Abuse, 36*(2), 130–133. doi:10.3109/00952991003734269.

Jin, X., Smith, K., Chen, R. Y., Ding, G., Yao, Y., Wang, H., ... & Wang, N. (2010). HIV prevalence and risk behaviors among male clients of female sex workers in Yunnan, China. *Journal of Acquired Immune Deficiency Syndromes, 53*(1), 131–135.

Jun, J., Ning, W., Lin, L., Yi, P., Guo, L., Wong, M., Zheng, L. & Xi, W. (2008). HIV and STIs in clients and female sex workers in mining regions of Gejiu City, China. *Sexually Transmitted Diseases, 35*(6), 558–556. doi:10.1097/OLQ.0b013e318165926b.

Kaufman, J., Kleinman, A. & Saich, T. (2006). Introduction: Social policy and HIV/AIDS in China. In J. Kaufman, A. Kleinman & T. Saich (Eds.), *AIDS and social policy in China* (pp. 3–14). Cambridge, MA: Harvard University Asia Center.

Kaufman, J. & Meyers, K. (2006). AIDS surveillance in China: Data gaps and research. In J. Kaufman, A. Kleinman & T. Saich (Eds.), *AIDS and social policy in China* (pp. 47–71). Cambridge, MA: Harvard University Asia Center.

Kettemann, M. C. (2006). The conceptual debate on human security and its relevance for the development of international law. *Human Security Perspectives, 1*(3), 39–52.

Knutsen, W. L. U. (2012). An institutional account of China's HIV/AIDS policy process from 1985 to 2010. *Politics & Policy, 40*(1), 161–192.

Kurth, A. E., Celum, C., Baeten, J. M., Vermund, S. H. & Wasserheit, J. N. (2011). Combination HIV prevention: Significance, challenges, and opportunities. *Current HIV/AIDS Reports, 8*(1), 62–72.

Li, H., Kuo, N. T., Liu, H., Korhonen, C., Pond, E., Guo, H., ... & Sun, J. (2010). From spectators to implementers: Civil society organizations involved in AIDS programmes in China. *International Journal of Epidemiology, 39*(suppl. 2), ii65–ii71.

Li, J., Ha, T. H., Zhang, C. & Liu, H. (2010). The Chinese government's response to drug use and HIV/AIDS: A review of policies and programs. *Harm Reduction Journal, 7*, 1–6. doi:10.1186/1477-7517-7-4.

Li, L., Liang, L. J., Lin, C., Wu, Z. & Rotheram-Borus, M. J. (2010). HIV prevention intervention to reduce HIV-related stigma: Evidence from China. *AIDS, 24*(1), 115–122.

Li, L., Lin, C., Wu, Z., Wu, S., Rotheram-Borus, M., Detels, R. & Jia, M. (2007). Stigmatization and shame: Consequences of caring for HIV/AIDS patients in China. *AIDS Care, 19*(2), 258–263. doi:10.1080/09540120600828473.

Li, L., Wu, S., Wu, Z., Sun, S., Cui, H. & Jia, M. (2006). Understanding family support for people living with HIV/AIDS in Yunnan, China. *AIDS and Behavior, 10*(5), 509–517. doi:10.1007/s10461-006-9071-0.

Li, X., He, G., Wang, H. & Williams, A. B. (2009). Consequences of drug abuse and HIV/AIDS in China: Recommendations for integrated care of HIV-infected drug users. *AIDS Patient Care & STDs, 23*(10), 877–884. doi:10.1089/apc.2009.0015.

Liao, S., Weeks, M. R., Wang, Y., Li, F., Jiang, J., Li, J., ... & Dunn, J. (2011). Female condom use in the rural sex industry in China: Analysis of users and non-users at post-intervention surveys. *AIDS Care, 23*, 66–74. doi:10.1080/09540121.2011.555742.

Lin, C., Li, L., Wu, Z., Wu, S. & Jia, M. (2008). Occupational exposure to HIV among health care providers: A qualitative study in Yunnan, China. *Journal of the International Association of Physicians in AIDS Care (JIAPAC), 7*(1), 35–41.

Lin, C., Wu, Z., Rou, K., Pang, L., Cao, X., Shoptaw, S. & Detels, R. (2010). Challenges in providing services in methadone maintenance therapy clinics in China: Service providers' perceptions. *International Journal of Drug Policy, 21*(3), 173–178.

Lin, C., Wu, Z., Wu, S., Rotheram-Borus, M., Detels, R. & Jia, M. (2007). Stigmatization and shame: Consequences of caring for HIV/AIDS patients in China. *AIDS Care, 19*(2), 258–263.

Liu, S. H. (2011). *Passage to manhood: Youth migration, heroin, and AIDS in Southwest China*. Stanford, CA: Stanford University Press.

Liu, Y. & Kaufman, J. (2006). Controlling HIV/AIDS in China: Health system challenges. In J. Kaufman, A. Kleinman & T. Saich (Eds.), *AIDS and social policy in China* (pp. 75–95). Cambridge, MA: Harvard University Asia Center.

Lu, L., Jia, M., Ma, Y., Yang, L., Chen, Z., Ho, D. D., ... & Zhang, L. (2008). The changing face of HIV in China. *Nature, 455*(7213), 609–611.

Mao, Y., Wu, Z., Poundstone, K., Wang, C., Qin, Q., Ma, Y. & Ma, W. (2010). Development of a unified web-based national HIV/AIDS information system in China. *International Journal of Epidemiology, 39*(suppl. 2), ii79–ii89.

Marukutira, T., Stoové, M., Lockman, S., Mills, L. A., Gaolathe, T., Lebelonyane, R., ... & Crowe, S. M. (2018). A tale of two countries: Progress towards UNAIDS 90-90-90 targets in Botswana and Australia. *Journal of the International AIDS Society, 21*(3), e25090.

McInnes, C. & Rushton, S. (2010). HIV, AIDS and security: Where are we now?. *International Affairs, 86*(1), 225–245.

McIntosh, M. & Hunter, A. (2010). Perspectives on human security: An emergent construct. In M. McIntosh & A. Hunter (Eds.), *New perspectives on human security.* Sheffield, UK: Greenleaf Publishing.

Merli, M. G. & Hertog, S. (2010). Masculine sex ratios, population age structure and the potential spread of HIV in China. *Demographic Research, 22*, 63–94.

Mishra, S., Sgaier, S. K., Thompson, L. H., Moses, S., Ramesh, B. M., Alary, M., ... & Blanchard, J. F. (2012). HIV epidemic appraisals for assisting in the design of effective prevention programmes: Shifting the paradigm back to basics. *PLoS ONE, 7*(3), e32324.

Naiqun, W. (2006). Flows of heroin, people, capital, imagination, and the spread of HIV in southwest China. In T. Oakes & L. Schein (Eds.), *Translocal China: Linkages, identities, and the reimagining of space* (pp. 193–212). New York, NY: Routledge.

NCAIDS, NCSTD & China CDC. (2017). Update on the AIDS/STD epidemic in China in December, 2016. *Chinese Journal of AIDS & STD, 23*, 93–94.

Needham, K. (2019). Blood plasma scandal latest stain on China's medical products image. *The Sydney Morning Herald,* February 7. Retrieved from www.smh.com.au/world/asia/blood-plasma-scandal-latest-stain-on-china-s-medical-products-image-20190207scandal-latest-stain-on-china-s-medical-products-image-20190207-p50wd3.html?fbclid=IwAR2ExaKQin_CygytCPZaXjJvEVRX1nVlYxobpnjhUW3-KhCPtt55znZ8pGg

Newman, E. (2010). Critical human security studies. *Review of International Studies, 36*, 77–94. doi:10.1017/S0260210509990519.

Nishikawa, Y. (2009). Human security in Southeast Asia: Viable solution or empty slogan? *Security Dialogue, 40*, 213–236. doi:10.1177/0967010609103088.

Ogata, S. & Sen, A. (2003). *Human security now.* New York, NY: Commission on Human Security.

Parish, W., L. & Pan, S. (2006). Sexual partners in China: Risk pattern for infection by HIV and possible interventions. In J. Kaufman, A. Kleinman & T. Saich (Eds.), *AIDS and social policy in China* (pp. 190–213). Cambridge, MA: Harvard University Asia Center.

Philbin, M. M. & Zhang, F. (2010). Exploring stakeholder perceptions of facilitators and barriers to accessing methadone maintenance clinics in Yunnan province, China. *AIDS Care, 22*(5), 623–629. doi:10.1080/09540120903311490.

Piot, P., Greener, R. & Russell, S. (2007). Squaring the circle: AIDS, poverty, and human development. *PLoS Medicine, 4*(10), e314.

Pirkle, C., Soundardjee, R. & Stella, A. (2007). Female sex workers in China: Vectors of disease? *Sexually Transmitted Diseases, 34*(9), 695–703.

Qian, H. Z., Schumacher, J. E., Chen, H. T. & Ruan, Y. H. (2006). Injection drug use and HIV/AIDS in China: Review of current situation, prevention and policy implications. *Harm Reduction Journal, 3*(1), 4. doi:10.1186/1477-7517-3-4.

Qin, L., Yoda, T., Suzuki, C., Yamamoto, T., Cai, G., Rakue, Y. & Mizota, T. (2005). Combating HIV/AIDS in mainland China: An epidemiological review of prevention and control measures. *Southeast Asia Journal of Tropical Medicine and Public Health, 36*(6), 1479–1486.

Rushton, S. (2010). AIDS and international security in the United Nations system. *Health Policy and Planning, 25*(6), 495–504. doi:10.1093/heapol/czq051.

Saich, T. (2006). Social policy development in the era of economic reform. In J. Kaufman, A. Kleinman & T. Saich (Eds.), *AIDS and social policy in China* (pp. 15–46). Cambridge, MA: Harvard University Asia Center.

Selgelid, M. J. & Enemark, C. (2008). Infectious diseases, security and ethics: The case of HIV/AIDS. *Bioethics, 22*(9), 457–465. doi:10.1111/j.1467-8519.2008.00696.x.

Sgaier, S. K., Claeson, M., Gilks, C., Ramesh, B. M., Ghys, P. D., Wadhwani, A., ... & Chandramouli, K. (2012). Knowing your HIV/AIDS epidemic and tailoring an effective response: How did India do it? *Sexually Transmitted Infections, 88*(4), 240–249.

Shaw, T., MacLean, S. J. & Black, D. R. (2006). Introduction: A decade of human security: What prospects for global governance and new multilateralisms? In S. J. MacLean, D. R. Black & T. M. Shaw (Eds.), *A decade of human security: Global governance and new multilateralisms*. Farnham, UK: Ashgate Publishing Company.

Skeldon, R. (2000). *Population mobility and HIV vulnerability in South East Asia: An assessment and analysis*. Bangkok, Thailand: UNDP South East Asia HIV and Development Project.

Stern, R. & O'Brien, K. (2011). Politics at the boundary: Mixed signals and the Chinese state. *Modern China, 38*(2), 174–198. doi:10.1177/0097700411421463.

Su, L., Liang, S., Hou, X., Zhong, P., Wei, D., Fu, Y., … & Yang, H. (2018). Impact of worker emigration on HIV epidemics in labour export areas: A molecular epidemiology investigation in Guangyuan, China. *Scientific Reports, 8*(1), 16046.

Sun, J., Liu, H., Li, H., Wang, L., Guo, H., Shan, D., … & Ren, M. (2010). Contributions of international cooperation projects to the HIV/AIDS response in China. *International Journal of Epidemiology, 39*(suppl. 2), ii14–ii20.

Tang, Y. & Hao, W. (2007). Improving drug addiction treatment in China. *Addiction, 102*(7), 1057–1063. doi:10.1111/j.1360-0443.2007.01849.x.

Thiesmeyer, L. (2005). *Gender, public health, and human security policy in Asia* (pp. 177–192). New York, NY: United Nations, Division for the Advancement of Women.

Tsai, T., Morisky, D. E. & Chen, Y. A. (2010). Role of service providers of needle syringe program in preventing HIV/AIDS. *AIDS Education & Prevention, 22*(6), 546–557. doi:10.1521/aeap. 2010.22.6.546.

Tucker, J. D., Peng, H., Wang, K., Chang, H., Zhang, S. M., Yang, L. G. & Yang, B. (2011). Female sex worker social networks and STI/HIV prevention in South China. *PLoS ONE, 6*(9), e24816.

Tuñón, M. (2006). Internal labour migration in China: Features and responses. Beijing, ILO, April, 1–51. Retrieved from www.ilo.org/wcmsp5/groups/public/--asia/--ro-bangkok/--ilo-beijing/documents/publication/wcms_158634.pdf

UN (United Nations). (2000). Security Council Resolution 1308 (2000) on the Responsibility of the Security Council in the Maintenance of International Peace and Security: HIV/AIDS and International Peace-keeping Operation. Resolution 1308 (2000*)*. Adopted by the Security Council at its 4172nd meeting, on 17 July 2000. Retrieved from: www. unaids.org/sites/default/files/sub_landing/files/20000717_un_scresolution_1308_en.pdf

UN (United Nations). (2010). General Assembly concludes human security debate, with some speakers saying idea too imprecise, while others describe it as forward-thinking, adaptable to UN. Press Release: General Assembly GA/10944, 21 May 2010. Department of Public Information, United Nations, New York. Retrieved from www. un.org/News/Press/docs/2010/ga10944.doc.htm

UN (United Nations). (2012). General Assembly calls for accelerated efforts to eliminate malaria in developing countries, particularly Africa, by 2015, in consensus resolution. Also adopts consensus text on human security, holds dialogue on macroeconomic policy, sustainable development. Press Release: General Assembly GA/11274, 10 September 2012. Department of Public Information, United Nations, New York. Retrieved from www.un.org/News/Press/docs//2012/ga11274.doc.htm

UNAIDS. (2011). *HIV in Asia and the Pacific: Getting to zero*. UNAIDS. Retrieved from www.unaids.org/en/media/unaids/contentassets/documents/unaidspublication/2011/20110826_APGettingToZero_en.pdf

UNAIDS. (2014a). *2014 China AIDS response progress report.* National Health and Family Planning Commission of the People's Republic of China. May. Retrieved from www.unaids.org/sites/default/files/documents/CHN_narrative_report_2014.pdf

UNAIDS. (2014b). 90–90–90 An ambitious treatment target to help end the AIDS epidemic. Geneva, Switzerland. Retrieved from: www.unaids.org/sites/default/files/media_asset/90-90-90_en_0.pdf

UNAIDS. (2015). *2015 China AIDS Response Progress Report.* National Health and Family Planning Commission of the People's Republic of China. May. Retrieved from www.unaids.org/sites/default/files/country/documents/CHN_narrative_report_2015.pdf

UNAIDS & China's Ministry of Health (CMOH). (2012). *2012 China AIDS response progress report.* Ministry of Health of the People's Republic of China. 31 March. Retrieved from www.unaids.org/sites/default/files/country/documents//file,68497,es..pdf

UNDP (United Nations Development Program). (1994). *Human development report 1994.* Oxford, UK: Oxford University Press.

Wang, H., Chen, R. Y., Ding, G., Ma, Y., Ma, J., Jiao, J. H., … & Wang, N. (2009). Prevalence and predictors of HIV infection among female sex workers in Kaiyuan city, Yunnan Province, China. *International Journal of Infectious Diseases, 13*(2), 162–169.

Wang, B., Li, X., Stanton, B., Fang, X., Lin, D. & Mao, R. (2007). HIV-related risk behaviors and history of sexually transmitted diseases among male migrants who patronize commercial sex in China. *Sexually Transmitted Diseases, 34*(1), 1–8.

Weiser, S. D., Young, S. L., Cohen, C. R., Kushel, M. B., Tsai, A. C., Tien, P. C., … & Bangsberg, D. R. (2011). Conceptual framework for understanding the bidirectional links between food insecurity and HIV/AIDS. *The American Journal of Clinical Nutrition, 94*(6), 1729S–1739S.

Wishnick, E. (2010). Dilemmas of securitization and health risk management in the People's Republic of China: The cases of SARS and avian influenza. *Health Policy and Planning, 25*(6), 454–466. doi:10.1093/heapol/czq065.

Wu, Z., Wang, Y., Detels, R. & Rotheram-Borus, M. J. (2010). China AIDS policy implementation: Reversing the HIV/AIDS epidemic by 2015. *International Journal of Epidemiology, 39*(suppl. 2), ii1–ii3.

Xiao, Y., Kristensen, S., Sun, J., Lu, L. & Vermund, S. H. (2007). Expansion of HIV/AIDS in China: Lessons from Yunnan Province. *Social Science & Medicine, 64*(3), 665–675.

Yang, C., Latkin, C., Luan, R. & Nelson, K. (2010). Condom use with female sex workers among male clients in Sichuan Province, China: The role of interpersonal and venue-level factors. *Journal of Urban Health, 87*(2), 292–303.

Yang, G. Y. & Le, T. (2008). Cultural and political factors in conducting qualitative research in China. *Qualitative Research Journal, 8*(2), 113–123.

Yang, L. H. & Kleinman, A. (2008). 'Face' and the embodiment of stigma in China: The cases of schizophrenia and AIDS. *Social Science & Medicine, 67*(3), 398–408. doi:10.1016/j.socscimed.2008.03.011.

Yang, X., Derlega, V. J. & Luo, H. (2007). Migration, behaviour change and HIV/STD risks in China. *AIDS Care, 19*(2), 282–288.

Yao, Y., Wang, N., Chu, J., Ding, G., Jin, X., Sun, Y., … & Smith, K. (2009). Sexual behavior and risks for HIV infection and transmission among male injecting drug users in Yunnan, China. *International Journal of Infectious Diseases, 13*(2), 154–161.

Yi, H., Mantell, J. E., Wu, R., Lu, Z., Zeng, J. & Wan, Y. (2010). A profile of HIV risk factors in the context of sex work environments among migrant female sex workers in Beijing, China. *Psychology, Health & Medicine, 15*(2), 172–187.

Yip, R. (2006). Opportunity for effective prevention of AIDS in China: The strategy of preventing secondary transmission of HIV. In J. Kaufman, A. Kleinman & T. Saich (Eds.), *AIDS and social policy in China* (pp. 177–189). Cambridge, MA: Harvard University Asia Center.

Yu, D., Souteyrand, Y., Banda, M. A., Kaufman, J. & Perriëns, J. H. (2008). Investment in HIV/AIDS programs: Does it help strengthen health systems in developing countries? *Globalization and Health, 4*(1), 8.

Zhang, F., Hsu, M., Yu, L., Wen, Y. & Pan, J. (2006). Initiation of the national free antiretroviral therapy program in rural China. In J. Kaufman, A., Kleinman & T., Saich (Eds.), *AIDS and social policy in China* (pp. 96–124). Cambridge, MA: Harvard University Asia Center.

Zhang, L., Chow, E. P., Jing, J., Zhuang, X., Li, X., He, M., … & Wang, L. (2013). HIV prevalence in China: Integration of surveillance data and a systematic review. *The Lancet, Infectious Diseases, 13*(11), 955–963.

Zhao, G. M. (2003). Trafficking of women for marriage in China: Policy and practice. *Criminal Justice, 3*(1), 83–102.

Zhao, R., Gao, H., Shi, X., Tucker, J. D., Yang, Z., Min, X., … & Wang, N. (2005). Sexually transmitted disease/HIV and heterosexual risk among miners in townships of Yunnan Province, China. *AIDS Patient Care & STDs, 19*(12), 848–852.

Zhou, F., Kominski, G. F., Qian, H. Z., Wang, J., Duan, S., Guo, Z. & Zhao, X. (2011). Expenditures for the care of HIV-infected patients in rural areas in China's antiretroviral therapy programs. *BMC Medicine, 9*(6), 1–10. doi:10.1186/1741–7015-9-6.

2   Human insecurity and non-traditional threats to security

'The Foolish Old Man' removes a mountain.

愚公移山

HIV/AIDS is a non-traditional threat to security at both a macro (state/governmental) level and a micro (individual) level. Epidemics damage states from the inside out. They cause problems between proximate states and damage national economies. At the macro level, there are several reasons for this, including

- cross-border migration increasing the probability of HIV infections;
- loss of economic revenue;
- over-burdened health systems;
- increasing costs, as HIV/AIDS becomes a chronic health issue.

Additionally, there has been continuing debate about the effect that HIV/AIDS epidemics have on state militaries. At the micro level, individuals suffer from:

- the fear of stigmatisation;
- poverty;
- harassment and imprisonment;
- lack of food;
- lack of shelter;
- inability to access the medicines needed to ensure their survival.

Non-traditional security is a concept that has continued to come to the fore in the present globalised world. Economics, governance and issues such as climate change, terrorism, disaster preparedness and pandemic disease have been elevated from being strictly a concern for nation-states and local communities to concerns for the global community. When an issue that does not respect state boundaries affects one state, then all states (particularly those in close proximity) must of necessity intervene in an attempt to protect themselves. These types of issues cannot be resolved or even effectively managed within state boundaries. Coordinated responses between states, global regimes and international donors become imperative.

Human security is a term that encompasses aspects of both development and human rights. It is concerned with the individual and ensuring that their basic needs are met. It is premised on the idea that everyone has certain expectations in life. Individuals should have their basic needs met. In human security frameworks, this is classified as being free from want. Human security frameworks also insist that individuals should also be free from fear and protected from harm. Additional to the basic tenets of freedom from fear and want, there are seven sub-provisions of security:

1   economic
2   food
3   health
4   environmental
5   personal
6   community
7   political security.

Finally, individuals should also have the freedom to live in dignity. Kofi Annan introduced this third pillar of human security in 2005 and it was reiterated in Resolution 60/1 of the World Summit Outcome in the same year (UN, 2005). It is apparent that these freedoms and seven tenets should be attainable for all people. This is even more imperative for key populations in HIV/AIDS epidemics due to the correlation between human security (or more specifically the results of insecurity which can be defined as the absence of human security) and the drivers of virus communicability.

Theoretical approaches to security: traditional and non-traditional

There are many schools of thought concerning securitisation. It is an evolving field of academic contemplation. As the world changes, so too does the need to understand the role that security plays in the global amphitheatre. This book concentrates on ideas of critical security, which focus on the referent of security, the nature of the threats, and whose interests are being served (Browning & McDonald, 2013). Securitisation has a performative power and is not only useful as a descriptor for a situation being securitised but can also have a transformative role (Balzacq, Léonard & Ruzicka, 2016). Ultimately, securitisation is concerned with how a security issue is determined; what should be done about it?; and what are the consequences of agreeing that something is a threat (Balzacq, Léonard & Ruzicka, 2016)? Irrespective of the differing schools of thought within securitisation theory, they share basic characteristics and are rather simply modulated by interpretations of power relations, context and agency (p. 6).

Thus, in order to grasp the foundations of non-traditional security, it is useful to briefly examine the trajectory taken by securitisation scholars. Differing schools of thought in the area of critical security have emerged in order to address the variations of aim and modes of analysis among scholars (Peoples & Vaughan-Williams, 2015). However, there are limitations to the categorisation of schools of security thought. The implication in such a rendering is that all scholars within the different schools are in accord. This is misleading, as scholars ascribing to the tenets of these schools are in diverse locations and many more do not fit within the parameters of thought at all. Rather, it may be more useful to think of them as networks of diverse thinkers from a range of disciplines whose scholarship and dialogue on security topics outweigh their contradictory thinking (Peoples & Vaughan-Williams, 2015).

For example, securitisation theory has a close affinity with the following:

• social constructivism and the role of language and the practice and power of argument in global politics;
• speech act theory;
• Foucault's theory of governmentality, which provides securitisation theory with an analysis of the conditions under which entities emerge, exist and change;
• Bourdieu's theories on sociology;
• Schmitt's theories of political realism (Balzacq et al., 2016).

Schmitt and Foucault in particular have had a continuing influence on the shaping of securitisation theory over the past decade. Understanding these complexities, the two schools of thought most appropriate as frameworks for understanding the theoretical underpinnings being used are what are called the Welsh (Aberystwyth) and Copenhagen Schools.

The Welsh or Aberystwyth School

The Welsh or Aberystwyth School of thought began with Ken Booth and Richard Wyn Jones proposing a brand of security studies that challenged existing definitions of security. Booth argued that entrenchment in traditional notions of security privileged the nation-state and preserved state regimes at the cost of the individual (Browning & McDonald, 2013). Instead of accepting previous notions of security as simply being military threats to the nation-state, they considered that security should be linked to the goal of human emancipation. The nation-state should be concerned with the well-being of its citizens and the means for their security rather than the referent object.

This is a normative approach that challenges the concept of state security and instead posits that consideration should be given to how individuals can be made secure from broader threats such as poverty, environmental degradation and political oppression (Peoples & Vaughan-Williams, 2015). However, while they attempt to use security to advance emancipation, they give less consideration to the possibility that other methodologies (such as the language of human rights, justice or economics) might be better suited to achieving such goals (Browning & McDonald, 2013). What is missing is an understanding that the goal of security is variable, depending on circumstance, place and time, and a singular reading fails to provide a useful ethical framework (foundational or procedural) and thus becomes ambiguous and inconsistent.

The Copenhagen School

Scholars at the Copenhagen Peace Research Institute (COPRI), prompted by socio-political events occurring at the time (such as the fall of the Berlin Wall, ethnic and interstate conflicts and the demise of the Soviet Union), began to question the sufficiency of existing security dialogues (Van Munster, 2005). The new concept of security moving away from military concerns with security sought to include the wide range of threats to human survival. They became known as the Copenhagen School. Unlike the Welsh School's explicitly normative approach, the Copenhagen School offers an analytical concept of 'securitisation' as a way to develop security dialogues (Peoples & Vaughan-Williams, 2015). Thus, in 1998, securitisation developed as a constructivist theory.

The securitisation of a particular issue from risk to security threat requires that it be established as something that is in urgent need of attention and should therefore take absolute priority (Buzan, Wæver & De Wilde, 1998). Therefore,

> [S]ecurity is about survival. It is when an issue is presented as posing an existential threat to a designated referent object (traditionally, but not necessarily, the state, incorporating government, territory and society). The special nature of security threats justifies the use of extraordinary measures to handle them.
>
> (p. 21)

Thus, the securitisation process involves a particular issue being declared as a present threat to security (Buzan et al., 1998; Lo, 2015). These declarations are considered to be speech acts and are directed towards a particular audience (Elbe, 2010; McDonald, 2008). They only become securitised once the audience has been convinced and has accepted that they are threats.

The Copenhagen School considers that the act of securitisation is a 'self-referential practice, because it is in this practice that the issue becomes a security issue – not necessarily because a real existential threat exists but because the issue is presented as such a threat' (Buzan et al., 1998, p. 24). Therefore, the securitisation process is based on the identification of particular problems affecting individuals, nation-states or the international community as a whole.

> Issues become 'securitized' when a threat exists or is believed to exist against some fundamental values that are held by some actor, be it an individual, a group, a community, a nation, a group of nations, or an international community.
>
> (Akaha, 2002, p. 1)

Predictably, the success of the securitisation process is not determined by the entity seeking securitisation but rather by the audience (whether citizens or other stakeholders) (Lo, 2015). However, the Copenhagen School is concerned with analysing the consequences of invoking security frameworks and are sceptical about whether issues such as poverty and environmental degradation should be considered threats to security (Peoples & Vaughan-Williams, 2015). Irrespective of their concerns about which issues should be securitised, they acknowledge that once a particular issue is accepted as a threat, then securitisation may occur.

Thus, the broadly constructivist approach of the Copenhagen School is used when explaining that securitisation identifies security threats as politically and socially constructed (Hameiri & Jones, 2015). Threats are not just bound in reality but constructed, spoken and accepted (Elbe, 2010). The Copenhagen School argues that 'to "securitise" an issue means identifying it as a threat to some cherished reference object, raising it to the top of, or even above, the political agenda and mobilising extraordinary measures and resources to combat the problem' (Hameiri & Jones, 2015, p. 1).

Elbe (2010) suggests: 'Security "is not interesting as a sign referring to something more real; it is the utterance itself that is the act. By saying the words something is done …"' (p. 11). Balzacq et al. (2016) suggest that:

> [T]he key idea underlying securitization is that an issue is given sufficient saliency to win the assent of the audience, which enables those who are authorised to handle the issue to use whatever means they deem most appropriate. In other words, securitization combines the politics of threat design with that of threat management.
>
> (p. 3)

Securitisation then is the identification of something as a security threat and its acceptance by others in such a manner that authorities are enabled to manage the threat.

Securing humanity: state and human security

Non-traditional threats to security can be defined as transboundary in nature rendering state-based governance inadequate to successfully address the challenges inherent in the global issues that have been contextualised as threats. The following useful interpretation of non-traditional security suggests: '[E]fforts to manage transboundary security threats do not simply involve empowering supranational organisations, but primarily seek to transform state apparatuses dealing with specific issue-areas and integrate them into multilevel, regional or global regulatory governance networks' (Hameiri & Jones, 2015, p. 4).

Non-traditional security solutions require collaboration between states. The nature of the threats being faced and the globalisation of society ensure that solutions are beyond traditional arguments of sovereignty. In the realm of non-traditional security, what affects one nation-state almost always results in a causal sequence of events occurring in another.

The world is a changing place. No longer is international travel the privilege of the elite or governmental representatives but rather it is increasingly accessible to everybody. As a result, rather than limited incidences of cross-border travel, hundreds of thousands of people are travelling from place to place on any given day. National borders are permeable. What affects one nation-state quite often has the ability to affect another, especially those in proximate areas. Nation-states wanting to engage on the global stage can no longer put up walls of sovereignty and isolate themselves from other stakeholders. Non-state actors, such as NGOs, INGOs and transnational corporations, are also growing in increased importance in global affairs (Swanström, 2010). Threats are no longer just external and an expanded concept of sovereignty denotes more than the conviction that threats from outside must be repelled but also that threats from inside must be dealt with.

Traditional forms of security are rooted in realist paradigms and operate on the premise that a nation-state's main threat comes from external forces (Akaha, 2002; Alkire, 2003). These paradigms have been in place since the Treaty of Westphalia of 1608 that formally established the concept of the nation-state and the sovereignty implicit to it (Swanström, 2010). As a result, the nation-state became the main actor and at the centre of international relations (Selgelid & Enemark, 2008). Accordingly, as proposed by Hans Morgenthau, with people being at the core egotistical and selfish, the international system is anarchic and geared towards war. In this arena, international relations are a struggle to maintain or obtain power, irrespective of ethical considerations (Donnelly, 2005).

Threats are dealt with in the arena of war. Success is conferred when one nation-state overcomes the oppressive advances of another. Realism considers that war is not only probable but acceptable (Donnelly, 2005). Within that framework, threats such as pandemic disease, economic collapse, state failure, environmental pollution and dealing with environmental disasters have been the purview of state governments. Sovereignty is unassailable and the attempts of other nation-states to interfere in national policies concerning these previously exclusively internal dilemmas are greeted with outrage and military force.

Therefore, traditional forms of security place the nation-state as the referent object with the express purpose of protecting its territory, political boundaries, population and interests against external attempts to seize power, whether military or economic (Akaha, 2002; Bernard, 2013). National policies within this traditional, realist framework are intended to meet the needs and values of the nation-state as a whole rather than the needs of individuals within the state. Buzan et al. (1998) conclude: 'Sovereignty can be existentially threatened by anything that questions recognition, legitimacy or governing authority' (p. 22). Threats are perceived as being external to the state and are most likely to manifest themselves as war or non-military coercion in the form of political and economic sanctions.

Conversely, the more liberalist, non-traditional security is concerned with state threats originating discrete from, or at least additional to, the sanctions and military conflicts that operate in the domain of traditional security. Significantly, non-traditional concepts of security, such as human security, are not implemented in place of traditional concerns but are rather mutually reinforcing and complementary in nature (Hayes & Qarluq, 2011; Swanström, 2010). Often they are transnational in nature and focus on non-military threats that affect multiple nation-states. As such, these threats may originate externally to or within a nation-state and generally involve natural threats or transnational activities (commonly criminal in nature). The salient point is that they are uncontainable and often asymmetrical in nature, thus requiring non-conventional solutions.

While nation-states will always protect themselves from eternal threats and perceived violations of sovereignty, issues of environmental degradation, terrorism, transnational crime, global pandemics, national economic collapse and state failure must be solved collaboratively. Since the end of the Cold War, there has been growing awareness of the need to widen the concept of security beyond traditional concepts (Swanström, 2010). This has had the effect of raising the profile of what have conventionally been viewed as 'soft' threats to national security (Swanström, 2010). This is essential in a world where many more people die from threats to their human security, such as food scarcity and disease, than through conventional warfare (De Waal et al., 2010b). In a globalised world, since the Cold War, the rapid growth in technology has forced security dialogues to be reframed. Weaker communities have become more disadvantaged and social inequality is more pronounced. The likelihood of new types of security threats becoming manifest continues to increase.

Thus, international spaces are increasingly influenced by events taking place within the sovereign borders of nation-states. A security threat for one nation-state becomes a security threat for another and is of global concern. In framing these global security issues, it is evident that in order for something to be considered a security threat, it must first be identified and agreed upon as posing a significant risk. This process must occur whether the issue is being resolved within a state or poses a threat to other nation-states or globally. The referent threatened must believe that they are threatened by a particular state of affairs or situation and convince others of that belief.

Human security

Within the context of globalisation the individual has become an important focus of security dialogues. As discussed, security agendas have been elevated beyond the confines of state-centric ideology to incorporate considerations of the pervasive threats faced by individuals. Issues such as poverty and infectious disease affect individuals within states and therefore, inevitably, the state itself. Within the realm of non-traditional security, human security frameworks have emerged to address the needs of individuals.

There are a number of different definitions of human security. In order to understand how it is applied, it is important to provide an overarching definition. In general, most definitions encompass many of the same concepts, with freedom from fear and want featuring prominently in the majority of definitions. Ramesh Thakur describes it as referring to the quality of life of a people or polity (Thakur, 1997, cited in Annan, 2001). Yukio Takasu (2000), the UN Under-Secretary-General for Management, has previously described human security as preserving and protecting the life and dignity of human beings. Van Ginkel and Newman (2000, cited in Annan, 2001) describe it as a comprehensive security that is both integrated and sustainable.

While all of these definitions are applicable, this book adopts the broad UN definition, presented in Chapter 1, stating that human security can be encapsulated as freedom from fear, freedom from want and the freedom to live in dignity. The rationale for doing so is that it is most applicable for comprehending the needs of marginalised and mobile populations in HIV/AIDS epidemics. This definition makes it apparent that human security is concerned with the individual and ensuring that they have the freedom to make their own choices and the opportunity to fulfil their potential. This definition was expanded (UNDP, 1994, pp. 24–25) to incorporate seven specific threats to human security: economic, food, health, environmental, personal, community and political.

Rather than simply addressing the rights of individuals and the threats they face, human security also seeks to incorporate an individual's development needs into discussions and action. It creates a framework for disparate communities to discuss concepts of security beyond traditional concerns (Christie, 2010). Therefore, human security shares conceptual space with ideas of human rights and human development (Alkire, 2003). Indubitably, for human security initiatives, they are parallel roads leading to the same desired outcome – the right of individuals to live free from fear and want.

The concept of human rights has existed for decades. As early as 1941, Theodore Roosevelt addressed the idea of human rights in his State of the Union speech, when he discussed four fundamental freedoms (Kettemann, 2006). He articulated that freedom means the supremacy of human rights universally and that people should be fighting for the rights of individuals everywhere (Burgers, 1992). He further expanded the concept to include the notion that true freedom means being 'free from fear and want' (Elbe, 2010). It was here that the term was first vocalised.

While Roosevelt was discussing human rights, it is also applicable to the realm of human security (human security incorporates notions of human rights). Later it became a foundational philosophy in defining human security's basic tenets, as introduced by Kofi Annan in his address to the UN Security Council in 2000. When presenting the concept to the UN Security Council, Annan built upon the understandings of President Roosevelt 59 years earlier. Moreover, the concept of human security has continued to be clarified and refined by the UN in the decades since Annan's declaration.

As a concept, human security is focused on creating feasible solutions that address the particular rights and needs of people rather than states. It is protective and normative and involves reshaping security dialogues around the individual. Newman (2010) suggests that human security 'seeks to challenge attitudes and institutions that privilege so-called "high politics" above individual experiences of deprivation and insecurity' (p. 79). When the people become the referent object, then security must be built from below at the level of the individual (Dahl-Eriksen, 2007). Additionally, human security dialogues provide opportunities to identify links between distinct factors and address issues that may have been neglected (Fukuda-Parr, 2003).

Ultimately human security should protect the individual from critical pervasive threats and enable long-term human fulfilment (Alkire, 2003). It is concerned with the sanctity of the individual and the community and the preservation of life (McIntosh & Hunter, 2010). Hudson (2005) advises, 'In this way, emphasis shifts from a security dilemma of states to a survival dilemma of people' (p. 163). Focus changes to the actual conditions that threaten insecurity in daily life and to sustaining the dignity of individuals (Martin & Owen, 2010). Thus, human security provides a crucial scaffold for shaping responses to the ever-present threats faced by states and individuals in current global environments. Because institutions and actors primarily implement policy, the focus is on top-down interventions whereas vulnerable populations face human insecurity from a bottom-up micro level (Lemanski, 2012).

Consequently, a more useful mode of delivery is a 'dual strategy of bottom-up empowerment balanced with top-down policies' (Chen & Takemi, 2015). Thus, unless the needs of individuals are paramount in creating policy, effective and sustainable change will remain elusive. Therefore, human security can serve three roles in shaping responses to health emergencies (Figure 2.1). First, it can be used as a philosophy that prioritises the attainment of human freedoms (freedom from want, freedom from fear and the freedom to live with dignity) in government policies; second, it can be used as a tool to generate policy at the governmental and institutional levels that will enable individuals to undertake actions that will allow them to fulfil their potential. Finally, it can be used by

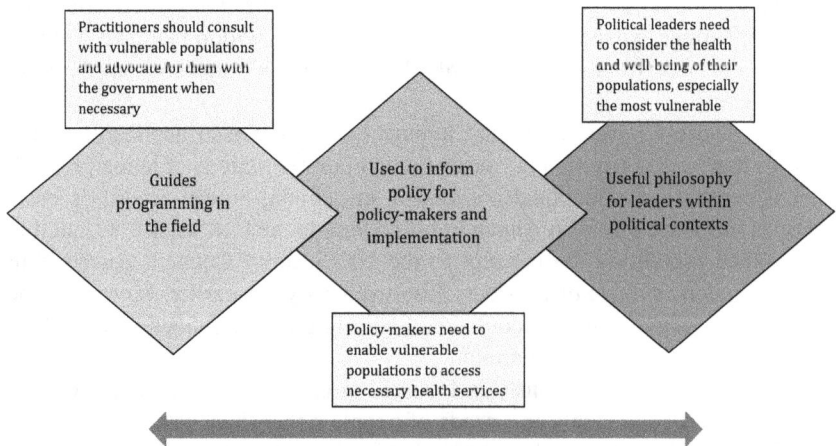

Figure 2.1 Human security's role in the health field.

practitioners to guide their programming in the field in order to reduce the sources of vulnerability and mitigate the threat to the lives of individuals (Korc, Hubbard, Suzuki & Jimba, 2016).

The idea that successful intervention can only be achieved by addressing the needs of individuals was tacitly promoted in the United Nations Development Programme (UNDP) *Human Development Report*, presented in 1994. In that report the margins of human security, under the umbrella of non-traditional security theory, were enlarged to identify seven main assumptions necessary for the realisation of human security for individuals (Nishikawa, 2009). In order for individuals to fully obtain human security they must be protected from threats affecting:

> economic security (poverty, unemployment, homelessness), food security (undernourishment, famine, hunger), health security (disease, infections, insufficient health care), environmental security (degradation, pollution, natural disaster), personal security (physical torture, war, crime, violence), community security (ethnic tensions, oppression, discrimination) and political security (repression, torture, ill treatment, human rights violations).
>
> (Gündüz, 2006, p. 53)

Significantly, while engagement in war does produce a substantial lack of human security, there are many situations having pronounced impacts on the safety and security of individuals that do not involve war. Additionally, many of these insecurities are interconnected and a lack of human security in one of these areas often leads to a lack of human security in other areas.

Importantly, many of the dialogues surrounding human security take note of the theory's express collocation to the many challenges faced by individuals. The UNDP report (1994) highlights the fact that 'For most people, a feeling of insecurity arises more from worries about daily life than from the dread of a cataclysmic world event' (p. 22). It stated that human security is people-centred and concerned with how they live (UNDP, 1994). All types of insecurity have an effect on people living with HIV/AIDs (PLWHA). Human (in)security and the vulnerability of individuals, particularly those who are marginalised and stigmatised, have a profound effect on health outcomes. The individual must be the main point of reference in order to effectively address epidemiological concerns. To reiterate, HIV is passed from individual to individual, therefore prevention efforts must concern the individual.

Conversely, in public health scenarios, the HIV+ individual remains important only as a vector for the spread of disease. The human security of individuals is subsumed under the overarching policy goals concerned with halting the spread of the disease, especially within the general population. This is the situation in China. While Beijing has made some inroads into dealing with HIV/AIDS, its focus remains on the disease rather than the individuals. While there are some indications that this may be changing, the human security needs of PLWHA are not paramount. Aside from some programmes run by (relatively) independent community-based organisations (CBOs) at a grassroots level, HIV/AIDS treatment and prevention services are offered mainly in relation to the greater public good. While this seems appropriate at the surface level, it does not deal with the underlying reasons for the spread of HIV/AIDS among populations.

China's concept of people's safety

Ideas of human security have been aired in China since the late 1990s and generally greeted with suspicion and wariness (Shen, 2014). They do not engage with the definitions emanating from Western schools of thought but rather couch their understanding in terms of broader concepts of 'people's safety' (Chu, 2002). The main reason for this is Beijing's insistence on maintaining the traditional prioritisation of sovereignty. Events occurring in China are therefore China's concern and outside forces should not interfere in sovereign issues. Additionally, China's past history and current challenges in managing the many disparate nationalities and ethnic groups within its borders have an impact on the breadth of its interpretations regarding human security (Chu, 2002). That being said, they do acknowledge the need to protect the safety of the people, which may be loosely compared with some of the precepts of human security.

At the sixty-fourth UN General Assembly, the Chinese representative, La Yifan, explained China's understanding of the concept of human security as a broad and abstract idea pertaining to many different fields that did not enjoy international consensus (UN, 2010). China considered it was governments that retained the primary responsibility for the security of their citizens (UN, 2010). However, due to international influences, they have undoubtedly begun to recognise the need to generate discussion concerning the idea of individual safety. Chu (2002) states: 'Human security means protecting people. The Chinese government and people have no problem accepting and following the idea of protecting their people, but they regard such human security issues as ones of human safety, not of "security"' (p. 9). When used in China, the language of human security has been translated to encompass a broad range, allowing for manoeuvrability and adaptation by Beijing. Xiao (2015) argues that China acknowledges that the security for people to develop and survive is fundamental to their notions of security and that this is well represented in the Chinese dream[1] (Xiao, 2015). It is probable that over the decades since the 1994 UNDP report that China has been incrementally engaging with notions of human security within political discourse (Shen, 2014). Thus, the scope of security is being widened to consider people's safety, the regime and system security, alongside the overarching concerns with national security (Chu, 2002).

This needs to be understood in terms of China's definitional application. What might be considered a legitimate incursion in the realms of human security according to Chinese definitions may not fully resemble generally held concepts. Basically, China follows a developmental approach to human rights. Rather than thinking in terms of 'freedom from fear' and 'freedom from want', Chinese leaders and academics promote a non-traditional, state-oriented approach (Shen,

2014). While it does have some comparable objectives with that of human security, they follow a modified approach that still places the state as the primary referent.

In attempting to understand China's use of people's safety concepts, it is helpful to consider the language of their security dialogues. Shen (2014) states that there are two distinct translations of human security in Chinese academic and policy literature. *Ren de an de quan* and *ren lei an quan* both refer to human security in general but have subtle differences, denoting the level of people-centredness. The first term is more ambiguous and can be interpreted in terms of both 'individuals' and 'people' in a collective sense (Shen, 2014). The second is more concentrated on more general renderings such as 'people', 'mankind' or 'humanity', meaning individual aspects of humanity should be more correctly understood in a 'universal' manner (Shen, 2014). The terms are somewhat interchangeable but it should come as no surprise that the latter, broader term is chosen for Chinese translations of the 1994 UNDP report (Shen, 2014).

In practical terms, in HIV/AIDS and other public health situations, China still operates from a collective people viewpoint. Their reasons for this appear to be twofold: the first is grounded in their broad people safety framework; the second is due to their greater political agendas concerning their expansion as a major economic power. China is a country seeking to perpetually increase economic development. It is a one-party authoritarian regime and therefore much of its legitimacy is derived from its successful attainment of economic growth (Lo, 2015).

Inevitably, compromises are made and pursuing short-term economic development may lead to the lower prioritisation of health and disease prevention (Lo, 2015). Beijing then is faced with hard choices for the management of risk (Wishnick, 2010). The moves towards increased economic growth and development that take the focus away from national health may be one of the main risk factors for the spread of HIV in China. This is because, for the main part, their public health infrastructure has been ignored. In such a situation, people's access to health services, and their right to health security, cannot be guaranteed, especially for those who are living in poverty (Chan, Lee & Chan, 2009). China's policies concerning external intervention in national affairs have meant that public health has been considered to be an exclusively domestic problem. As has been shown in the past epidemics, such as SARS, China has consistently played down the international implications of emerging health emergencies within its borders. While this has changed somewhat now, it would be premature to consider that they have adopted an attitude of transparency in the international arena; their health governance has remained state-led (Chan et al., 2009). As yet, the human security concerns of individuals have gained no traction in state dialogues.

Health security into the twenty-first century

The securitisation of disease is generally performed within the framework of human security. Seeking to understand and frame threats are rarely undertaken by individuals but, rather, are pursued through dialogue or speech acts between governments (Elbe, 2010). However, the referents of these speech dialogues are individuals. In acknowledging the individual as the referent, it has become possible to reframe security to identify those things that most hinder the ontogenesis of freedom from fear and want for individuals in global contexts. Thus, the securitisation of infectious disease is not a new phenomenon.

During outbreaks of disease, such as the bubonic plague and influenza, nation-states have rallied to address the urgent need to halt their spread throughout communities and lessen their impact on state economies and institutions (Peterson, 2002). It is beyond the scope of this chapter to consider all aspects of the securitisation of disease (including biological terrorism) or comment on the many differing viewpoints throughout the field of security studies. Rather, it focuses on the more pertinent aspects of securitisation of disease as related to infectious disease and HIV/AIDS in particular.

As presented previously, a seminal change has occurred in recent decades with the securitisation of specific diseases and their link to the core interest of nation-states (Elbe, 2012; Fidler, 2015). This is particularly the case in today's world of high mobility, predominantly via air travel, resulting in shared risk and the fear of the rapid presentation of pathogens or biological agents, whether intentional or unintentional (Tappero, Thomas, Kenyon & Frieden, 2015). Infectious diseases clearly represent transnational threats to security (Campbell, 2012). This change has been driven by the securitisation of HIV/AIDS and successive infectious diseases, such as SARS and H5N1 influenza.

While the securitisation of disease means that extraordinary resources are allocated and directed towards treatment, this may not be universally perceived as positive. Moves towards the securitisation of disease mean that the agents of disease, or the referent and external threat source (in this case, disease as external to the traditional workings of a nation-state and possibly the state itself), are locked into the logic of securitisation (Davies, 2008). Consequently, the simple presentation of a disease as a threat makes it a security issue, whether a real existential threat exists or not (Davies, 2008). This has implications for the manner in which disease is contextualised and thus approached. As a result, there are extant debates about whether or not disease should be securitised at all and it has become a disputed concept.

In general, securitisation theory, when applied to disease and global health, focuses on the normative and methodological aspects: should health be securitised and how is the success of securitising moves to be measured (Balzacq et al., 2016)? In general, scholars and practitioners assessing the benefits of the securitisation of disease agree that there are both positive and negative consequences. While the negative consequences are real, they are alleviated by the positive outcomes, or usefulness, of mobilising resources to address the challenges of disease.

Critics of the securitisation of disease

Critics of the securitisation of disease generally object to either the process or the outcome of securitisation (Roe, 2012). Among security scholars there are those who believe that the securitisation of disease, particularly in human security scenarios, opens up the possibility of creating flaws in policy. The question of whether or not health problems actually comprise a security threat is important, as are guidelines for how they correspond with other security concerns (Peterson, 2002). In the context of securitisation, silence and speed are preferred to debate, deliberation and consideration of the rules and procedures of normal government (Roe, 2012). In essence, securitisation is bad for democracy. There are also concerns that the securitisation of HIV/ADS will activate the 'threat-defence logic' where the members of the armed forces would receive the highest priority in health services and medical treatment (Balzacq et al., 2016).

In this scenario some people fear that health is perceived as less important, and justifiable only in terms of its impact on national security (Davies, 2008; Gündüz, 2006). The referent becomes the disease and its impact on the state, rather than the individual living with disease. In essence, bodies become the battlefield rather than the reason for battle to take place (Elbe, 2012). In this situation, the political effects of health security may lead to the sacrifice of an individual's human security in the name of the greater good or collective security (Nunes, 2014; Selgelid & Enemark, 2008; Stephenson, Davis, Flowers, MacGregor & Waller, 2014; Vieira, 2007). Yet, there is some concern that without a link between epidemic disease and national security, elites will pay little attention to the problem.

Aldis (2008) and Kettemann (2006) question whether framing a disease as a threat to human security is helpful, arguing that the outcome of securitisation can lead to an us:them binary. Roe (2012) argues that securitisation pushes responses to disease away from the transparency of civil society towards the opaque workings of military and intelligence organisations, which creates the potential for violations of human rights and civil liberties. A direct result of these misunderstandings may be the discrimination of individuals, refusal to share data and restrictions on civil liberties (Wishnick, 2010). Additionally, there are some fears that an extreme focus on a particular threat may leave nation-states open to other threats as their bureaucratic organisations, and human and financial resources are consumed by the issue considered the highest priority (Balzacq et al., 2016).

Aldis (2008), Newman (2010) and Pitsuwan and Caballero-Anthony (2014) also argue that all definitions of human security are contested, therefore human security is analytically weak and too broad to be functionally appropriate. Elbe (2010) and Hindmarch (2016) posit that when applying human security frameworks, everything considered detrimental to an individual's ability to achieve personal fulfilment becomes a threat to their human security and thus loses analytical usefulness. Having such a broad focus can possibly lead to misunderstandings and breakdown of global collaborations and dialogues (Aldis, 2008). It is clear that some of the arguments presented by the critics are valid, but while acknowledging the negative concerns, it is essential that they be weighed against the positive outcomes.

Proponents of the securitisation of disease

The proponents of securitisation of disease within a human security framework are concerned with the benefits conferred by being placed in the global spotlight. A positive securitisation approach embraces the concept that securitisation need not be militaristic and dismissive of due process but rather that human connectedness and shared values, such as compassion, justice and dignity cut across existing social and political divisions (Booth, 2007). When diseases such as HIV/AIDS become securitised, they attract attention as urgent problems and therefore receive proportionate resources for addressing the problem (Wishnick, 2010). Concerns about the potential of infectious diseases to incur high rates of mortality also come to the fore in securitised frameworks (Peterson, 2002).

As a result of this, surveillance mechanisms are improved and there is an added focus upon early warning and prevention efforts (Fukuda-Parr, 2003). Korc et al. (2016) advise:

> The Institute of Development Studies in the United Kingdom suggested that adopting a human security framework would improve the post-2015 agenda by acknowledging interactions among different threats, promoting more cross-disciplinary thinking, addressing in-country inequalities, creating more linkages between people and their governments, and transcending borders of all types.
>
> (p. 10)

With an increased focus on infectious disease due to securitisation, there also emanates an increased will to address issues of stigmatisation and maintain sustainable budgets (Lo, 2015).

Ultimately, for many who are interested in promoting the usefulness of human security frameworks in addressing infectious disease, academic debates are somewhat superfluous and incidental. They are more concerned with the functionality of human security in protecting individuals from fear and want. In this context, addressing the needs of those who are perilously insecure is paramount (Newman, 2010). Significantly, since the release of the 1994 UNDP Development Report, understandings of human security have continued to expand to become holistic and more development-orientated (Lisk, Šehović & Sekalala, 2015). When the basic human security needs of individuals are dealt with, they become more likely to become actively involved in contributing to sustainable long-term security solutions within their communities, their nations, and, eventually, within the global commons.

The securitisation of HIV/AIDS

The idea that AIDS posed a threat to security was being debated as early as 1987 (McInnes & Rushton, 2010), but it was not until July 2000 that HIV/AIDS formally became securitised with the passing of Resolution 1308 at the UN Security Council. Al Gore addressed the Security Council, introducing AIDS as a combatant in a field of war – the war against AIDS was to begin in earnest (Gore, 2000). In the act of securitising AIDS, he used realist language and traditional concerns with security to highlight the serious nature of the threat being presented by the AIDS epidemic. For the first time, AIDS became a focus of the UN within the context of a non-traditional threat to security. Previously it had been solely contextualised as a medical problem to be dealt with by sovereign states.

HIV/AIDS was presented as an immediate threat to military and peace-keeping forces (Singer, 2002). At the time of its securitisation, it was believed that AIDS would contribute to instability by wreaking devastating losses on security forces (Rushton, 2010). Security forces were perceived to have higher infection rates than other cohorts and that peacekeepers, through high-risk behaviours, could be implicated in the spread of HIV/AIDS. Essentially, claimed Fourie and Schönteich (2001): 'War is an instrument for the spread of HIV/AIDS' (p. 35). Annan (2000b) proposed that the destructive nature of AIDS was no less destructive than warfare itself and that in some ways it was worse. He claimed that it overwhelmed health services, cause economic crisis and threatened political stability.

Significantly, there is evidence that HIV/AIDS may contribute to the instability of states, particularly those more vulnerable due to other factors (Feldbaum, Lee & Patel, 2006). In addition, it is also argued that it poses 'diverse threats to human security and to national and international security' (De Waal et al., 2010b, p. 25). Singer (2002) argues that the presentation of HIV/AIDS as a security threat strengthens reactions to the disease, not simply due to altruism but in the pursuit of self-interest. In securitising HIV/AIDS through the UN Security Council, it is hoped that, due to its high profile and status in international law, the UN will be able to apply political pressure and encourage governments to address the issue through early and prompt responses to the pandemic (Elbe, 2006).

With the adoption of Resolution 1308, the securitisation of HIV/AIDS was assumed to have been accepted unanimously. However, Fourie and Schönteich (2001) queried its classification as a security threat (although conceding that in terms of post-Cold War human security regimes, it did pose a pervasive and non-violent threat to the existence of individuals), because it did not fit into the traditional military framework of security. McInnes and Rushton (2013) agree with this stance, commenting, 'it is not obviously a security issue, at least not in the narrow national/international security sense' (p. 17). Nevertheless, the belief that HIV/AIDS affects the security of states has been widely accepted and requires exceptional responses (McInnes & Rushton, 2013).

Conclusion

Non-traditional threats to security have emerged on global political agendas in response to the identification of ever-expanding threats in a globalised world. Traditional security approaches, while still of paramount importance, are no longer the sole preoccupation of state governments. Non-traditional issues, such as pandemic disease, environmental degradation, transnational crime and terrorism, have been catapulted onto political security schedules. As a result of these expanded concepts of threat, human security frameworks have been developed and implemented in order to understand the confluence of dangers apparent in contemporary transboundary circumstances.

The concept of human security was introduced internationally with the release of the UNDP (1994) *Human Development Report.* Having generated a scaffold to explain, and attempt to address, the myriad of insecurities faced by individuals in a globalised context, it serves to entwine concepts of human rights and development in practical ways. The seven subclauses that extrapolate on the basic principles of 'freedom from fear' and 'freedom from want' include; economic security, food security, health security, environmental security, personal security, community security and political security.

HIV/AIDS was securitised by the UN Security Council in 2000 and has undergone subsequent refining processes over the intervening decades. While debates still remain concerning its veracity as a securitised concept, there seems little disagreement concerning the very real threats to human attainment inherent in the disease. Securitisation of HIV/AIDS, while initially implemented using traditional security language focusing on the threats to states rather than the threats to individuals, considers individuals as the referent object. However, due to the military repercussions of burgeoning HIV/AIDS epidemics being prioritised, the day-to-day human security of PLWHA and other stakeholders has been of secondary concern.

In order for issues to become securitised, they must be communicated to an audience who then agrees with their identification as a threat. The Copenhagen School describes this as a speech act and explains that the securitisation occurs at the moment it is elucidated as a threat rather than its basis in any real threat. A threat is a threat because a collective group of people agree that it is. This can cause stakeholders to debate issues of definition and application when responding to problems, particularly when using broad human security definitions about what constitutes a threat.

This has been an issue of contention among scholars for decades. Both the critics and the proponents of the securitisation of disease have put forward valid arguments for their position. The acceptance of human security frameworks lies in the belief that the positive outcomes for the securitisation of threats, such as pandemic disease, greatly outweigh negative considerations. While it is possible that securitisation may concentrate attention on the nation-state rather than on the individual, it does highlight that there is an issue. It also attracts resources and can result in dialogue between stakeholders. Within securitisation frameworks, human security serves to draw attention to the needs of the individual as a way to positively affect the actions of the nation-state.

However, in China, the concept of human security has not been embraced. Rather, they believe that the state is the progenitor of security understandings and thus is solely responsible for ensuring the collective safety of its citizens. People's safety does share some conceptual space with human security discourse but has at its core a predisposition to reference individual security within broader, universal security frameworks. This has been exacerbated by China's push for economic progress, resulting in their focus being drawn away from meeting the health needs of the population in the pursuit of economic ascendancy.

Without sustained political will in health settings, there is little chance of effective engagement in the health security of individuals. China has yet to fully accept the securitisation of HIV/AIDS. However, they have begun to more fully engage with, and acknowledge the need for, non-governmental and international participation. However, they still hold to the belief that dealing with the HIV/AIDS epidemics within their borders is ultimately the internal responsibility of the state.

Therefore, the lack of transparency that currently results in a lack of data, particularly data that fully identifies the extent of the epidemic within their borders, is deemed justifiable. Despite China's stance, when the non-traditional threats are not containable within national borders, they must be discussed and dealt with at a global level. This is particularly the case for pandemic disease. Ultimately, HIV passes from person to person and it is in those spaces that real impact must happen so that the disease may be defeated as a global security threat.

Case study 2.1 Lily's story

Lily is a female sex worker (FSW) and sex worker advocate, who worked along the Myanmar/China border. Her story highlights the problems associated with human insecurity for a key population in HIV/AIDS epidemics. Stigmatisation, lack of access to adequate health care and resources, and lack of personal, community and economic security all contribute to the difficulties faced by Lily and her cohorts. As a result of these insecurities, FSW often feel compelled to operate their business in a manner that poses high risks for the transmission of HIV.

When I met Lily, she was quiet and reserved but seemed happy to be talking to me about her life. For my part, I just wanted to listen and learn and absorb as much about her history as I could. Her life had been challenging and yet she had such an upbeat attitude towards everything. Lily is from Myanmar and with her long black hair and infectious smile, she radiated beauty. When I met her, she was working as a sex worker in Myanmar in an area close to Yangon. She said that this was so that she could be close to her family but she had worked in brothels on both sides of the Chinese border. She told me that she had been in the industry for a long time.

She did not tell me how or why she had become a sex worker and I did not ask. I was not focused on her reasons for becoming a sex worker (although in cases of coercion and hopelessness, it is a valid research point of interest); I wanted to know the challenges that she faced daily to obtain the tools and services necessary to stay healthy. And so, Lily told me her story. Parts of it were what I had expected, based on the existing literature, but she also revealed some troubling aspects to the sex trade in Yunnan's national border areas that had not been represented in any of the literature that I had previously read.

Lily told me that many of the girls struggled with their daily reality but work was work, and sex work gave them a good opportunity to make decent money. She did not feel that there were many other options. She told me, 'It's just a job like any other. I don't know why there is such a problem with it. We pay our bills and take care of ourselves. We are not a burden to anyone.' But it is not an easy job. There are challenges, and when I asked her if she was concerned about HIV, she assured me that she was and that the girls all took what precautions they could. She herself is HIV+. She started sex work as a teenager and had contracted the disease through the course of doing business.

She told me that it was best for the girls to travel from one area to another. This was not only to avoid being arrested but also because the brothel owners preferred to have a high turnover of women as their customers liked to see new faces. She said that many girls like her had worked on both the Myanmar and China sides of the border. Lily revealed that the borders are so porous that girls travel and set up operations from one country to another with great ease. I knew this to be true because when I had been in Ruili, I had decided to see for myself how easy it was to cross the border. The place I went to was on the Ruili River near to where it joins the Shweli River (known as *Nam Mao* in Shan and *Lung Chuan Chiang* in Chinese) that serves as the border between Myanmar and China. There was a small shack that operated as a waiting area and I was told that boats went back and forth with great regularity. I would not have to wait long the owner told me and it would only cost me 10 yuan for the journey. And so I waited for the boat to return.

As I sat there waiting, groups of people began to show up. I do not know if there was an advertised timetable for boat crossings or whether the boats just came and went with such regularity at certain times of the day that people had become familiar with when they might have the least amount of time to wait. Near where I sat waiting, there was a steep concrete ramp that disappeared into the water. As I watched, a flat-bottomed boat backed up to the ramp and dropped a rudimentary gangplank. I was fascinated to see young women in impossibly high heels totter down the ramp clutching the arms of the men assisting them. When the young women had embarked, the men returned and started to drive motorbikes down the ramp and right up onto the boat. Then the owner turned to me and asked if I was ready to go. I declined and told him that I was really just there to find out how easy it would be to make the journey but that as a foreigner I did not want to cross into Myanmar without the correct authorisations.

The same river that is used to transit people between Myanmar and China is also used to transit illicit drugs and other goods and services. Yunnan is well known for having border towns and villages used as transit points on the drug trafficking routes originating in both the Golden Triangle and the Golden Crescent drug production areas. Ruili is one such area but there are many others. Lily explained to me that the girls often set themselves up in these areas or have been trafficked into these areas due to the trade in illicit drugs. Where there is a trade for drugs, there is trade for sex. She went on to explain to me that the sex and drug trades are very closely connected.

In a startling revelation that I had not come across in any of the literature, Lily told me that sex workers are given a monetary fine by the brothel owners/madams if they do not entice the clients to partake of drugs when engaging in sexual services. I asked her whether the sex workers were beaten when they failed to convince their clients to take the drugs and she assured me that they were not, they simply had a fine deducted from their takings. She said that this places a great deal of pressure on the sex workers to push so-called party drugs, such as ketamine and methamphetamines and ecstasy (in particular) on clients. She told me that the sex workers and clients took the drugs together and that the clients paid a lot extra for the privilege. When asked, she said that injection drugs such as heroin were not pushed onto clients but that many of the girls were themselves injection drug users.

Apart from the challenges associated with having to push drugs onto their clients, Lily recounted an event to me that sheds light on some of the discrimination faced by sex workers. Condom distribution is considered to be a benchmark in global best practice (GBP) for key populations in HIV/AIDS epidemics. Barrier protection is considered paramount between sex workers and clients in an attempt to halt the bidirectional contagion of HIV. Many condom programmes are available and most areas have at least some kind of distribution process. However, many of the key populations are hard to reach and closed to non-peers. Lily explained to me that she had arranged to meet a worker from an NGO who was involved in condom distribution to sex workers in Myanmar. The NGO worker had a supply of condoms to be distributed to sex workers within the district.

When Lily described the events to me, she admitted that it had made her feel shamed and unclean. The NGO worker who had brought the boxes of condoms contacted Lily and told her that she was in town and asked her to come and collect the supplies from a nearby hotel where the NGO worker was staying for the night. The meeting was scheduled for the next morning but when Lily arrived at the hotel to collect the condoms, the NGO worker had simply left the supplies there and departed. The result was that Lily had to negotiate receipt of the condoms from the hotel manager. When he found out that his hotel had been used as a collection point for condom distribution, he was livid. I asked her if that was normal procedure. She told me that sometimes the person delivering the condoms did not want to interact with the sex workers. However, it was the first time that they had just been left at the hotel when she was collecting them and that it had made her very angry and scared that she had to plead with the hotel manager to get the condoms. She told me that she had only persisted because she had to get them for all of the girls in her peer network.

Condoms are delivered to the area for distribution once every three months. In the more remote rural areas they are brought less often and it is harder to get supplies. Lily told me that the allocation of condoms per person totalled 60 free condoms for a three-month period (five condoms per week). I asked her if she thought that this allocation was sufficient to protect sex workers from HIV and other STIs. She told me that it was not enough. Sometimes they might have six or seven clients in a night and that in general most girls had used their free condom supplies within the first two or three weeks. I asked her what happened when the condoms ran out. Lily divulged to me that many times the sex workers were forced to provide services to clients without using condoms, adding that they had no choice as there were not enough condoms to go round.

I asked her whether sex workers were able to purchase their own supplies and she stated that often the girls did try to do that but the costs involved with having to buy condoms made it difficult. In addition, particularly in the more rural areas, it was often difficult to obtain them, even if they did want to pay for them. She said that she knew that she could transmit HIV to her clients if she did not use a condom but that she was given little choice. She told me that they all needed to work and could not afford to be without the income from sex work.

The case study involving Lily shows that there is very little human security for sex workers along the China/Myanmar border area. Research has shown that the story of Lily is also representative of the situation for sex workers in the China/ Vietnam and China/Laos border regions. Sex work is still highly stigmatised even among medical and NGO workers who claim they are providing assistance. Sex workers do not have sufficient access to the numbers of condoms needed to provide sexual services without risking infection with HIV or other STIs. Their vulnerability also forces them to become drug pushers and be constantly mobile in search of work. Finally, in addition to being unable to access condoms easily in different areas, their mobility often prevents them from gaining access to sufficient health care. GBP clearly indicates that sex workers are a key population in HIV epidemics. They need to be a focus for increased human security in order to address the current shortfalls of services within this population.

Note

1 In his first month of office, Chinese President Xi Jinping proposed the *China Dream*, calling for a great rejuvenation of the Chinese nation resulting in: prosperity, the strengthening of society and the military, and a common dream for all Chinese people under the socialist party rule.

References

Akaha, T. (2002). Non-traditional security: Issues in Northeast Asia and prospects for international cooperation. Paper presented at 'Thinking Outside the Security Box: Non-traditional Security in Asia: Governance, Globalization, and the Environment'. United Nations University Seminar, United Nations, New York, March (Vol. 15). Retrieved from http://archive.unu.edu/ona/seminars/securityinasia/akaha.pdf

Aldis, W. (2008). Health security as a public health concept: A critical analysis. *Health Policy and Planning, 23*(6), 369–375. doi:10.1093/heapol/czn030.

Alkire, S. (2003). A conceptual framework for human security. Working Paper no. 2. Centre for Research on Inequality, Human Security and Ethnicity (CRISE). Oxford University.

Annan, K. (2000). Secretary-General salutes international workshop on Human Security in Mongolia. Ulaanbaatar, 8–10 May. Press release SG/SM/7382. Retrieved from www.un.org/News/Press/docs/2000/20000508.sgsm7382.doc.html

Annan, K. (2001). Definitions of human security. United Nations definitions, Retrieved from www.gdrc.org/sustdev/husec/Definitions.pdf

Balzacq, T., Léonard, S. & Ruzicka, J. (2016). 'Securitization' revisited: Theory and cases. *International Relations, 30*(4), 494–531.

Bernard, K. W. (2013). Health and national security: A contemporary collision of cultures. *Biosecurity and Bioterrorism: Biodefense Strategy, Practice, and Science, 11*(2), 157–162. doi:10.1089/bsp.2013.8522.

Booth, K. (2007). *Theory of world security* (vol. 105). Cambridge, UK: Cambridge University Press.

Browning, C. S. & McDonald, M. (2013). The future of critical security studies: Ethics and the politics of security. *European Journal of International Relations, 19*(2), 235–255.

Burgers, J. H. (1992). The road to San Francisco: The revival of the human rights idea in the twentieth century. *Human Rights Quarterly, 14*(4), 447–477. Retrieved from http://humanrightsinitiative.ucdavis.edu/files/2012/10/burgerroadtosf.pdf

Buzan, B., Wæver, O. & De Wilde, J. (1998). *Security: A new framework for analysis.* Boulder, CO: Lynne Rienner Publishers.

Campbell, J. R. (2012). Human health threats and implications for regional security in Southeast Asia. In B. T. C. Guari (Ed.), *Human security* (pp. 173–191). New York, NY: Springer.

Chan, L. H., Lee, P. K. & Chan, G. (2009). China engages global health governance: Processes and dilemmas. *Global Public Health, 4*(1), 1–30.

Chen, L. & Takemi, K. (2015). Ebola: lessons in human security. In D. L. Heymann, L. Chen, K. Takemi, D. P. Fidler, J. W. Tappero, M. J. Thomas, … & R. P. Rannan-Eliya (Eds.), Global health security: The wider lessons from the West African Ebola virus disease epidemic. *The Lancet, 385*(9980), 1885–1888.

Christie, R. (2010). Critical voices and human security: To endure, to engage or to critique? *Security Dialogue, 41*(169). 169–190. doi:10.1177/0967010610361891.

Chu, S. (2002). China and human security. North Pacific Policy Papers No. 8. Northeast Asia Cooperation Project. Institute of Asian Research. Vancouver, Canada: University of British Columbia.

Dahl-Eriksen, T. (2007). Human security: A new concept which adds new dimensions to human rights discussions? *Human Security Journal, 5*(Winter), 16–27.

Davies, S. E. (2008). Securitizing infectious disease. *International Affairs, 84*(2), 295–313. doi:10.1111/j.1468-2346.2008.00704.x.

De Waal, A., Klot, J. F. & Mahajan, M. (2010a). HIV/AIDS, security and conflict: New realities, new responses. *Forced Migration Review, 6.*

De Waal, A., Klot, J. F., Mahajan, M., Huber, D., Frerks, G. & M'Boup, S. (2010b). *HIV/AIDS, security and conflict: New realities, new responses AIDS, security and conflict initiative.* New York, NY: Social Science Research Network.

Donnelly, J. (2005). Realism. In S. Burchill (Ed.), *Theories of international relations,* (pp. 29–54). New York, NY: Palgrave Macmillan.

Elbe, S. (2006). Should HIV/AIDS be securitized? The ethical dilemmas of linking HIV/AIDS and security. *International Studies Quarterly, 50,* 119–144.

Elbe, S. (2010). *Security and global health.* Cambridge, UK: Polity.

Elbe, S. (2012). Bodies as battlefields: Toward the medicalization of insecurity. *International Political Sociology, 6*(3), 320–322.

Feldbaum, H., Lee, K. & Patel, P. (2006) The national security implications of HIV/AIDS. *PLoS Medicine, 3*(6): e171, 0774–0778. doi:10.1371/journal.pmed.0030171.

Fidler, D. P. (2015). The Ebola outbreak and the future of global health security. In D. L. Heymann, L. Chen, K. Takemi, D. P. Fidler, J. W. Tappero, M. J. Thomas, … & R. P. Rannan-Eliya (Eds.), Global health security: The wider lessons from the West African Ebola virus disease epidemic. *The Lancet, 385*(9980), 1888–1889.

Fourie, P. & Schönteich, M. (2001). Africa's new security threat: HIV/AIDS and human security in Southern Africa. *African Security Review, 10*(4), 29–42. http://dx.doi.org/10.1080/10246029.2001.9627950

Fukuda-Parr, S. (2003). New threats to human security in the era of globalization. *Journal of Human Development, 4*(2), 167–179. doi:10.1080/1464988032000087523.

Gore, A. (2000). Remarks prepared for delivery by Vice President Al Gore U.N. Security Council session on AIDS in Africa. Washington, DC: The White House. Retrieved from http://clinton4.nara.gov/WH/EOP/OVP/speeches/unaid_health.html

Gündüz, Z. (2006) The HIV/AIDS epidemic: What's security got to do with it? Retrieved from http://sam.gov.tr/wpcontent/uploads/2012/02/ZuhalYesilyurtGunduz.pdf (accessed 9 October 2015).

Hameiri, S. & Jones, L. (2015). *Governing borderless threats: Non-traditional security and the politics of state transformation.* Cambridge, UK: Cambridge University Press.

Hayes, A. & Qarluq, A. (2011). Securitising HIV/AIDS in the Xinjiang Uyghur autonomous region. *Australian Journal of International Affairs, 65*(2), 203–219. doi:10.1080/10357718.2011.550104.

Hindmarch, S. (2016). *Securing health: HIV and the limits of securitization.* New York, NY: Routledge.

Hudson, H. (2005). 'Doing' security as though humans matter: A feminist perspective on gender and the politics of human security. *Security Dialogue, 36*(2), 155–174.

Kettemann, M. C. (2006). The conceptual debate on human security and its relevance for the development of international law. *Human Security Perspectives, 1*(3), 39–52.

Korc, M., Hubbard, S., Suzuki, T. & Jimba, M. (2016). Health, resilience, and human security: moving toward health for all. AIDS Data Hub. Retrieved from www.aidsdatahub.org/health-resilience-and-human-security-moving-toward-health

Lemanski, C. (2012). Everyday human (in)security: Rescaling for the southern city. *Security Dialogue, 43*(1), 61–78. doi:10.1177/0967010611430435.

Lisk, F., Šehović, A. B. & Sekalala, S. (2015). Health and human security: A wrinkle in time or a new paradigm?. *Contemporary Politics, 21*(1), 25–39. doi:10.1080/13569775.2014.993908.

Lo, C. Y. P. (2015). *HIV/AIDS in China and India: Governing health security.* Basingstoke, UK: Palgrave Macmillan.

Martin, M. & Owen, T. (2010). The second generation of human security: Lessons from the UN and EU experience. *International Affairs, 86*(1), 211–224.

McDonald, M. (2008). Securitization and the construction of security. *European Journal of International Relations, 14*(4), 563–587. doi:10.1177/1354066108097553.

McInnes, C. & Rushton, S. (2013). HIV/AIDS and securitization theory. European Journal of International Relations, 19(1), 115–138.

McIntosh, M. & Hunter, A. (2010). Perspectives on human security: An emergent construct. In M. McIntosh & A. Hunter (Eds.), *New perspectives on human security.* Sheffield, UK: Greenleaf Publishing.

Newman, E. (2010). Critical human security studies. *Review of International Studies, 36*, 77–94. doi:10.1017/S0260210509990519.

Nishikawa, Y. (2009). Human security in Southeast Asia: Viable solution or empty slogan? *Security Dialogue, 40*, 213–236. doi:10.1177/0967010609103088.

Nunes, J. (2014). Questioning health security: Insecurity and domination in world politics. *Review of International Studies, 40*(05), 939–960. doi:10.1017/S0260210514000357.

Peoples, C. & Vaughan-Williams, N. (2015). *Critical security studies: An introduction* (2nd ed.). London, UK: Routledge.

Peterson, S. (2002). Epidemic disease and national security. *Security Studies, 12*(2), 43–81.

Pitsuwan, S. & Caballero-Anthony, M. (2014). Human security in Southeast Asia: 20 years in review. *Asian Journal of Peacebuilding, 2*(2), 199–215.

Roe, P. (2012). Is securitization a 'negative' concept? Revisiting the normative debate over normal versus extraordinary politics. *Security Dialogue, 43*(3), 249–266.

Rushton, S. (2010). AIDS and international security in the United Nations system. *Health Policy and Planning, 25*(6), 495–504. doi:10.1093/heapol/czq051.

Selgelid, M. J. & Enemark, C. (2008). Infectious diseases, security and ethics: The case of HIV/AIDS. *Bioethics, 22*(9), 457–465. doi:10.1111/j.1467-8519.2008.00696.x.

Shen, W. (2014). New wine in an old bottle? The Chinese perspective on human security: Implications for EU-China security cooperation. *Policy, 15*, 1–13.

Singer, P. W. (2002). AIDS and international security. *Survival, 44*(1), 145–158.

Stephenson, N., Davis, M., Flowers, P., MacGregor, C. & Waller, E. (2014). Mobilising 'vulnerability' in the public health response to pandemic influenza. *Social Science & Medicine, 102*, 10–17. http://dx.doi.org/10.1016/j.socscimed.2013.11.031

Swanström, N. (2010). Traditional and non-traditional security threats in central Asia: Connecting the new and the old. *China and Eurasia Forum Quarterly, 8*(2), 35–51.

Takasu, Y. (2000). Statement by Director-General Takasu Yukio at 'International Conference on Human Security in a Globalized World', Ulan-Bator, 8 May. Retrieved from www.mofa.go.jp/policy/human-secu/speeeh0005

Tappero, J. W., Thomas, M. J., Kenyon, T. A. & Frieden, T. R. (2015). Global health security agenda: Building resilient public health systems to stop infectious disease threats. In D. L. Heymann, L. Chen, K. Takemi, D. P. Fidler, J. W. Tappero, M. J. Thomas, ... & R. P. Rannan-Eliya (Eds.), Global health security: the wider lessons from the West African Ebola virus disease epidemic. *The Lancet, 385*(9980), 1884–1887.

UN (United Nations). (2005). Resolution adopted by the General Assembly on 16 September 2005. Sixtieth session Agenda items 46 and 120. 60/1. 2005 World Summit Outcome. Retrieved from www.un.org/en/development/desa/population/migration/ generalassembly/docs/globalcompact/A_RES_60_1.pdf

UN (United Nations). (2010). General Assembly concludes human security debate, with some speakers saying idea too imprecise, while others describe it as forward-thinking, adaptable to UN. Press release: General Assembly GA/10944, 21 May 2010. Department of Public Information, United Nations, New York. Retrieved from www. un.org/News/Press/docs/2010/ga10944.doc.htm

UNDP (United Nations Development Program). (1994). *Human development report 1994.* Oxford, UK: Oxford University Press.

Van Munster, R. (2005). *Logics of security: The Copenhagen School, risk management and the war on terror.* Copenhagen, Denmark: Syddansk Universitet.

Vieira, M. A. (2007). The securitization of the HIV/AIDS epidemic as a norm: A contribution to constructivist scholarship on the emergence and diffusion of international norms. *Brazilian Political Science Review, 1*(2), 137–181. Retrieved from www.bpsr.org.br/english/arquivos/BPSR_v1_n2_feb2008_05.pdf

Wishnick, E. (2010). Dilemmas of securitization and health risk management in the People's Republic of China: The cases of SARS and avian influenza. *Health Policy and Planning, 25*(6), 454–466. doi:10.1093/heapol/czq065.

Xiao, R. (2015). Human security in practice: The Chinese experience. JICA-RI Working Paper no. 92, 1–26. Retrieved from http://jica-ri.jica.go.jp/publication/assets/ JICA-RI%20WP%20No. 92.pdf

3 HIV/AIDS overview

Disease comes like a fall from a mountain but leaves like coiling silk.

病来如山倒病去如抽丝

The examination of HIV/AIDS as a non-traditional security threat provides a foundation for understanding the threat that HIV/AIDS poses to both individuals and nation-states. Lack of human security adds to the complexities inherent in the management of HIV/AIDS epidemics. This chapter considers the main drivers of the HIV/AIDS epidemic in relation to the pathogenesis and epidemiological functions of the virus. Its value lies in the provision of a clear understanding of the complexities involved in dealing with the disease on a political, social and individual level. Understanding the various challenges inherent in dealing with a virus of such adaptability and diversity provides a foundation for understanding the need for non-traditional security viewpoints, and human security dialogues, to be implemented in continuing discussions concerning treatment and prevention.

A rudimentary, but sufficient, representation of the molecular mechanisms used by the HIV-1 virus to enter the body and begin the process of infection is helpful at this point. This is important because the way the virus uses the human body to progress its own replication has a direct correlation with the behaviours of individuals. Knowing the 'how' enables researchers to provide the general population with the information required to make informed decisions about their own health. It also enables governments and civil service institutions to focus prevention efforts on programmes that are likely to be most efficacious in rendering the HIV's incursion methods ineffective.

In addition, knowing the 'how' enables researchers to develop drug treatment regimes that are specifically targeted at stopping the replication of the virus by preventing, among other things, fusion between the envelope and target cell receptors. In order to counteract viral drug resistance, recombination between different sub-types (or clades) and reduce viral shedding, epidemiologists and other researchers must attempt to comprehend not only the myriad of reactions occurring within the virus but also the distinct immunological reactions implemented by the host. The ultimate goal of such efforts is the development of an effective vaccine functional across the many types, sub-types and recombinants.

The global context for HIV/AIDS and the spread of the disease over the past almost 30 years since it was first identified will provide an understanding of the similarities and differences of HIV/AIDS epidemics, within the context of a global pandemic.[1] There are challenges in all HIV epidemics; on an individual level, people may be dealing with problems of cultural practices, low adherence to complex drug regimens, delays in initiating antiretroviral therapy (ART) or a limited ability to access services. Other problems might arise from drug toxicity, pill fatigue and drug resistance (Eisinger & Fauci, 2018). Sometimes the challenges are due to lack of commitment by central governments to swiftly address the spread of HIV within their borders. While China has made some significant progress in its HIV/AIDS programming over the last two decades, there are areas still requiring attention.

Identification of the HIV-1 strains common to China's epidemics, and the ongoing burden of sexually transmitted infections (STIs) will help in understanding the changing dynamics of the spread of HIV/AIDS from people who inject drugs (PWID), female sex worker (FSWs) and mobile populations into the general population. Men who have sex with men (MSM), mother-to-child transmission (MTCT), former plasma donors (FPDs), although worthy of mention, will only briefly be considered in the context of their impact upon other key populations and when providing valuable information on China's overall HIV epidemiology. Understanding the pathogenesis of different strains of HIV allows policy-makers and researchers to trace the epidemics back to the source and provide valuable information on the behavioural drivers and the required ART regimes.

The HIV virus is adaptable, efficient and lethal. Without effective intervention agendas, it will continue to spread throughout populations. In attempting to gain a solid understanding of the challenges of the virus, the next section discusses the pathogenesis of HIV-1 and the mechanisms used by the virus to enter and exploit the host's immune system. The diversity, rapid rate of reproduction, ability to form new recombinant strains, and defences against the body's immune system make it a formidable adversary.

Pathogenesis and epidemiology of HIV/AIDS

In order to understand the practicalities of dealing with the HIV virus in a global context, it is essential to gain an understanding of the pathogenesis and epidemiology of the virus. Detailing the different strains of HIV and the transmission mechanisms of HIV/AIDS allows understanding of its impact on individuals and populations. Epidemiologists are able to trace the distinct trajectory of various strains back to their source to understand the main drivers of the spread in a specific community. This section provides elementary information on the molecular and immunological function of the virus in order to aid the understanding of the complex nature of the virus's immunological functions once it has breached the defence systems of the host.

In addition to identifying the molecular structures of the virus, understanding how HIV works allows researchers to ascertain what types of behaviours might be considered 'high risk' in HIV epidemics. A comprehensive appreciation of the virus's entry points into the body enables researchers to inform programming efforts geared towards creating physical barriers and addressing cultural and behavioural change. It also allows researchers to work towards creating the drugs necessary to assist the immune system to form chemical barriers. Understanding how the HIV virus progresses to AIDS allows researchers to work towards developing a vaccine. Ultimately, as HIV/AIDS moves from a guaranteed death sentence to a chronic health issue, it becomes crucial for a vaccine to be developed as national economies are unlikely to be able to sustain the current treatment and prevention practices.

The pathogenesis of HIV/AIDS

HIV enters the human body through an exchange of bodily fluid (semen, vaginal fluids, blood and breast milk). In this way, transmission of HIV can occur during birth or when breast-feeding; through sexual contact; and due to needle-sharing practices of PWID. However, most HIV epidemics are sexually driven and more than 90 per cent of infections are through heterosexual intercourse (Andreoletti et al., 2007). Considering that it has the highest infection percentage rate, this section will concentrate on sexual transmission of HIV. The transmission of HIV through sexual activity occurs when the HIV virus contained in genital secretions (semen and vaginal fluid) breaches the epithelial barrier, due to tearing, inflammation and micro-abrasions of the rectal mucosa or cervico-vaginal or penile epithelium in the vagina or anal cavity (Geise & Duerr, 2009, p. 55).

Interestingly, transmission of HIV during sexual contact is not overly efficient (Anderson, 2009). Research suggests that only one in every hundred exposures will lead to infection (Geise & Duerr, 2009). Reasons for this include the generally inhospitable environment for pathogens due to immune system responses within the mucosal lining of the genital area, and the low or acidic pH-levels of the vagina in its normal state (Anderson, 2009; Tyssen et al., 2018). HIV-1 is inactivated at low pH levels (Anderson, 2009). Unfortunately, bacterial infections can elevate pH levels and semen (which is alkaline) creates an almost instant pH-neutral environment in the vagina during unprotected sexual intercourse; which can last for up to an hour after sexual contact, allowing a brief window of opportunity for HIV-1 virons to infect target cells (Anderson, 2009). Additionally, the transmission rates increase during pregnancy due to increased hormonal levels. Of course, this defence does not apply to anal sex or during sexual encounters between MSM.

HIV is more easily transmitted to a recipient partner due to the higher likelihood of the recipient epithelium tearing during sexual activity. This is particularly the case during unprotected anal sex (McGowan, 2009). However, the risk factor is increased bidirectionally in the presence of STIs, which not only add to the likelihood of viral shedding but also cause a higher number of target cells to be found at the site (Anderson, 2009; McGowan, 2009), and both the inserting and recipient partner are at higher risk of contracting HIV regardless of which partner is HIV+ (Anderson, 2009).

The epithelial layers in the genitalia vary in thickness depending on their location. The skin lining the outer genital areas and the inner genital surfaces in both men and women are multi-layered and may be up to 45 epithelial cells thick, making it a forbidding barrier for HIV pathogens (Anderson, 2009). However, the epithelium changes and becomes single-layered and columnar at the cervical opening (for women) and penile urethra (for men), which means that HIV virons are more easily able to penetrate (Anderson, 2009; McGowan, 2009). As mentioned, tearing or inflammation makes the multi-layered squamous epithelium of the outer genital tract breachable.

Infection rates are likely to increase when sexual activity occurs within two months of seroconversion and within the acute infection stage. This is due to higher viral loads and the increased presence of HIV-1 R5 phenotype (or R5-tropic HIV strain)[2] (González et al., 2010). R5-tropic HIV-1 strains are particularly efficient at causing infection in mucosal environments, are not neutralised by HIV-specific antibodies (Anderson, 2009), and R5 phenotypic strains may increase HIV replication (Locher, Witt, Kassel, Dowell, Fujimura & Levy, 2005). There may also be a mixed population of HIV virons with diverse molecular genotypes and phenotypes occurring simultaneously within infected persons (Locher et al., 2005).

Additionally, research suggests that both the female genital tract (Andreoletti et al., 2007) and the male genital tract act as both reservoirs and compartments for the production of HIV (Anderson, 2009; Gay, Kashuba & Cohen, 2009). A reservoir can be defined as tissue that is able to both produce and release the virus and has a continuous inflow of virus (Anderson, 2009, p. 33). Since they act as compartments, this means the genital tracts are environments where HIV viral reproduction can occur independently of other tissues (Anderson, 2009). There may be a diversity of HIV-1 species (quasi-species), phenotypes and molecular genotypes, within and between the blood and semen or vaginal mucosae (Locher et al., 2005; Simon, Ho & Karim, 2006).

There are also latent cellular reservoirs of macrophages and CD4 T memory cells (anatomical sanctuary sites) where the virus can ingress a cell and become integrated into the DNA, becoming almost impossible to remove (Autran, Hamimi & Katlama, 2014; Geise & Duerr, 2009; Simon et al., 2006). In this instance, the virons are resting and non-active in contributing to the infectiousness of the host but are 'replication-competent' (Autran et al., 2014, p. 172). These cell populations, particularly the T cell lymphocytes, are long-lived and resistant to eradication by current ART (Simon et al., 2006).

In the initial infection stage it is thought that Langerhans or dendritic cells catch HIV-1 virons in the genital mucosae and transport them to the draining lymph nodes where the infection cycle starts (Anderson, 2009; Geise & Duerr, 2009; McGowan, 2009). In unprotected sex, the high levels of HIV target cells in the genital area provide HIV virons with a greater chance of breaching a target cell and being carried further into the body. Both cell-associated HIV (cells that have been infected with HIV virons) and cell-free HIV virons can be found in the genital secretions of HIV+ men and women and both are infectious (Anderson,

2009). HIV-infected cells such as macrophages can traverse through mucus and cell-free virons can diffuse through mucus in the absence of HIV-specific antibodies (Anderson, 2009).

Once infected, there are likely to be a number of different pathways for the mucosal transmission of HIV particularly in the presence of epithelial disruption and inflammation (McGowan, 2009). Once the virus has managed to penetrate the epithelium (or been transmitted through blood or breast milk), it targets host cells containing HIV receptors (Figure 3.1). These types of cells include macrophages, Langerhans and dendritic cells found in the mucous and subepithelial layer (Anderson, 2009; McGowan, 2009).

The HIV-1 virons gain entry to the host cell through interacting with two major receptors (R5 and X4) and fusion of the viral envelope with the cell membrane (González et al., 2010). These host cells then carry, or shuttle, HIV to the target cells (Geise & Duerr, 2009). In particular, HIV attacks the CD4+ lymphocytes (also known as T cells and T helper cells) that are a main component of the body's immune system. It does this by replicating and then destroying the CD4+ T cells (Kanki, 2013). These cells then rapidly transport the virus into even deeper tissues. HIV virons are particularly successful at taking advantage of cellular pathways while neutralising and avoiding components of the immune system (Simon et al., 2006).

While ethical considerations prevent research on human subjects, according to modelling done on animals, once HIV virons have been taken up by the target cells, infection can occur within an hour and dissemination of the virus (systemic infection) within 24 hours (McGowan, 2009, p. 86). HIV-1 can be discovered in regional lymph nodes within two days of infection and in the blood within seven days (Geise & Duerr, 2009). The body has not yet been able to generate HIV-specific immune responses and HIV-specific antibodies, thus the virus replicates at a high rate unconstrained (Gay, Kashuba & Cohen, 2009). In infected individuals, HIV progeny are generated at a rate of one billion viral particles a day (Santos & Soares, 2010). Therefore, even though an individual is unlikely to know they are infected, the rapid rate of infection and high numbers of virons in the host mean that high-risk sexual behaviours undertaken during this time are more likely to result in infection.

There is a particularly high viral build-up in areas of the gastrointestinal and genital areas. One of the reasons for this is that gut-associated lymphoid tissues (GALT) have the highest number of CD4+ T cells, particularly memory T cells. This means that this area is a significant reservoir, contains tissue with HIV flowing in and also being produced and released (Anderson, 2009; Kononchik et al., 2018), and is thus a highly active region for the HIV virus. The result of the destruction of CD4+ T cells in the body is the crippling, or severe compromising, of the immune system, making it susceptible to the opportunistic infections that are characteristic of AIDS, which the body no longer has the ability to fight (Arthos et al., 2018; Geise & Duerr, 2009; Kononchik et al., 2018). While ART does cause viral suppression, it has no capacity to restore or restructure this GALT tissue and the damage is apparently irreversible even in individuals who initiate ART within two weeks of infection (Arthos et al., 2018).

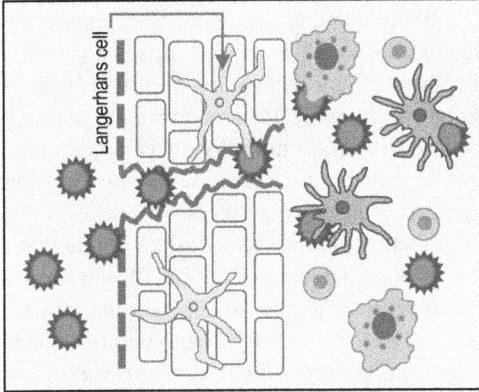

The mucosal tissue of the vaginal wall is layered but the cells are loosely connected making it possible for HIV to pass through (unlike normal skin).

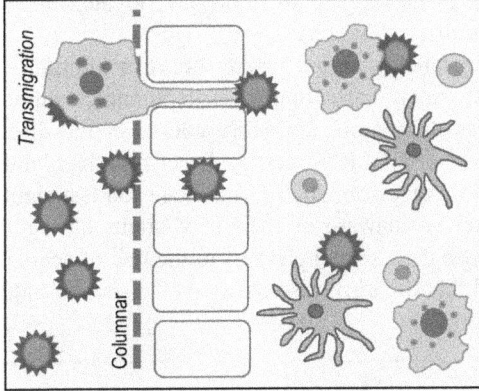

The anus is also lined with mucous membrane but is only a single layer thick (with column-shaped cells), making it even easier for HIV to pass through and why unprotected sex is riskier for the receptive partner.

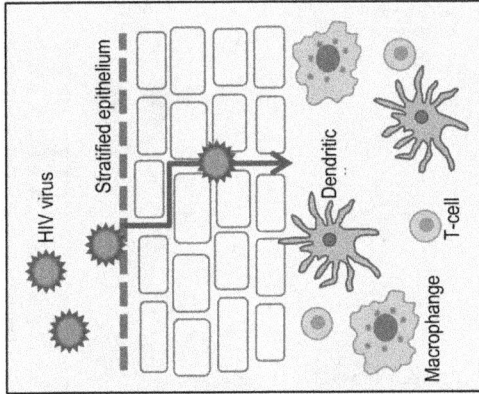

When there is a tear in the skin or micro-abrasion in the mucosal tissue HIV passes through more easily. When an STI is present, the body sends immune cells to fight infection. These are the cells HIV needs to target and they use them to establish infection.

Figure 3.1 Transmission of HIV virus via the epithelium.

The progression of the virus occurs in three different phases, with each phase being either symptomatic or asymptomatic (Figure 3.2). It is important to understand these different phases when grappling with the unique challenges of HIV/AIDS epidemics. One reason for this is that people in the first two stages show no ongoing external indications of infection and as such may misdiagnose themselves and unknowingly spread the disease to others. In fact, this is a problem in HIV/AIDS epidemics with an estimated 50 per cent of people living with HIV and AIDS (PLWHA) being unaware of their HIV seroconversion status. An essential component of HIV prevention is educating individuals concerning the exposure risks and risk behaviours in order to incline those having engaged in high-risk behaviours to seek testing and counselling services.

The initial or acute stage of the infection presents as a flu-like illness that can often be dismissed as a severe cold or a simple bout of the flu. During this time the virus is abundant with very high rates of viral loads in both the blood and genital fluids (Anderson, 2009) and has free reign until the activation and recruitment of CD8+ T cells; which create antibodies to fight the virus (seroconversion) (Zhang et al., 2018). At this stage HIV+ individuals have greater potential to transmit HIV to their sexual partners.

The next phase is the clinical latency period where the virus continues to destroy CD4+ T cells. However, many cases appear asymptomatic, although HIV-1 viral replication continues throughout the entire course of the disease (Simon et al., 2006), and little trace of HIV RNA can be detected in the blood or genital mucosae and seminal fluid (Anderson, 2009). This stage can last eight to ten years. If an HIV+ individual is unaware of their HIV status during this period, they can continue to expose their sexual partners to the risk of acquiring the virus. It is during this period that the virus also develops the sites of hidden

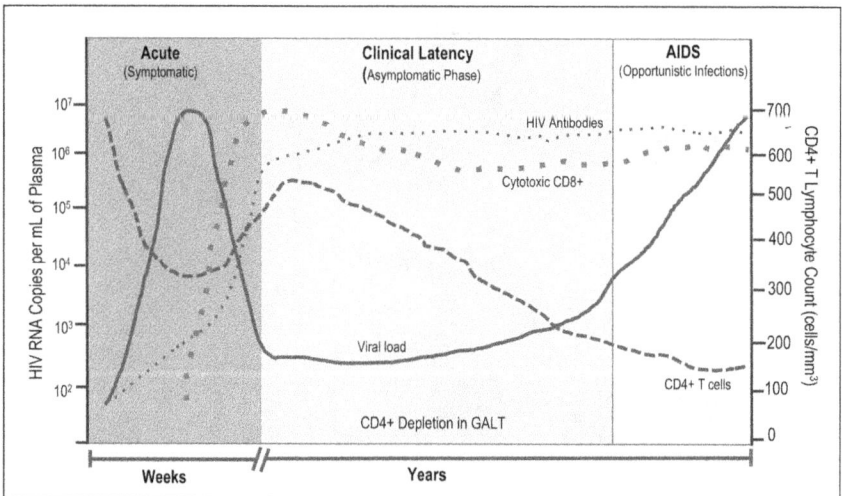

Figure 3.2 The course of HIV-1 infection defined by the level of viral replication.

infection or persistent virus reservoirs. These reservoirs are particularly problematic as they prevent ART from completely eradicating the virus. As yet, no
successful strategies have been developed to flush out these reservoirs but
research continues with the ultimate goal of a cure or long-term control of HIV
without the need for ART (Autran et al., 2014).

As a result of the new treatment as prevention (TasP) guidelines, ART
regimes are initiated when a HIV+ individual acquires a CD4 count <350 cells/
mm^3 (WHO, 2016). Some of the reasons for early initiation of ART include the
preservation of immune cells; limiting the establishment of cell reservoirs;
prevent ongoing immune activations within the body; and to control the inflammation caused by high numbers of HIV viremia occurring in ongoing systematic
infections (Autran et al., 2014). However, even cases where an individual has
received optimal treatment, chronic immune activity can persist, resulting in a
continuous low, undetectable level of virus production (p. 177).

Early implementation of ART may prevent individuals from progressing to
the last phase of the disease: the development of the acquired immunodeficiency
syndrome (AIDS). At this stage of the disease the body's immune system is
severely compromised through a gradual destruction of naïve and memory CD4+
T-lymphocyte cells and HIV viral levels are again elevated in the blood and
semen and the person is no longer able to fight off infection (Simon et al., 2006).
If left untreated, in most cases, this will eventually result in death (Kanki, 2013).

As has been demonstrated, HIV-1 is a particularly effective virus. It has
several defence mechanisms against the formidable arsenal of immune responses
launched by the body and an uncanny ability to use the host cells to further its
replication. Simon et al. (2006) state: 'Mammalian cells are not welcoming
micro-environments, but rather deploy a defensive web to curb endogenous and
exogenous viruses. HIV-1's ability to circumvent these defences is as impressive
as its efficiency to exploit the cellular machinery' (p. 493).

In addition, high rates of viral replication; genetic variability through the
mutation and recombination rates of the reverse transcriptase enzyme (Hemelaar, Gouws, Ghys & Osmanov, 2011); the ability to form recombinants and
quasi-species; and the ability to create compartments and reservoirs allowing
HIV to remain undetectable within some CD4+ memory cells (Autran et al.,
2014) all present a daunting challenge for researchers attempting to create vaccines and ART regimes (Geise & Duerr, 2009; Simon et al., 2006).

This overview of HIV pathogenesis and transmission clearly shows the com-
plexity involved in dealing with ongoing treatment and transmission of the
disease. HIV is adept at hiding in cells of the body, resulting in asymptomatic
presentation of the infection. People often do not realise that they are even
infected. The virus's ability to use the body to create reservoirs and compartments, the high rates of viral production and the ability to generate recombinant
forms add to the challenges of vaccine production and ART. When added to the
complications surrounding STIs and their increased infectiousness, a combination of initiatives is needed to make a real impact.

The role of STIs in exacerbating the spread of HIV

An added risk for HIV transmission within these populations is the presence of STIs. There is much evidence to suggest that individuals who have a pre-existing STI are more prone to becoming infected with HIV in what has been termed an 'epidemiological synergy' (Fleming & Wasserheit, 1999; Xu, Leontyev, Kaul & Gray-Owen, 2018). Equally, infection with HIV may also make individuals more susceptible to STIs (Kilmarx et al., 2018). In addition to their facilitation of HIV seroconversion, the majority of STIs manifest no symptoms (Fleming & Wasserheit, 1999). STIs are rampant globally, particularly in developing nations. Therefore, a combination of high-risk behaviours, STIs and ignorance of HIV status creates an epidemic confluence that exacerbates HIV transmission in both key and general populations.

Ulcerative and non-ulcerative STIs increase the risk of HIV infection through a number of biological mechanisms but primarily through facilitation of HIV shedding in the genital tract, which disrupts the normal epithelial barrier and promotes HIV infectiousness; and through the activation and deployment of HIV-susceptible inflammatory cells, creating an increased vulnerability to HIV infection (Fleming & Wasserheit, 1999; Risbud, 2005). Additionally, immunosuppression due to HIV can add to the complications, alter the course of STIs and impact on their response to treatment (Rein, 2000).

Genital ulcers, such as acute herpes simplex virus (HSV-2), are thought to increase the risk of transmitting HIV-1 bidirectionally (from male to female or female to male) as infected persons frequently bleed during intercourse and HIV has been detected in these ulcer exudates (Fleming & Wasserheit, 1999, p. 10; Rein, 2000; Simon et al., 2006). Non-ulcerative STIs, such as gonorrhoea and chlamydia, are thought to primarily increase the risk for the receptive partner and contribute to HIV transmission through facilitation of HIV shedding and increased viral loads in the HIV+ individual's seminal fluid and genital mucosa. Significantly, gonorrhoea has been associated with a five-fold increase in the possibility of HIV seroconversion (Fleming & Wasserheit, 1999; Xu et al., 2018).

Moreover, the presence of STIs in the insertive or recipient sexual partner increases the risk of HIV transmission bidirectionally (in the case of ulcerative STIs) and to the recipient partner (in non-ulcerative STIs) through the facilitation of HIV shedding and increased viral loads in genital fluids (Zhu et al., 2019). In addition to adding to the risk of HIV, receptive anal intercourse adds to the risk of contracting human papilloma virus (HPV) infection of the anus (Rein, 2000). Significantly, percentage rates of anal HPV infection among homosexual men are extremely high with 93 per cent of HIV+ homosexual men carrying multiple types of HPV and 61 per cent of HIV-negative men infected with a single type (p. 87). When considering the 'epidemiological synergy' between STIs and HIV, this is of some concern.

Regardless of the defence systems deployed by the body and the many technological and biological advances being made in attempts to halt HIV/AIDS epidemics, the disease continues to spread. This is particularly the case in the most vulnerable and difficult to reach populations. Behavioural interventions have also yielded results but cultural and situational environments mean that these may also be limited in success. Women are particularly vulnerable to STI infections due to gender inequalities and gender-based violence; they are more likely to engage in transactional sex; and they more often have asymptomatic STI infections leading to delayed diagnosis and treatment (Medina-Perucha, Family, Scott, Chapman & Dack, 2019). Essentially, it is necessary for policy-makers and those implementing HIV initiatives to understand the precise nature of the epidemic they are dealing with.

STIs in China

China currently has a high burden of STI infections, particularly in FSW, MSM and PWID cohorts. While STIs were once virtually eliminated in China, they have been on the rise since the opening up and reform period of China, beginning in 1978. A relaxation of sexual cultural prohibitions and norms has meant that many more young people are engaging in sex earlier and with multiple partners. When added to the high volume of drug use (both injection and non-injection), alcohol consumption and lack of education about preventing STIs, the probability of incidences of STIs is inevitable. While HIV is considered to be an STI, it is not considered in this section concerning China's STI burden. Rather this section provides information as an addendum to the previous section in order to understand China's epidemiological synergy for HIV and STI infections.

It is difficult to obtain information on the current figures for STIs in China. Available figures, which may be underestimated, show that since the 1980s there has been a dramatic 36-fold increase in the number of infections, with figures suggesting 23,534 in 1986 rising to 859,040 in 2000 (Zheng, Guo, Padmadas, Wang & Wu 2014). Apart from HIV, only syphilis and gonorrhea have mandatory reporting in China, therefore little is known about the extent of other infections, such as HSV-2 (genital herpes), chlamydia infection, genital warts or urethral infection (Zheng et al., 2014).

The incidences of the various types of infection vary across different populations. STIs are found throughout the general population and in the HIV/AIDS key populations. FSWs and MSM communities are most likely to have higher infection rates of specific and highly contagious STIs, such as syphilis, chlamydia, HSV-2 and gonorrhea. Data suggest that there is a much higher incident rate of STIs in commercial sex workers (CSWs), clients of CSWs and individuals engaging in high-risk sex (Zheng et al., 2014). The ulceration due to syphilis and the HSV-2 is implicated in exacerbating HIV transmissibility due to its disruption of the epithelium (Zhu et al., 2019). Other STIs add to infectiousness due to inflammation, chemical changes and the attraction of HIV target cells to the genital area.

In 1991, gonorrhea was the most dominant STI in China but this has changed over the past decades and data now suggest that syphilis is the main STI (Zheng et al., 2014). Prior to 1949, syphilis was dominant but was virtually eliminated due to Chairman Mao's national STI control campaign of the 1950s (Zhang et al., 2014). The STI control campaign entailed shutting down brothels, treatment and screening programmes, and the use of the mass media to provide education on prevention (Zhang et al., 2014).

However, since that time and the move from a socialist to a more market-oriented economy, there has been a substantial increase in commercial sex, drug trafficking and drug addiction. This is particularly problematic with the high numbers of mobile populations in China. As has already been discussed, this mobility, coupled with high-risk behaviours, generates a high probability of these populations exacerbating the spread of STIs in China; in particular, their role as clients of FSWs. In 2012, 68 per cent of STIs in China were thought to be from heterosexual transmission, with transmission through FSWs of particular burden (Zhang et al., 2014).

While Beijing has implemented a number of health initiatives addressing harm reduction, there is still a significant dearth of interventions required. Condom distribution, education and prevention efforts are in place, but as can been seen by the rapid and exponential increase in STIs since 1986, there is vast room for improvement. The challenges for health care and lack of human security in vulnerable populations increase susceptibility to high-risk behaviours and therefore transmission opportunities. It is essential to provide more grassroots-level interventions that address the ongoing human security issues in order to be effective in reaching these populations.

Having discussed the pathogenesis of HIV and the function played by STIs both in global epidemics and the specific context of China, the next section examines the epidemiology of HIV/AIDS epidemics. In order to understand the implications of current prevention and education efforts, it is useful to compre-hend the manner in which the disease has spread and the lessons learned from previous interventions. It also provides a brief framework for understanding the epidemiological considerations for disease outbreaks, particularly within a national and global context.

Global assessment of HIV/AIDS

While there are two types of HIV (HIV-1 and HIV-2), this section concentrates upon understanding and examining the various strains of HIV-1 and its different strains and quasi-species, including circulating and unique recombinant forms of the virus as the main type responsible for global epidemics. This happens in the realm of molecular epidemiology. As such, a definition of epidemiology is useful and so are the reasons why it is essential to halt and ultimately reverse HIV/AIDS epidemics. Significantly, as previously explained and reiterated in this section, identification of the different strains of the HIV virus enables research-ers to follow its trajectory (epidemiology) throughout populations.

Definition and purpose of epidemiology

To assess the scope of the global pandemic and the ways that it progresses through populations, it is beneficial to understand how different strains travel between individuals and populations. These strains are identified using a toolkit of genetic sequencing mechanisms. This chapter does not delve into the specific molecular mechanisms, such as phylogenetic sequence analysis, Gag-pol sequencing, bootstrap analysis and other molecular and genomic identification systems, which are then compared against a library of full-length genomic sequences in public sequence databases, such as that in Los Alamos. Suffice to say that these mechanisms for identifying the different HIV-1 sub-types or strains and the various circulating and unique recombinant forms are essential on both an individual and a societal level. On an individual level, optimal ART is conditional on the correct identification of a particular strain of the virus. On a societal level, correct identification is important because it is essential to understanding the specific drivers contributing to the transmission of HIV-1 throughout key populations and their convergence with the general population.

Current global HIV/AIDS epidemics have been ongoing for more than 30 years and yet the disease continues to elude efforts to bring about its drug-independent control or demise. The complex array of measures that can presently be combined and adapted to meet the needs of specific HIV epidemics are a demonstration of the cooperation and determination of the global community to arrest the further spread of the disease. Much of this nascent success in the global HIV/AIDS pandemic can be traced to epidemiological efforts in the development and assessment of ART and public health initiatives (Amon, 2014). Additionally, epidemiology has contributed to understanding molecular underpinnings of infections and their history, prevalence and trends.

Epidemiology is the practice of tracing the trajectory of diseases through populations. Essentially, it backtracks through the molecular data to find the source of an outbreak and to look at present situations in order to best focus interventions that will provide optimal impact in epidemics. Primarily, it does this by examining specific strains of disease and mapping their movement through specific populations. It is concerned with the biological aspects of disease and employs a portfolio of molecular tools to understand the biological aspects of specific virus and bacteria. Epidemiologists then disseminate this information to assist in formulating methods to halt the disease spread, such as vaccines and drug therapy regimes. Less stridently, it also scrutinises some of the social drivers for epidemics.

There are other aspects of epidemiology that should be considered, such as political and social epidemiology. These have come to the forefront in recent years as the 30+-year lifespan of HIV/AIDS has shown that regardless of how effective molecular mechanisms are in tracing disease and informing public health initiatives, they are insufficient on their own. It is essential to trace the patterns of behaviour and political will, as they are applied to epidemics. Many epidemiologists have highlighted the need to go beyond the molecular determinants to adopt a more ethnographic people-centred approach that considers the consequences of certain behaviours upon epidemics (Amon, 2014).

As such, social epidemiology has contributed significantly to efforts to deal with the ongoing HIV/AIDS pandemic overall and to understandings of situation-specific epidemics. Social epidemiology examines the social and structural determinants for the spread of epidemics (Amon, 2014). It is therefore concerned with the impact of mobile populations, poverty, gender inequity, conflict, stigma and marginalisation. Understanding the macro-social and economic determinants of HIV/AIDS prevalence is essential. Human beings live in communities and therefore the way they are perceived and treated will have a direct impact on disease outcomes. Regardless of how effective the molecular interventions are, they will be useless if an individual cannot afford to see the doctor administering it or if they are afraid of being stigmatised by others.

Additionally, political epidemiology is required for epidemiological approaches to be more consequential. Political epidemiology recognises that political decisions have consequences and long-lasting impacts on disease outcomes. Effective and sustainable interventions in HIV/AIDS epidemics must be backed by strong political will. Governmental policies, law enforcement practices (including police harassment), discriminatory laws, and a weak public health sector have a direct impact on health-related behaviours and the efficacy and outcomes of interventions (Amon, 2014).

As well as mitigating poor HIV/AIDS outcomes through highlighting deleterious discriminatory practices and out-dated law enforcement paradigms, political epidemiology provides other positive contributions. Often, there are limited resources available for allocation of resources, particularly in middle- and low-income countries, and political epidemiology is able to ascertain which HIV strategies are most cost-effective, best suited to the situation and accessible by the populations being targeted (Amon, 2014). Without this analysis, HIV/AIDS programmes are likely to be unsustainable, and unable to address the human rights (as a component of human security) needs of populations, regardless of how effective they may be in other environments.

Political leadership and top-down policy initiatives can have either positive or negative contributions to efforts to halt HIV/AIDS epidemics. Additionally, the criminalisation of sex work, same-gender consensual sex, and drug usage has had a direct influence on the spread of HIV/AIDS globally. There is a dearth of engagement in this area of epidemiology, regardless of the possible benefits it would provide in understanding the human rights/health outcome correlation (Amon, 2014). In HIV/AIDS epidemics, the overwhelming trend is still to concentrate on molecular interventions.

Therefore, in a specific HIV/AIDS context, the practice of epidemiology studies the propagation, transmission patterns and distribution of HIV throughout different geographical areas and key populations. Epidemiology has two main functions: 'examining the distribution and determinants of health, and acting on this knowledge to promote health' (p. 2). In general, epidemiology is concerned with the molecular epidemiologic features of a virus in the context of the risk practices and behavioural trends of populations (Thomson & Nájera, 2005). Quintessentially, it attempts to answer the 'when', 'how', 'why' and 'who' questions. In an HIV/AIDS context, doing so provides essential information for policy-makers and researchers developing prevention interventions, ART and possible vaccines (Amon, 2014). In elucidating the biological mechanisms for transmission, it provides illumination on the behaviours involved in the increase in transmission of the virus.

When tracing the HIV/AIDS pandemic back to its origins, it was discovered that in the early 1900s the original virus jumped species through a number of zoonotic transmissions of Simian Immunodeficiency Virus (SIV) (Hemelaar et al., 2011). As a consequence, the virus adapted and developed to contend with the biological milieus of the new host. In recognising the blood-borne nature of the virus, suppositions were made that the slaughter and eating of non-human primates (namely, chimpanzees and sooty mangabeys) led to the virus being introduced into humans through entry in open wounds on the skin (Mayer & Pizer, 2009). HIV-1 M, from Simian Immunodeficiency Virus Chimpanzee (SIVcpz), is the strain that began the global pandemic but it began to diversify into genetic sub-types (A–D, F–H and J–K) soon after transmission (Hemelaar et al., 2011; Santos & Soares, 2010).

The global HIV/AIDS situation broadly encompasses two transmission configurations: that of generalised epidemics due to heterosexual transmission within the general population; and that within key populations such as CSWs, MSM, and PWID (Kilmarx, 2009). These transmission patterns are characterised by specific strains of HIV, including the original clades, circulating recombinant forms (CRFs) and unique recombinant forms (URFs). Epidemiology reveals that while these sub-types and CRFs can be divergent globally, there are often specific sub-types and CRFs within geographic areas and specific key populations. The next section goes into a more detailed rendering of the global dispersal of the different strains of HIV.

HIV sub-type diversity and why it matters

HIV is an incurable retrovirus (belonging to the *Retroviridae* family, and to the Lentivirus genus) (Santos & Soares, 2010) that can be distinguished genetically and antigenically and exists as two distinct types: HIV and HIV-2 (Lashley, 2006). HIV and HIV-2 both originated in simian species as SIV, notably chimpanzees (SIVcpz) and sooty mangabeys (SIVsm) (Santos & Soares, 2010). HIV-2 is found in West Africa but is rarely found elsewhere, and this is most likely due to its lower infectivity when compared to HIV-1. As previously noted, the genetic diversity, virulence and high transmission rates of HIV-1 have facilitated its dispersion and evolution into a global pandemic.

In addition to the main types, there are four sub-groups within the HIV-1 strain. These are M (main or major) which is responsible for more than 95 per cent of the HIV pandemic; N (new), which is epidemiologically rare, was traced to a recombinant event between the ancestor of group M and SIVcpz (Santos &

Soares, 2010); O (outlier), which is the most divergent group; and P (discovered in 2009 with only one identified case to date). These are all variations arising from the distinct introduction of SIVcpz into human populations (Santos & Soares, 2010).

The M group is the most prevalent among the four groups with nine sub-types, all originating in Central Africa (Kandathil, Ramalingam, Kannangai, David & Sridharan, 2005) and 99 CRFs (Reis, Guimarães, Bello & Stefani, 2019). Within the main sub-group (the M sub-type) there are at least 10 viral isolates, referred to as sub-types or clades, the first nine are classified as A–D, F–H and J–K (Figure 3.3) and the remaining viral isolate grouped as CRFs. Classification of these sub-types is based on percentage differences in the viral envelope nucleotide sequences (Kandathil et al., 2005). There can also be mosaics or CRFs and URFs between different sub-types due to simultaneous or subsequent infection by two or more different sub-types infecting a single cell, causing strand transfer during reverse transcription (Hankins, 2013; Hunt, 2012; Kanki, 2013; Santos & Soares, 2010).

A recombinant is deemed to be a CRF when it is identified through full-genomic sequencing as infecting more than three epidemiologically unlinked individuals (Kandathil et al., 2005; Thomson & Nájera, 2005). URFs are found in epidemiologically linked persons and are thought to be due to a secondary recombination of CRFs (Kandathil et al., 2005). Additionally, 'superinfection' is caused when individuals have a primary HIV infection and are later infected with a different strain from a subsequent transmission event (Kilmarx, 2009). Apart from the possibility of new recombinants, individuals with dual infection

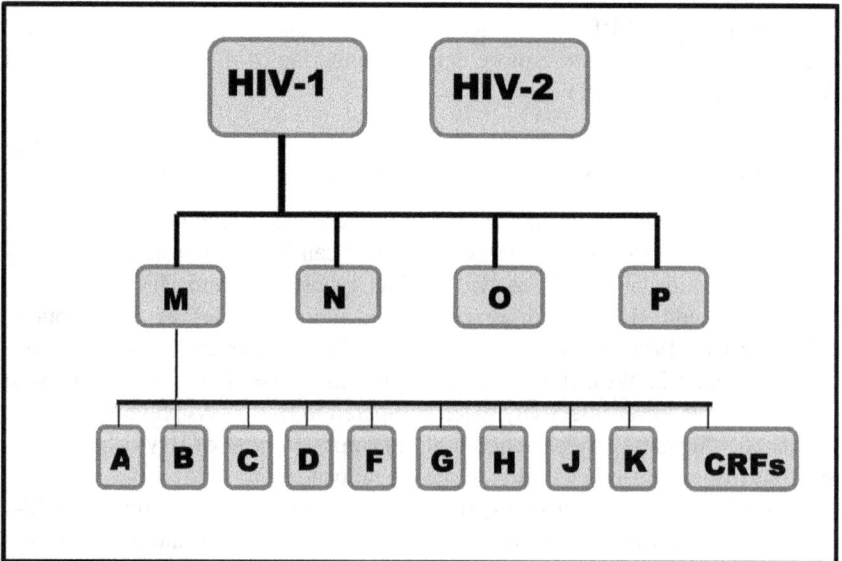

Figure 3.3 Levels of HIV genotypic diversity.

challenge the notion that initial HIV infection confers immunity against future infections; they may also progress to AIDS more quickly (Simon et al., 2006).

Interestingly, the CRFs are numbered in order of discovery and to reflect their originating strains. For example CRF01_AE was the first recombinant form discovered and was a combination of the A and E sub-types. HIV-1 M group sub-types occur globally with different regional variants and recombinant forms. Globally, sub-type C is the strain most commonly predominating in Sub-Saharan Africa, the East African countries, Asia and Brazil (Santos & Soares, 2010), India and Ethiopia (Kandathil et al., 2005). Sub-type B is the most widely disseminated variant and occurs in the USA, the countries of South-East Asia, Australia and Japan. It is also referred to as Thai-B and, along with CRF01_AE, is responsible for the majority of epidemics in South-East Asia. Sub-types D, F, G, H, J and K have less incidences than the two main sub-types (Chang et al., 2018).

Recombinant forms such as CRF01_AE in South-East Asia can also have huge impacts in HIV/AIDS epidemics (Santos & Soares, 2010). Although the majority of infections in East Africa are caused by sub-type A, there are many AC and AD CRFs due to the circulation of sub-types A, D and C (Kandathil et al., 2005). In fact the greatest diversity is found in Central Africa with all sub-types and many of the CRFs and URFs found in the population (Hemelaar et al., 2011). The global diversity and spread of HIV are one of the main challenges faced in the production of ART and vaccines (Hemelaar et al., 2011). The distribution of sub-types and recombinants is complex and their high frequency appears to be a major mechanism for the global diversity (Thomson & Nájera, 2005). Another factor leading to the diffusion of the virus is its ability to counteract the body's immune system and efficiently replicate.

HIV/AIDS in the People's Republic of China

As mentioned, sub-types and recombinant forms of HIV can be traced to areas of origin and allow experts to understand the epidemiology of HIV as it spreads between populations. By understanding which sub-types are active in different populations, it is possible to ascertain changes such as when new strains enter different groups. Generally, the higher the percentages of particular strains in a population, the longer a specific genotype has been active. Additionally, in keeping with 'know your epidemic, know your response' mandates, it is essential to understand which strains are being treated in order to effectively administer TasP initiatives.

China has several different epidemics with different sub-types dominating in different provinces and key populations. HIV-1 sub-type B (found in the USA and Europe) and B' (also referred to as Thai-B) were the first outbreaks to be reported in Yunnan in China but in the years 1995–1997 the virus spread rapidly and accounted for 50 per cent of infections in PWID outside of the province (Beyrer, Razak, Lisam, Chen, Lui & Yu, 2000; Lu et al., 2008; Yang et al., 2005). Currently, there are at least seven HIV-1 sub-types and three major circulating recombinant forms that are active in China. The main sub-types are A, B/B', C, D, E, F and G and the main recombinants are CRF01_AE, CRF07_BC, and CRF08_BC (Qian, Schumacher, Chen & Ruan, 2006).

In the years since the epidemic began, researchers have been able to identify how HIV spread throughout the different provinces of China. An example of this is early HIV virus sequencing that took place in Xinjiang, Sichuan and Guangxi showing many identical gene sequences, but at lower genetic divergence than those identified in Yunnan, suggesting that the virus originated in Yunnan and subsequently spread throughout China (Xiao, Kristensen, Sun, Lu & Vermund, 2007). Therefore, Yunnan, as the origin of China's patient zero, is an essential site for understanding the dispersal of HIV/AIDS throughout China. In China, CRF01_AE has been an important driver of the epidemic and is still the main type transmitted in PWID populations.

In China, HIV sub-types and recombinant forms are found in each region and epidemic cohort. One research study was undertaken to map the HIV-1 genotypes in risk groups and regions of China (He et al., 2012). Their data indicate that there are different strains of HIV found in PWID and MSM populations and that where the genotypes are the same, the percentage rates of infection differ between PWID and MSM populations. They found that, within PWID populations, the highest percentage of genotype is CRF07_BC (48.5 per cent). Among MSM populations, the highest percentage of genotype is CRF01_AE (55.8 per cent), which is different from the US/European B sub-type that predominated in the initial stages.

Their research in heterosexual populations, including FSWs and their clients, indicated a high genotypic diversity (He et al., 2012). In these populations, the main sub-type is CRF01_AE (39.8 per cent) but all 12 HIV-1 genotypic categories are found. The predominant sub-type in mother-to-child transmissions is B' (34.1 per cent), but as with the heterosexual populations, there is high genotypic diversity. However, they found that this was not the case in FPD and blood transfusion recipients where sub-type B' accounted for 92.5 per cent of all infections (He et al., 2012).

Tracing the strains within particular cities has allowed researchers to understand more fully the role of the floating populations in the spread of HIV-1. One study located in Guangyuan City found the genotypic sub-types CRF07_BC and CRF01_AE were the dominant strains in migrant workers. When geographic network analysis was applied, they found that these strains were circulated by multiple lineages (linked to different provinces) exhibiting different characteristics (Su et al., 2018). Molecular transmission network analysis found that those with a migrant history had more sequences linked to other provinces than non-migrant workers (Su et al., 2018). This clearly outlines the movement of workers from one location to the other as a key factor in HIV epidemics in China.

This is mirrored in a study that was undertaken over a 9-year period testing cross-border travellers from neighbouring states into Yunnan Province (B. Wang et al., 2015). They found infection rates across the border points differed but of the 280,961 total number of travellers recruited, 2,380 were found to be HIV+

with 76.22 per cent of those being between the ages of 21–40 (B. Wang et al., 2015). What was even more troubling was that of the 22,699 individuals tested at the gates in the Dehong prefecture, 12.80 per cent of those who tested HIV+ were found to have drug-resistant strains of HIV-1 (Xuan et al., 2018). Of all the individuals tested in Dehong, 298 individuals were ART-naïve and 35 individuals of that cohort were found to exhibit 45 different mutations associated with drug resistance (Xuan et al., 2018). This means that rather than developing drug resistance through taking ART, individuals are being infected with drug-resistant strains from ART-active populations (Xuan et al., 2018).

Of those tested, 12.80 per cent became infected through unsafe sexual practices, 33.20 per cent through IDU and the remainder did not know how they had become infected (Xuan et al., 2018). This is significant when considering the genotypic diversity found in the heterosexual (general) population seems to indicate that infection has spread into the general population through sexual contact with various vectors (Shan et al., 2014). In the transmission of HIV, the impact of geographical communities is weaker than that of behavioural communities (He et al., 2012). An obvious reason for this is that people generally interact within specific cohorts and form communities of like-minded people. HIV spreads when members of these communities interact with non-members, as in the case of clients and non-commercial partners of sex workers, and wives or girlfriends of MSM and PWID populations.

As highlighted by examining the current strains of HIV, in China and globally, the diversity and infectiousness of the HIV virus have considerably added to the spread of the global pandemic since its identification in 1985. Since its inception through the cross-species infection in 1908, the virus has continued to diversify and adapt. An overview of the history of the spread of the virus globally is presented in order to gain an insight into the epidemiology of the disease on a large scale. Broadly painting the picture of the trajectory of the disease will provide a solid grounding in understanding the implementation of GBP.

Overview of the HIV/AIDS pandemic

This section provides an overview of the progression of HIV/AIDS from the beginning of the pandemic until the present day. It places the information concerning the molecular characteristics and routes of transmission of the disease into the pandemic context. Thus, we highlight the rapid spread and efforts undertaken to halt the disease in order to comprehend not only the current challenges, but also the ongoing issues that have plagued epidemiologists since the disease's inception.

The world first became aware of a devastating new infection in mid-1981. Several homosexual men presented with a form of pneumonia at three different Los Angeles hospitals in the USA (Eisinger & Fauci, 2018). Medical staff noted that the men showed marked depletion of the T-lymphocytes. These initial patients were soon followed by a number of other previously healthy young homosexual men presenting with opportunistic infections and rare malignancies, such as kaposi's sarcoma (Eisinger & Fauci, 2018; Sharp & Hahn, 2011). These health scenarios had never been seen before and initially medical practitioners were not aware that they were seeing a new disease threat.

It soon became apparent that they were in the early stages of an epidemic of unknown cause that they were unable to identify. Fear became rampant in the homosexual community with every new infection and it soon became known as the 'gay plague' (Greene, 2007). It was a new type of infection and it invariably led to death. In the initial stages of the spread of the disease, it was named the Gay Related Immunodeficiency Deficiency (GRID) in the USA (Hung, 2018; Lo, 2015). However, after infections began to spread to non-homosexual cohorts, the Centers for Disease Control (CDC), in September of 1982, named it AIDS (Greene, 2007). It soon became apparent that it was not confined to the homosexual community when PWID started to become infected. Due to its absence in the general community at that time, it was considered to be a lifestyle disease caused by the risky behaviours of those infected (Greene, 2007; Mann & Tarantola, 1998).

Over the course of 1982, information concerning infection among partners, and a national case study, suggested that it was sexually transmitted (De Cock, Jaffe & Curran, 2012). By January 1983, the major transmission routes, that of blood, sexual contact and MTCT, had been established. The causative agent was still unknown at that time as such cases were identified at the end stage of the disease once an individual had progressed to AIDS (De Cock et al., 2012).

The US epidemic is understood to have resulted from an infected individual, or individuals, entering the USA from Haiti. It is believed that infection in Haiti was spread from Africa in the 1960s (De Cock et al., 2012). At the time of discovery in the USA the new disease attacking the immune system had not been reported anywhere in the world. What was then unknown but soon to be discovered was that the disease had been running unchecked throughout the African continent and was present in other countries. Places that were apparently free from the disease soon showed visible evidence of the disease and the death resulting from it (De Cock et al., 2012). As a result, when testing began, incidences of AIDS went from an epidemic limited to the USA to millions affected globally within a decade.

The beginnings of the HIV/AIDS pandemic has been traced back to four unique cross-species zoonotic episodes and correspond to the different main strains: M, O, N and P. Epidemiologic backtracking has been accomplished through historical records, genetic sequencing and the use of molecular clocks (Korber et al., 2000). This has allowed an estimation of the three main crossover infections (M, O, N) as occurring around 1908 (M), 1920 (O) and 1963 (N) (Tebit & Arts, 2011). It is believed that the HIV-1 sub-groups originated from the equatorial forests of the Cameroon in West Africa (Tebit & Arts, 2011). From there they spread to Zaire (now the Democratic Republic of the Congo) and from there through the rest of Africa. The epidemic began its spread in Central Africa in the 1970s and by the mid-1980s, the majority of sex workers in Kenya were infected (De Cock et al., 2012; Greene, 2007). The virus then continued to spread through the continent and at the present time Sub-Saharan Africa bears the majority of the global HIV/AIDS burden.

The causative agent HIV was discovered during the period from 1983 to 1984 and in 1986 became known as HIV. Once that became known, efforts to understand the virus and attempts to create a way to identify it in infected persons were implemented. This was achieved in 1985 with the first blood test (Greene, 2007). Attempts to discover a treatment and vaccine began in earnest. Since the early years of the pandemic, there has been ongoing attempts to understand the drivers of HIV in diverse populations. Behavioural interventions, from those highly stigmatising initiatives of the early years to more sensitive initiatives of recent years, have progressed alongside the molecular interventions that have continued to improve since the discovery of HIV as the causative agent.

The spread of HIV/AIDS has been dynamic and over the past 30+ years epidemics have manifested in all countries. There are diverse epidemics with differing sub-types driving them but they all share common themes. MSM, PWID, MTCT, and CSWs have been key populations since the epidemic first appeared. Fortunately, understandings of these cohorts' impacts on HIV/AIDS epidemics has moved from the inflammatory blaming dialogues of the early years and being labelled as high-risk populations, to the more current understanding of them as having key roles in HIV epidemics. When AIDS first emerged on the scene, it was something that had never been faced by the medical community and there was a lot of fear surrounding the disease. There were no existing protocols or understandings of how to treat such a disease.

Since that time, amazing progress has been made and the world is on the cusp of changing HIV/AIDS from a death sentence to a chronic disease. In high-income countries, this has all but occurred. Regardless of significant medical breakthroughs, HIV/AIDS is still a death sentence in many countries due to a lack of access to human security initiatives. Nevertheless, the history of the HIV/AIDS epidemic has revealed that while advances in technology have enabled many HIV+ people to live almost full-term life expectancies, these advances have also resulted in certain complacencies. Particularly in countries where access to ART (including pre-exposure prophylaxis (PrEP) and post-exposure prophylaxis (PEP)), microbicides and good medical services lull communities into believing that contracting HIV is not as horrendous as it once was. In low- and middle-income countries, such as China, preventing the spread of HIV/AIDS is still an enormous economic and political challenge.

Conclusion

Having examined the mechanisms by which HIV enters the human body, it is clear that protection through the use of a barrier, such as condoms, is an essential mechanism for prevention. Yet, there are high rates of non-condom usage throughout key populations due to behavioural norms and misunderstandings about the effectiveness of ART and microbicides as stand-alone prevention measures. When considering the pathogenesis of HIV, is obvious that there are extreme challenges in dealing with a virus of such high diversity, rapid rate of production and ability to adapt and form new strains. As of 2019, there are now some 99 CRFs in circulation throughout the different epidemics globally and there are likely to be many more before HIV becomes a thing of the past. The high rates of STIs within societies and in particular key populations highlight that there is an epidemiological synergy in place. STIs are proven to exacerbate HIV infectiousness through an increase of viral shedding in the genital tracts; inflammation causing higher levels of HIV target cells; and disruption to the integrity of the epithelial layers of the genital area. In general, the human body is effective at repelling pathogens but when there are already suboptimal health conditions, HIV takes advantage of the opportunities provided and slips through the defences.

The situation for HIV/AIDS and STIs in China reveals that there is a high possibility of HIV rapidly expanding if complacency becomes the norm. There are new CRFs in circulation in China as well as the continued spread of existing strains. Beijing's sustained political will and determination to support the most vulnerable within China's expanding population will be an overarching require-ment for any real success in the continuing HIV/AIDS epidemic. When added to the challenges inherent in dealing with human beings and their cultural and behavioural biases and norms, HIV/AIDs constitutes a formidable adversary. In China and globally, high-risk behaviours in key populations continue to be problematic.

As shown in the brief history of the pandemic, the news is not all negative. While at the beginning of the epidemic there were deleterious attitudes and modes of addressing the disease, these are becoming things of the past. Conten-tious understandings and imputations of responsibility towards populations have now given way to more deliberate attempts to be inclusive rather than marginal-ising. Stigmatisation has been recognised to add to the challenges of HIV/AIDS epidemics. There are new discourses emerging that call for an acknowledgement that in dealing with HIV/AIDS, it is paramount to deal with the cessation of behaviours that further push vulnerable populations underground. Only then will the true nature of the epidemic be revealed and efficiently addressed by interventions.

Case study 3.1 Daiyu's story

The case study of Diayu highlights how stigmatisation, food insecurity, economic insecurity, community insecurity and health insecurity can have impacts on HIV+ individuals who might seem, at first rendering, to be sufficiently resourced. Although Diayu owns a home and has the potential to use it to gain an income, this has proved impossible within her community due to her HIV+ status.

I did not quite know what I was going to see and hear when I went to a village less than a day's drive from Kunming. We were going to meet seven families who had become vulnerable due to the complications of HIV/AIDS and its related stigma. I was travelling with a contact who worked closely with an NGO that was providing services to PLWHA, and he informed me that on this journey we would be trying to assess whether or not a micro-loan would be beneficial to the individuals we would be meeting. All the people we would be visiting had dreams of making a living and rising above the poverty that they had fallen into due to supporting (or losing a HIV+ family member), or contracting the disease themselves.

It was the first opportunity I had been given to meet people in their own homes. I would be able to experience what life was really like for them rather than simply making observations at a drop-in centre. The individuals we were meeting were receiving some assistance and were accessing the available programmes so I had hopes that their situations would be positive examples of how China was getting it right.

We arrived in the village and met our village contact. He was a PWID peer worker undertaking a methadone maintenance programme. He informed us that the village's network had indicated that some of the people we would meet were in dire straits.

Daiyu's house was the second stop on our trip. We had just spent an hour listening to one family talk about the difficulties they were facing after their middle-aged son contracted HIV through injection drug use and I was feeling a little overwhelmed. In China, sons are traditionally expected to care for their parents in their old age and the fact that the situation had been reversed and they had to care for him also caused them to worry for the future. Their home had been small, cluttered and in need of repair so I was surprised when we arrived at Daiyu's home and found the situation to be very different. She opened the door to her home and we stepped into a central courtyard with an open roof and potted plants. We stayed there as the interview took place, sitting bundled in our overcoats and scarves with the sun warming us through the winter cold.

The house we were sitting in was large and had two storeys. The interior was old but in reasonably good repair. Daiyu lived there alone and had found that the upkeep was getting more and more difficult. I asked her which room was hers and she told me that the entire building belonged to her. It was the family home. My contact asked her to share her story. I speak Chinese but I asked him to translate into English to ensure that my understanding of what she was saying was correct. Daiyu was a petite woman who spoke in a gentle voice and had us mesmerised by her life story. The house had been in Daiyu's family for a number of generations and had operated as a bustling boarding house when her parents were alive.

She had inherited it along with her sister. Like Daiyu, her sister had been an injection drug user and had contracted HIV. She had recently died of an AIDS-related infection and Daiyu no longer had any family left. Daiyu was 30 years old. She had known her HIV+ status for a number of years and she was still using drugs. Heroin was her main habit and she told us that while she knew she should stop, she was not able to. In addition, she acknowledged to us that her heroin habit had cost her everything. All she had left was the house that her parents had left to her. We asked her why she did not rent out rooms in the same way that her parents had done. 'I can't,' she said. 'Since I was diagnosed as being HIV+ no one will rent the rooms. They are all afraid that they might catch the disease from being in my home.'

Her response was sombre but she seemed very resigned to people's attitudes. Nevertheless, she said she was optimistic that there were fewer stigmas than there used to be surrounding HIV/AIDS and anticipated that if the NGO gave her a micro-loan, she might be able to make a living. She felt hopeful that some people might be more willing to rent from her. There had been some education about HIV and perhaps people might understand that it was not possible to get the disease just from being in the same house as someone HIV+.

We asked her how she had been managing to make an income and support herself in the meantime. She told us that she had become a sex worker. Being known as someone who was HIV+, she did not make a lot of money but it was enough for her to buy the drugs she needed and a meal each day. I was surprised at this and asked for clarification. She replied that after buying her drugs and paying for other expenses, she lived on 5 Yuan per day. It was enough for her to buy one meal at the local market. She did not elaborate on her sex work and we did not question her further concerning that or whether she used condoms with clients. We already knew that there was a high likelihood that Daiyu has not used condoms with clients at some time or another. This is supported by the research both from China but also that of sex workers globally (Chen et al., 2012; Li, He, Wang & Williams., 2009; Peng et al., 2012; Wang et al., 2010; Yang, Latkin, Luan & Nelson, 2010; Yi, Mantell, Wu, Lu, Zeng & Wan, 2010). While the cultural circumstances are different, the drivers are the same. Daiyu does what she feels she must to survive.

Thus, questioning Daiyu further on the topic of condom usage was unnecessary as Daiyu is not the main problem in HIV/AIDS epidemics. This chapter has examined the pathogenesis and epidemiology of HIV/AIDS and demonstrated that a barrier method is effective in preventing transmission of the disease (UNAIDS, 2013). However, the real problem driving continuing rates of HIV transmission is a lack of education, a lack of human security and a lack of alternate solutions. China is making great strides forward in its HIV/AIDS programming but there are still situations needing improvement. Presently, many of the new initiatives are rolled out in the form of pilot trials and these programmes often end after the trials have finished. As Chen told me, there are a lot of 'pop-up' NGOs working in the area of HIV/AIDS in China. They run a programme and exist while the funding is available and then disappear when the money has run out (Chen, pers. comm., 2014).

This situation is exacerbated by a lack of education about HIV/AIDS. While the situation does seem to be improving with the use of television advertising and advertising spaces in subway stations, these presentations are insufficient to change the deeply rooted negative attitudes that are leading to stigmatisation of PLWHA, people like Daiyu (Burki, 2011; Hood, 2012; Sun et al., 2010). In China, apart from the billboards and television advertising, most HIV/AIDS education slated towards the general public is presented on World AIDs Day. This is problematic when, as happened during my field research in 2013, there are few World AIDs Day activities in Yunnan. The main opportunity for disseminating information is missed as a result. Lack of clear and correct HIV information continues the stigma, and this stigma causes people like Daiyu to find themselves devoid of community support networks and increases their insecurity.

These problems are compounded by the ongoing human insecurity faced by PLWHA. Not only does human insecurity impact PLWHA in terms of lack of employment, food insecurity, community insecurity and health insecurity, when these deficits remain not only do they drive the high-risk behaviours of key populations, they make it difficult to treat those who do come forward for assistance. The ultimate result of this is that there are continuing sub-optimal outcomes for PLWHA (Kalichman, Hernandez, Cherry, Kalichman, Washington & Grebler, 2014).

As we left Daiyu's house and prepared to go to the next house on our list, I looked at her standing in the doorway, her small figure wrapped in a coat to keep the cold at bay. I do not know the outcome of that visit. I never heard whether Daiyu was granted her micro-loan or whether, if she was, the venture was successful. Her hope that the stigmatising attitudes of the community she lived in would soon be a thing of the past is one that we all shared. I felt that there was still a long journey ahead for China in overcoming that obstacle but I admired Daiyu's courage to try regardless of all the stigmatisation that she had already endured.

Notes

1 Hereafter pandemic will refer to the global HIV/AIDS burden and epidemic will refer to country- or population-specific HIV/AIDS situations.
2 Depending on which chemokine receptor is used by the HIV-1 virus envelope, the two major receptors are CCR5 (R5) and CXCR4 (X4), an HIV-1 strain will be classified as either R5 or X4-tropic or in cases of dual-tropic strains (which can enter the cell through either receptor) R5X4-tropic (González et al., 2010).

References

Amon, J. J. (2014). The political epidemiology of HIV. *Journal of the International AIDS Society*, *17*(19327). Retrieved from www.jiasociety.org/index.php/jias/article/view/19327

Anderson, D. J. (2009). Understanding the biology of HIV-1 transmission: The foundation for prevention. In K. H. Mayer & H. F. Pizer (Eds.), *HIV prevention: A comprehensive approach*. London, UK: Academic Press.

Andreoletti, L., Skrabal, K., Perrin, V., Chomont, N., Saragosti, S., Gresenguet, G., ... & Mammano, F. (2007). Genetic and phenotypic features of blood and genital viral populations of clinically asymptomatic and antiretroviral-treatment-naive clade-A human immunodeficiency virus type 1-infected women. *Journal of Clinical Microbiology*, *45*(6), 1838–1842.

Arthos, J., Cicala, C., Nawaz, F., Byrareddy, S. N., Villinger, F., Santangelo, P. J., ... & Fauci, A. S. (2018). The role of integrin $\alpha_4\beta_7$ in HIV pathogenesis and treatment. *Current HIV/AIDS Reports*, *15*(2), 127–135.

Autran, B., Hamimi, C., & Katlama, C. (2014). One step closer to HIV eradication? *Current Treatment Options in Infectious Diseases*, *6*, 171–182. doi:10.1007/s40506-014-0017-1.

Beyrer, C., Razak, M. H., Lisam, K., Chen, J., Lui, W. & Yu, X. F. (2000). Overland heroin trafficking routes and HIV-1 spread in south and south-east Asia. *AIDS*, *14*(1), 75–83.

Burki, T. K. (2011). Discrimination against people with HIV persists in China. *The Lancet*, *377*(9762), 286–287.

Chang, D., Sanders-Buell, E., Bose, M., O'Sullivan, A. M., Pham, P., Kroon, E., ... & Chomchey, N. (2018). Molecular epidemiology of a primarily MSM acute HIV-1 cohort in Bangkok, Thailand and connections within networks of transmission in Asia. *Journal of the International AIDS Society*, *21*(11), e25204.

Chen, G., Li, Y., Zhang, B., Yu, Z., Li, X., Wang, L. & Yu, Z. (2012). Psychological characteristics in high-risk MSM in China. *BMC Public Health, 12*(1), 1.

De Cock, K. M., Jaffe, H. W. & Curran, J. W. (2012). The evolving epidemiology of HIV/AIDS. *AIDS, 26*(10), 1205–1213.

Eisinger, R. W. & Fauci, A. S. (2018). Ending the HIV/AIDS pandemic. *Emerging Infectious Diseases, 24*(3), 413–416.

Fleming, D. T. & Wasserheit, J. N. (1999). From epidemiological synergy to public health policy and practice: The contribution of other sexually transmitted diseases to sexual transmission of HIV infection. *Sexually Transmitted Infections, 75*(1), 3–17.

Gay, C. L., Kashuba, A. D. & Cohen, M. S. (2009). Using antiretrovirals to prevent HIV transmission. In K. H. Mayer & H. F. Pizer (Eds.), *HIV prevention: A comprehensive approach* (pp. 107–145). London, UK: Academic Press.

Geise, R. E. & Duerr, A. (2009). HIV vaccines. In K. H. Mayer & H. F. Pizer (Eds.), *HIV prevention: A comprehensive approach* (pp. 53–84). London, UK: Academic Press.

González, N., Pérez-Olmeda, M., Mateos, E., Cascajero, A., Alvarez, A., Spijkers, S., … & Alcami, J. (2010). A sensitive phenotypic assay for the determination of human immunodeficiency virus type 1 tropism. *Journal of Antimicrobial Chemotherapy, 65*(12), 2493–2501. doi:10.1093/jac/dkq379.

Greene, W. C. (2007). A history of AIDS: Looking back to see ahead. *European Journal of Immunology, 37*(S1), S94–S102.

Hankins, C. (2013). Overview of the current state of the epidemic. *Current HIV/AIDS Report, 10*, 113–123. doi:10.1007/s11904-013-0156-x.

He, X., Xing, H., Ruan, Y., Hong, K., Cheng, C., Hu, Y., … & Takebe, Y. (2012). A comprehensive mapping of HIV-1 genotypes in various risk groups and regions across China based on a nationwide molecular epidemiologic survey. *PloS ONE, 7*(10), e47289.

Hemelaar, J., Gouws, E., Ghys, P. D. & Osmanov, S. (2011). Global trends in molecular epidemiology of HIV-1 during 2000–2007. *AIDS (London, England), 25*(5), 679. doi:10.1097/QAD.0b013e328342ff93.

Hood, J. (2012). HIV/AIDS and shifting urban China's socio-moral landscape: Engendering bio-activism and resistance through stories of suffering. *IJAPS, 8*(1), 125–144.

Hung, J. (2018). HIV-positive gay community in Hong Kong: Sexual and health stigmatization puts lives at stake. *The Yale Review of International Studies, February.* Retrieved from http://yris.yira.org/comments/2279

Hunt, R. (2012). Virology – chapter seven. Human immunodeficiency virus and AIDS, part six, Types, sub-types and co-receptors. Retrieved from http://pathmicro.med.sc.edu/lecture/hiv6.htm

Kalichman, S. C., Hernandez, D., Cherry, C., Kalichman, M. O., Washington, C. & Grebler, T. (2014). Food insecurity and other poverty indicators among people living with HIV/AIDS: Effects on treatment and health outcomes. *Journal of Community Health, 39*(6), 1133–1139. doi:10.1007/s10900-014-9868-0.

Kandathil, A. J., Ramalingam, S., Kannangai, R., David, S. & Sridharan, G. (2005). Molecular epidemiology of HIV. *Indian Journal of Medical Research, 121*, 333–344.

Kanki, P. J. (2013). HIV/AIDS global epidemic. In P. J. Kanki & D. J. Grimes (Eds.), *Infectious Diseases* (pp. 27–62). New York, NY: Springer.

Kilmarx, P. H. (2009). Global epidemiology of HIV. *Current Opinion in HIV and AIDS, 4*, 240–246.

Kilmarx, P. H., Gonese, E., Lewis, D. A., Chirenje, Z. M., Barr, B. A. T., Latif, A. S., … & Rietmeijer, C. A. (2018). HIV infection in patients with sexually transmitted infections in Zimbabwe: Results from the Zimbabwe STI etiology study. *PloS ONE, 13*(6), e0198683.

Kononchik, J., Ireland, J., Zou, Z., Segura, J., Holzapfel, G., Chastain, A., ... & Kano, D. (2018). HIV-1 targets L-selectin for adhesion and induces its shedding for viral release. *Nature Communications, 9*(1), 2825.

Korber, B., Muldoon, M., Theiler, J., Gao, F., Gupta, R., Lapedes, A., ... & Bhattacharya, T. (2000). Timing the ancestor of the HIV-1 pandemic strains. *Science, 288*(5472), 1789–1796.

Lashley, F. R. (2006). Transmission and epidemiology of HIV/AIDS: A global view. *Nursing Clinics of North America, 41*, 339–354.

Li, X., He, G., Wang, H. & Williams, A. B. (2009). Consequences of drug abuse and HIV/AIDS in China: Recommendations for integrated care of HIV-infected drug users. *AIDS Patient Care & STDs, 23*(10), 877–884. doi:10.1089/apc.2009.0015.

Lo, C. Y. P. (2015). *HIV/AIDS in China and India: Governing health security.* Basingstok, UK: Palgrave Macmillan.

Locher, C. P., Witt, S.A., Kassel, R., Dowell, N. L., Fujimura, S. & Levy, J.A. (2005). Differential effects of R5 and X4 human immunodeficiency virus type 1 infection on CD4+ cell proliferation and activation. *Journal of General Virology, 86*(pt. 4), 1171–1179. doi:10.1099/vir.0.80674-0.

Lu, L., Jia, M., Ma, Y., Yang, L., Chen, Z., Ho, D. D., ... & Zhang, L. (2008). The changing face of HIV in China. *Nature, 455*(7213), 609–611.

Mann, J. & Tarantola, D. (1998). Responding to HIV/AIDS: A historical perspective. *Health and Human Rights, 2*(4), 5–8.

Mayer, K. H. & Pizer, H. F. (2009). Introduction. In K. H. Mayer & H. F. Pizer (Eds.), *HIV prevention: A comprehensive approach* (pp. 1–8). London, UK: Academic Press.

McGowan, I. (2009). Microbicides. In K. H. Mayer & H. F. Pizer (Eds.), *HIV Prevention: A comprehensive approach* (pp. 85–106). London: Academic Press.

Medina-Perucha, L., Family, H., Scott, J., Chapman, S. & Dack, C. (2019). Factors associated with sexual risks and risk of STIs, HIV and other blood-borne viruses among women using heroin and other drugs: A systematic literature review. *AIDS and Behavior, 23*(1), 222–251.

Peng, Z., Yang, H., Norris, J., Chen, X., Huan, X., Yu, R., ... & Chen, F. (2012). HIV incidence and predictors associated with retention in a cohort of men who have sex with men in Yangzhou, Jiangsu Province, China. *PloS ONE, 7*(12), e52731.

Qian, H. Z., Schumacher, J. E., Chen, H. T. & Ruan, Y. H. (2006). Injection drug use and HIV/AIDS in China: Review of current situation, prevention and policy implications. *Harm Reduction Journal, 3*(1), 4. doi:10.1186/1477-7517-3-4.

Rein, M. F. (2000). The interaction between HIV and the classic sexually transmitted diseases. *Current Infectious Disease Reports, 2*(1), A87–A95.

Reis, M. N., Guimarães, M. L., Bello, G. & Stefani, M. (2019). Identification of new HIV-1 circulating recombinant forms CRF81_cpx and CRF99_BF1 in Central Western Brazil and of unique BF1 recombinant forms. *Frontiers in Microbiology, 10*, 97.

Risbud, A. (2005). Human immunodeficiency virus (HIV) and sexually transmitted diseases (STDs). *Indian Journal of Medical Research, 121*(4), 369.

Santos, A.F. & Soares, M. A. (2010). HIV genetic diversity and drug resistance. *Viruses, 2*(2), 503–531. doi:10.3390/v2020503.

Shan, D., Sun, J., Khoshnood, K., Fu, J., Duan, S., Jiang, C., ... & Liu, H. (2014). The impact of comprehensive prevention of mother-to-child HIV transmission in Dehong prefecture, Yunnan province, 2005–2010: A hard-hit area by HIV in Southern China. *International Journal of STD & AIDS, 25*(4), 253–260.

Sharp, P. M. & Hahn, B. H. (2011). Origins of HIV and the AIDS pandemic. *Cold Spring Harbor Perspectives in Medicine, 1*(1), a006841.

Simon, V., Ho, D. D. & Karim, Q. A. (2006). HIV/AIDS epidemiology, pathogenesis, prevention, and treatment. *The Lancet, 368*(9534), 489–504.

Su, L., Liang, S., Hou, X., Zhong, P., Wei, D., Fu, Y., ... & Yang, H. (2018). Impact of worker emigration on HIV epidemics in labour export areas: A molecular epidemiology investigation in Guangyuan, China. *Scientific Reports, 8*(1), 16046.

Sun, X., Lu, F., Wu, Z., Poundstone, K., Zeng, G., Xu, P., ... & Liau, A. (2010). Evolution of information-driven HIV/AIDS policies in China. *International Journal of Epidemiology, 39*(suppl. 2), ii4–ii13.

Tebit, D. M. & Arts, E. J. (2011). Tracking a century of global expansion and evolution of HIV to drive understanding and to combat disease. *The Lancet Infectious Diseases, 11*(1), 45–56.

Thomson, M. M. & Nájera, R. (2005). Molecular epidemiology of HIV-1 variants in the global aids pandemic: An update. *AIDS Reviews, 7*, 210–224.

Tyssen, D., Wang, Y. Y., Hayward, J. A., Agius, P. A., DeLong, K., Aldunate, M., ... & Tachedjian, G. (2018). Anti-HIV-1 activity of lactic acid in human cervicovaginal fluid. *mSphere, 3*(4), e00055–18.

UNAIDS. (2013). *Global report: UNAIDS report on the global AIDS epidemic 2013*. Retrieved from www.unaids.org/sites/default/files/media.../UNAIDS_Global_Report_2013_en_1.pdf

Wang, B., Liang, Y., Feng, Y., Li, Y., Wang, Y., Zhang, A. M., ... & Xia, X. (2015). Prevalence of human immunodeficiency virus 1 infection in the last decade among entry travelers in Yunnan Province, China. BMC Public Health, 15(1), 362.

Wang, L., Zeng, G., Luo, J., Duo, S., Xing, G., Guo-wei, D., ... & Ning, W. (2010). HIV transmission risk among serodiscordant couples: A retrospective study of former plasma donors in Henan, China. *Journal of Acquired Immune Deficiency Syndromes, 55*(2), 232.

WHO (World Health Organization). (2016). Consolidated guidelines on the use of antiretroviral drugs for treating *and preventing HIV infection: R*ecommendations for a public health approach. Geneva, Switzerland: World Health Organization.

Xiao, Y., Kristensen, S., Sun, J., Lu, L. & Vermund, S. H. (2007). Expansion of HIV/ AIDS in China: Lessons from Yunnan province. *Social Science & Medicine, 64*(3), 665–675.

Xu, S. X., Leontyev, D., Kaul, R. & Gray-Owen, S. D. (2018). Neisseria gonorrhoeae co-infection exacerbates vaginal HIV shedding without affecting systemic viral loads in human CD34+ engrafted mice. *PloS ONE, 13*(1), e0191672.

Xuan, Q., Liang, S., Qin, W., Yang, S., Zhang, A. M., Zhao, T., ... & Xia, X. (2018). High prevalence of HIV-1 transmitted drug resistance among therapy-naïve Burmese entering travelers at Dehong ports in Yunnan, China. *BMC Infectious Diseases, 18*(1), 211.

Yang, C., Latkin, C., Luan, R. & Nelson, K. (2010). Condom use with female sex workers among male clients in Sichuan province, China: The role of interpersonal and venue-level factors. *Journal of Urban Health, 87*(2), 292–303.

Yang, H., Li, X., Stanton, B., Liu, H., Liu, H., Wang, N., ... & Chen, X. (2005). Heterosexual transmission of HIV in China: A systematic review of behavioral studies in the past two decades. *Sexually Transmitted Diseases, 32*(5), 270–280.

Yi, H., Mantell, J. E., Wu, R., Lu, Z., Zeng, J. & Wan, Y. (2010). A profile of HIV risk factors in the context of sex work environments among migrant female sex workers in Beijing, China. *Psychology, Health & Medicine, 15*(2), 172–187.

Zhang, L., Liang, S., Lu, W., Pan, S. W., Song, B., Liu, Q., ... & Ruan, Y. (2014). HIV, syphilis, and behavioral risk factors among female sex workers before and after implementation of harm reduction programs in a high drug-using area of China. *PloS ONE, 9*(1), e84950. doi:10.1371/journal.pone.0084950.

Zhang, X., Lu, X., Moog, C., Yuan, L., Liu, Z., Li, Z., ... & Su, B. (2018). KIR3DL1-negative CD8 T cells and KIR3DL1-negative natural killer cells contribute to the advantageous control of early human immunodeficiency virus type 1 infection in HLA-B Bw4 homozygous individuals. *Frontiers in Immunology, 9.*

Zheng N, Guo Y, Padmadas S, Wang B, Wu Z. (2014). The increase of sexually transmitted infections calls for simultaneous preventive intervention for more effectively containing HIV epidemics in China. *BJOG, 121*(suppl. 5), 35–44.

Zhu, Z., Yan, H., Wu, S., Xu, Y., Xu, W., Liu, L., ... & Detels, R. (2019). Trends in HIV prevalence and risk behaviours among men who have sex with men from 2013 to 2017 in Nanjing, China: A consecutive cross-sectional survey. *BMJ Open, 9*(1), e021955.

4   Global best practice

How does the world do it?

Distant water won't help to put out a fire close at hand.

远水救不了近火

Global best practice (GBP) is an evolving methodology that informs prevention and treatment strategies; which can then be applied to specific HIV epidemics. It is not only comprised of information found to be effective in regional epidemics but also serves as a useful standard to measure the appropriateness of a country's response to HIV/AIDS epidemics within their borders. It is not mandatory for nation-states to adopt HIV/AIDS GBP but if they are serious about making a concerted effort to halt the spread of HIV, then embracing the wisdom of those who have dealt with similar issues seems intuitively sensible.

In general, these GBPs have been presented through UN agencies that work with researchers and other governmental and non-governmental agencies trialling different HIV/AIDS programmes worldwide. They have been refined throughout the almost 40 years since HIV/AIDS was first identified in the USA and have been adapted and developed as new research into the biomedical, social and governance aspects of the disease have been established. Consequentially, along with the changes in GBP methodologies, there has been a change in the language used to refer to different cohorts or key populations.

One reason for this changing language is a growing sensitivity to the ways that the general population may perceive and stigmatise people who live with HIV/AIDS (PLWHA). Recently the term for cohorts who inject drugs was changed from injection drug user (IDU) to people who inject drugs (PWID).[1] While the distinction may be subtle, the first term defines them as a person; the second explains one aspect of their lives. In a similar way, high-risk populations are now referred to as key populations. The first stigmatises their behaviour, and, by extension, them, as being generally responsible for the spread of HIV. The second acknowledges that while they have an influence, there are a multitude of sociological and biological extractions exacerbating the growth of HIV epidemics.

Stigma reduction efforts form a basis for the GBP needed to achieve sustainable and long-term treatment efficacy. The Millennium Development Goals

(MDGs) relating to HIV/AIDS[2] acknowledge that simply 'knowing your epidemic and knowing your response' is insufficient. It is equally important to understand the ways that HIV/AIDS interacts with human security threats such as stigma, poverty, income inequality, gender, education and other structural drivers in order to reduce the rate of new infections to zero (Kim, Lutz, Dhaliwal & O'Malley, 2011).

One of the main foci of policies such as the MDGs is the determination to provide antiretroviral therapy (ART) to all eligible PLWHA. ART has a tremendous impact on the spread of HIV and in countries where ART is affordable or free, the disease has moved from a guaranteed death sentence for the vast majority of PLWHA to a chronic health issue. Some of the countries with the greatest prevalence have the least resources to deal with it. AIDS continues to take the lives of more than a million people globally each year. Additionally, ART regimes are not a 'magic bullet' for the eradication of HIV. The disease must be considered holistically, with both medical and behavioural initiatives focused at fulfilling the human security needs of every population through which it passes.

This is particularly the case in China where cultural norms have created an environment where the needs of the masses trump the needs of the vulnerable. Arguably, this is done regardless of their individual human security needs and generally in order to mitigate their impact on the general population. When considering the potential magnitude of the threat, as explored in the UNAIDS (2000) report, *HIV/AIDS: China's Titanic Peril*, the human security of PLWHA needs to be among the government's main security priorities.

While issues of human security, especially those of PLWHA, will be explored in the Conclusion, at this point it is essential to understand once HIV becomes a generalised epidemic (and some scholars argue that it already has in parts of China), then the methods considered sufficient for eradicating it in specific key populations become inadequate. One of the key functions of GBP is to prevent epidemics from becoming generalised. Significantly, it is no longer possible to deal only with vulnerable populations as disease bridges needing to be closed off to protect general populations; rather, grassroots interventions that meet their needs as individuals must become dominant. At that point meeting the needs of the vulnerable becomes a valuable tool for inhibiting the spread of disease into the general population.

China has made some progress in implementing some of the GBPs but it is prudent to say that there are improvements to be made before those programmes generate a genuine and lasting impact on the overall epidemic in China. When compared to other countries that have been dealing with long-term epidemics and informing GBP through their experiences; China still needs to accelerate measures to deal with key populations – particularly those with extremely high percentage rates of infection. Again, this can be achieved best by addressing the human security needs of these vulnerable populations. Strategies dealing with poverty reduction, employment, education, affordable medical services target the problem at its nexus with HIV/AIDS.

In general, China has attempted to adopt and adapt GBP, however, there is a breach between the existence of programmes and their adequacy in dealing with the magnitude of the problem being addressed. The main forms of GBP adopted by China include condom programmes, methadone maintenance treatment (MMT) and syringe exchange, stigma reduction programmes, and HIV education programmes for key populations. In China, most HIV/AIDS education initiatives aimed at the general public are presented on World AIDS Day. Whether this is adequate is debatable and considering that the epidemic is now sexually driven, it becomes essential to ensure that those engaging in sexual activities, particularly high-risk sexual activities, are well informed about prevention measures.

What works best?

The sharing of GBP is the responsibility of the UNAIDS Secretariat. Information is gathered and considered with the support of co-sponsors such as the United Nations Office on Drugs and Crime (UNODC), the United Nations Children's Emergency Fund (UNICEF) and the World Health Organization (WHO). The original mandate for the collection of GBP was made in 1994 by the Economic and Social Council that established UNAIDS (Funnell, 1999). GBP is established through making judgements about information received from researchers, NGOs, INGOs, state governments, PLWHA and other sources.

Two procedures assist with this task; first, the documentation of anecdotal evidence about successful interventions, whether fully or partially successful; and, second, through a thorough analysis of the information using set criteria (UNAIDS, 2000). These criteria are effectiveness, efficiency, relevance, ethical soundness and sustainability. Using these criteria, UNAIDS are able to ascertain a programme's strengths and weaknesses and efficacy and shortfalls. This information is then made available and used by HIV/AIDS practitioners to further their existing programmes or implement new ones. They in turn, make the results of these ongoing initiatives available to UNAIDS to be considered as candidates for GBP.

GBP might be considered a depository of information and documentation concerning the lessons that have been learned by practitioners at the forefront of HIV epidemics – what worked and what did not work. As such, they are not comprised of exactitudes nor do they inculcate 'one-size fits all' paradigms. Rather, their aim is to identify and disseminate knowledge about the most effective responses in different HIV epidemics, in a variety of contexts (UNAIDS, 2000). As such, they are applicable at a global policy level. According to Hankins and Zalduondo (2010), the 2005 global policy guidelines called for 'strategic, simultaneous implementation of a combination of evidence-informed policies, and programmatic actions, including biomedical and behavioural approaches, promoting gender equality and protection of human rights, to reduce HIV risk, vulnerability, and impact' (p. 71).

Using GBP allows countries to benefit from understandings gained in ongoing HIV/AIDS epidemics and pool that knowledge together with the situational variables of their individual epidemics to promote best outcomes in both prevention and treatment. Even so, something that might work in one situation might be totally ineffective in another or may need to be adapted to be even partially successful. Consequently, GBP is about saving time and learning from the successes, and mistakes, occurring in different contexts and cultural environments. As the HIV/AIDS epidemic continues, procedures and policies are analysed and reanalysed over time in a type of cyclical distillation process (Figure 4.1).

Characteristically, successful intervention efforts are not simply dependent on being conversant with the commonalities of HIV/AIDS epidemics but rather the differences (culturally, environmentally, politically) specific to each situation. Ultimately, regardless of the cultural situation, there are commonalities in all HIV/AIDS epidemics, such as key populations, high-risk behaviours, and the need for successful treatment and education programmes. Understanding these commonalities is the starting point for any treatment and prevention efforts.

An important aspect of GBP, and in order to gain a comprehensive understanding of the epidemic in general, is to engage with communities of PLWHA. These communities are uniquely situated to provide inclusive understanding of the needs and challenges that they are facing on a daily basis. Many past HIV programmes have been discriminatory, stigmatising and alienating due to lack of

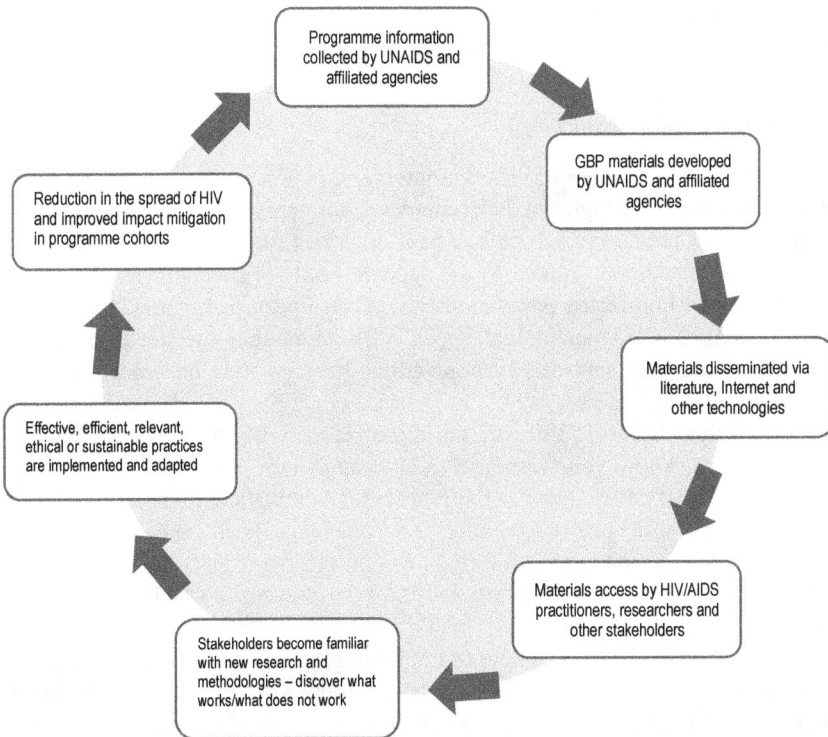

Figure 4.1 Cycle of GBP.

consultation. Likewise, GBP acknowledges the need to seek advice and under-standing from a broad cross-section of the members of key populations (regard-less of their HIV status). As mentioned previously, these populations are often impermeable to outsiders and are thus hard to reach and difficult to understand.

Key populations (FSWs, PWID MSN, migrants, MTCT) are common to all HIV/AIDS epidemics globally. As such, there are arrays of GBP dealing with the methodologies to curtail HIV in these populations and prevent them func-tioning as bridging populations into the general community. Often these pro-grammes and policies need to be adapted for specific cultural environments. Some GBP, such as the use of condoms, are practical intervention methods applicable in all HIV/AIDS epidemic contexts.

Just as there are different HIV/AIDS epidemics, there is a diverse range of GBP. The scope of this book does not permit all of them to be considered; and their non-inclusion should not be perceived as a commentary on their effective-ness or value. As such, even though the GBP are discussed in a global context, only the most widely used and most applicable to the HIV/AIDS operational environment in China are considered in the following section. While there is comprehensive evidence pointing to the value of male circumcision and pre-exposure prophylaxis (PrEP) and post-exposure prophylaxis (PEP), these interventions are not commonly being undertaken in China. Additionally, as they are also outside the scope of this book, GBP concerning the safety of blood sup-plies, MTCT and children are also not considered.

Recently implemented GBP

There have been a number of different intervention processes tested since it first became apparent that high-risk behaviours were a part of the cycle of infection. As knowledge has increased, so too have interventions and GBP has become more sophisticated and tailored to the specific needs of populations. While the need to protect uninfected populations has always been paramount, there is an increasing acknowledgement that specifically addressing the needs of HIV+ individuals and members of key populations has an effect on epidemics as a whole.

This section discusses three of the more recent GBP strategies: (1) 'know your epidemic, know your response'; (2) treatment as prevention (TasP); and (3) the cascade of care. Together these are often labelled combination treatment and prevention strategies. Essentially, the knowledge of the specific epidemic works in collaboration with ART regimes and the ongoing cascade of care to help ensure that PLWHA maintain ART to both prevent mortality and prevent further spread of the disease.

Accordingly, in order to be able to implement the most effective defence. it is essential to know your epidemic in order to know your response. You cannot implement efficacious interventions if you do not understand the drivers of the epi-demic being targeted. GBP must be adapted, refined and made sustainable in order to have any hope of having a substantive impact. A part of GBP is recognising that different epidemics may have similar drivers but none of them are exactly the same. Cultural norms, physical environment and national governance and priorities all have a role in the unique way that HIV/AIDS epidemics spread throughout different communities. To reiterate, what worked successfully in one epidemic with similar features may be less effective in another.

TasP has been developed to embrace observations that not only does ART have a life-sustaining effect on the PLWHA, but it can also drop their HIV infectiousness to a point where it is useful as a prevention measure. Although drug trials have been implemented for many years and there was evidence of this occurring, it has only been in the past two years, as evidence has demonstrated its efficacy and sustainability, that TasP has been fully advocated as a GBP. Along with the efficacy and sustainability of TasP as a prevention measure, the continued advances in ART have refined drug regimes in order to make them easier to maintain.

In a symbiotic synergy it has been acknowledged that along with long-term drug regimes and TasP, more comprehensive and holistic health care environments should be embraced. TasP only works if PLWHA continue to adhere to the correct regimes. The cascade of care GBP recognises that PLWHA need sustained and empathetic health care delivery and programmes. The ART drug regimes can be brutal on the body and many patients drop out before getting through the most difficult initial period. Additionally, with the threat of drug resistance always in the background, monitoring PLWHA on ART is essential. Combined, these three initiatives form a part of current strategies to address the HIV/AIDS pandemic.

Know your epidemic, know your response

Understanding the epidemiology of HIV is essential for the successful implementation of HIV/AIDS GBP. UNAIDS advocates a 'know your epidemic, know your response' methodology as advantageous in responding to HIV/AIDS epidemics. Consequently, the WHO, UNICEF and UNAIDS (2011) report states:

> The selection of which HIV prevention programme components to deploy for which priority populations must be based on a clear understanding and mapping of the national epidemiology of HIV – who is acquiring HIV, where, how and why – to design the appropriate mix of prevention programmes. To successfully limit transmission, effective prevention services must reach the areas and populations where HIV is spreading most rapidly. Achieving population-level impact requires that programmes be implemented at the necessary scale and intensity.
>
> (p. 62)

The main reason for this is that many countries face mixed epidemics and may have varied infection rates within different subpopulations and a range of different strains of HIV being spread. Without understanding the dynamics within the separate epidemics, it is impossible to know which programmes work best and what level of population coverage is required to make a long-term impact both on the spread of HIV within these groups and externally into different population cohorts.

Ultimately, when the programmes are implemented without a comprehensive understanding of disease drivers, precise HIV strains and detailed challenges within a specific epidemic, 'back doors' are left open and the response is likely to be ineffective or at best diminished. Thus, understanding the 'who', 'where', 'how' and 'why' of HIV infection in China is important. When these questions are answered, it becomes clear that a lack of human security for individuals is influencing the epidemic in China.

The 'who' (key populations, and increasingly, the general population) have specific human security needs that are not being met (such as economic security, political security, community security, health security and food security) often leading them to perform high-risk behaviors that impact the 'how' and 'why' of transmission. The 'where' intuitively refers to geographical locations but could also refer to the spaces of infection. The intimate spaces where HIV is transmitted; the hard-to-reach spaces where key populations congregate; the political spaces where decisions are made; and the medical facilities where infections are treated. This book expands upon current understandings in order to clearly identify the unique challenges faced by the key population cohorts (the who and why) and Beijing's present shortfalls in addressing those needs (the where and how).

Undertaking to 'know your epidemic' enables stakeholders to gain an understanding of where the next 1,000 infections will occur; while 'know your response' is useful for identifying existing programme gaps and analysing where resources can be allocated for maximum impact in epidemics (Hankins & Zalduondo, 2010). This is not only essential for providing viable treatment programmes but also for understanding and implementing successful prevention programmes. The 'know your epidemic, know your response' methodology is necessary for all HIV/AIDS epidemics but is particularly applicable when undertaking combination care for PLWHA. Optimal treatment with ART is facilitated through understanding which specific strain, or strains in the case of multiple infections, of HIV have been contracted. In addition to which, simply engaging in ART is not an assurance of success in the management of HIV/AIDS as a chronic disease.

Knowing, and understanding, the environmental and behavioural conditions engaging PLWHA can enable doctors and other health care workers to provide the necessary assistance for maintenance of ART regimes. The needs of PWID vary considerably, from those engaged in commercial sex work or pregnant women to labour migrants. While acknowledging that many PLWHA who could legitimately be undertaking ART are unable to access the required drugs (for a myriad of reasons, including poverty, stigma, ignorance of status and prosecution for illegal activities), ART has emerged as one of the most essential tools in the box of programme measures. The next section considers ART not only in its long-term function of obviating mortality but also in more recent years as a prevention method in and of itself.

TasP

Present thinking on GBP suggests that while ART is primarily concerned with preventing mortality and morbidity, it may be an efficient manner of preventing new infection (Montaner, 2014). ART has been used for more than 20 years. Since the identification of HIV and with advances in drug therapies, there have been significant improvements in long-term outcomes. It has long been understood that ART has the potential to be effective in preventing transmission of HIV in various contexts (Slavin, 2015). As a result of this understanding, trials have been undertaken for a number of years with comprehensive results indicating that the implementation of TasP strategies is both viable and sustainable (Cohen et al., 2011).

Consideration of the biomedical and immunological data concerning treatment regimes is beyond the scope of this book. However, the research has concluded that current ART regimes are effective in obtaining viral suppression in treatment-naïve individuals regardless of the type of strain being treated (Bangsberg, 2010; Santos & Soares, 2010). With ART, the immune system can recover and viral suppression virus loads can become minimised in blood and genital mucosal secretions, therefore, resulting in a decreased risk of ongoing transmission (Cohen et al., 2011).

Interestingly, there is little longitudinal information concerning the ramifications for different first- and second-line treatments on drug resistance across different clades of HIV and therefore more research needs to be done in this area (Santos & Soares, 2010). Additionally, ART is unable to completely eradicate HIV infection and thus leads to perpetual (lifelong) expenditures and increased toxicity and susceptibility to health complications, such as non-AIDS morbidity or premature ageing (Autran, Hamimi & Katlama, 2014; Deeks, Lewin & Havlir, 2014; Nakagawa, May & Phillips, 2013). However, what is indicated is that ART is effective regardless of epidemic setting and therefore presents a viable approach, combined with behavioural and educational strategies, for the prevention of ongoing transmission.

In order to maximise the benefits of ART in TasP contexts, it is essential to administer ART drug regimes in an efficient and sustainable manner. As mentioned in the previous section, this cannot be done without a comprehensive understanding of the main drivers for the spread of various HIV sub-types and clades throughout communities. Additionally, considering the limited number of eligible PLWHA accessing ART, there must be a scale-up of existing efforts. In order for TasP initiatives to have an optimal impact on global epidemics, the majority of ART-eligible HIV+ individuals must be initiated into TasP regimes and retained in treatment.

One of the main difficulties in TasP initiatives is the ongoing inequality of access to ART for key populations. Although specific data remain severely limited, it has been well established that HIV disproportionately affects key populations (such as sex workers, MSM and PWID), who are also mobile, marginalised and stigmatised. As a result of fears concerning the illegal nature of their activities, coupled with legal and human rights complications, many individuals in key populations, regardless of eligibility for ART, do not seek early access to ART (many presenting only after entering the AIDS phase where low CD4 counts allow opportunistic infections) or have high attrition rates due to mobility or complications due to lack of human security. When health and human security disparities, such as food insecurity, are not addressed, the full benefits of ART are not realised (Kalichman, Hernandez, Cherry, Kalichman, Washington & Grebler, 2014).

In accelerating the availability of ART globally, it has become obvious that a comprehensive clinical care and monitoring system must be in place. As HIV/AIDS moves towards becoming a chronic medical condition globally, previous programmes dealing with HIV as an acute and emerging threat must be adapted to cater for ART maintenance stretching into decades, with the probability of younger HIV+ individuals likely to be receiving treatment for three or four decades due to increased life expectancy (Nakagawa, May & Phillips, 2013). In addressing the changing nature of HIV life expectancy, the cascade of care has emerged as an essential tool for understanding the long-term attrition and sustainability of ART regimes.

Cascade of care

The 'cascade of care' or treatment cascade (hereafter referred to as the cascade) is a relatively new initiative that considers the spectrum of interventions that might be undertaken by PLWHA. It provides a quantitative delineation of the discrete (yet synergistic) steps an individual passes through along the HIV care continuum. As discussed, in recent years, studies have discovered that ART has implications not only for reduced mortality but also to aid prevention efforts. With this new understanding, it becomes essential to ensure that individuals become aware of their HIV status and be routed into programmes and health initiatives that lead to sustained retention on ART programmes.

Currently, only a small percentage of individuals eligible for ART are actively engaged in treatment programmes. For example, in Sub-Saharan Africa, more than three-quarters of PLWHA have not achieved viral suppression due to gaps and shortfalls in the HIV care continuum (UNAIDS, 2013). In the assessment of the cascade of care, considering the significant costs and challenges of providing ART, the optimisation of treatment through attention to the cascade provides a promising framework for ongoing ART programme (Hallett & Eaton, 2013). Significantly, it is a useful concept for linking PLWHA's eventual outcomes with the processes along the timeline from diagnosis through to viral suppression. This is regardless of the fact that PLWHA may not have undertaken ART until many years after becoming aware of their status (Hallett & Eaton, 2013).

Therefore, the cascade is recommended as an essential interpretive tool for the analysis and identification of 'leakage' points, or attrition from treatment occurring along the HIV care continuum and as such it is a focal point for TasP initiatives (Kilmarx & Mutasa-Apollo, 2013; Lourenço, Colley, Nosyk, Shopin, Montaner & Lima, 2014; Nosyk et al., 2014). Significantly, the cascade has become a focal point in order to effectively manage, maximise efforts and increase the beneficial effects of HIV treatments, as well as acting as the premier assessment and monitoring metric for global TasP response and reporting (Nosyk et al., 2014, p. 42).

The cascade emphasises that HIV+ individuals need ongoing and sustained care from the point of diagnosis and that the provision of ART alone does not guarantee successful treatment for PLWHA. The cascade is an important methodology that graphically demonstrates the key transitions along the HIV treatment continuum and their impact on viral suppression (UNAIDS, 2013). In addition to identifying the leakage points, it is a useful tool for determining the types of care individuals should be receiving and ascertaining the treatment that PLWHA are actually receiving (Hallett & Eaton, 2013).

There are five specific points on the cascade continuum. The individual stages range from testing for HIV through to all steps leading to the ultimate goal of virologic (HIV-1 RNA viral load) suppression, preferably before the development of HIV-related complications (Alvarez-Uria, Pakam, Midde & Naik, 2013). The specific steps are as follows: (1) testing to ascertain HIV status; (2) linking HIV+ individuals to clinical care; (3) retaining HIV+ individuals in pre-ART care for monitoring, leading to ART eligibility (this stage may continue for years before a HIV+ individual manifests decreased CD4 counts); (4) the initiation of ART; and (5) viral load suppression through ART adherence and retention in clinical care (Hallett & Eaton, 2013; Kilmarx & Mutasa-Apollo, 2013; Mugavero, Amico, Horn & Thompson, 2013; UNAIDS, 2013).

Without complete adherence to the cascade, the long-term outcomes of ART regimes are likely to be suboptimal, resulting in late or no initiation of ART, high attrition rates, and poor viral load suppression (Alvarez-Uria et al., 2013). This is applicable not only to the individuals undertaking therapies, but also to the cessation of ongoing HIV transmission in a wider societal context, as evidenced by increased risk of HIV-related morbidity, transmission and ultimately, individual mortality (Lourenço et al., 2014; Nosyk et al., 2014). The cascade is therefore useful for identifying problems related to programme deficits such as late diagnosis of HIV status, deficits in linkage and retention of individuals, poor treatment adherence and low levels of ART coverage (Hallett & Eaton, 2013; Nosyk et al., 2014).

To fully represent the cascade and identify points of weakness, large amounts of data must be collected and collated in order to identify the numbers and demographic characteristics of HIV-infected persons either lost to care at 'leaky' points on the continuum or (where possible) discrete from the cascade. Additionally, the cascade's identification and tracking of HIV-related health disparities and inequalities should identify existing challenges and inform future planning by provincial bodies (and assist in assessing their methodology and efficacy); and allow the potential redistribution of resources, thereby improving efficiency, population coverage, quality of care, and reducing health disparities (Nosyk et al., 2014).

The cascade indicates that its use in non-clinical settings may also be appropriate, given the right training of individuals and specific reporting and follow-up procedures. This has immense implications in settings for highly mobile and marginalised populations, as they would be able to access ART in settings where issues of stigma and the illegal nature of their activities would be inconsequential to obtaining care. In the context of China, it would mean that PLWHA would not have to live with the fear of having to access medications at government-run facilities.

To reiterate, each point of the cascade has been recognised as essential for ART programmes to achieve optimal results in the treatment of individuals (resulting in reduced mortality and morbidity) as well as contributing towards long-term positive impacts on HIV/AIDS epidemics (due to reductions in ongoing HIV transmission as evidenced by TasP initiatives). Vast amounts of data must be collected at all points on the care continuum in order for the cascade to correctly identify attrition trouble spots. In many countries eligible persons are not receiving treatment. This has enormous implications for countries such as China, where the health systems and data surveillance capacities are generally overburdened and inefficient.

In terms of GBP, the cascade offers a clear road map for stakeholders to follow in assessing the current challenges and shortfalls in retention of HIV+ persons on the HIV care continuum. When used in combination with other HIV treatment and prevention strategies comprising existing GBP the cascade is a valuable tool for HIV/AIDS programming efforts. Other strategies have been used for many decades and are essential, regardless of knowledge of HIV status or ART eligibility. These GBP (stigma reduction, MMT and condom distribution) address the behavioural and situational implications of HIV epidemics.

Longer-term GBP

Educating people on the causes and effects of HIV/AIDS is paramount in dealing with persistent epidemics. If people do not know how to prevent themselves from acquiring HIV they do not know what measures to take. There are a number of existing strategies that have been in place and adapted for various epidemics since the early appearance of HIV. The mainstays of all HIV epidemics (although policies and application parameters differ) are the distribution and education of stakeholders about the benefits of condom usage for the prevention of transmission; MMT and needle-sharing programmes aimed at mitigating the sharing of needles and reducing the high-risk behaviours attached to injection drug use; and lastly, stigma reduction efforts due to the enormous effect that feelings of stigma and shame have on PLWHA preventing them from accessing treatment programmes and ascertaining their HIV status.

The effects of stigma on people

The stigma of PLWHA is a relentless global problem. The ramifications of the high stigmatisation of these key populations lead to enduring effects in HIV epidemics. People who suffer from stigma or discrimination are disinclined to put themselves in positions of suffering. When a person knows they will be punished and treated badly because of their HIV+ status, they would rather not know that they are living with the disease. Even if that means that they cannot access support networks, medical interventions and life-saving ART. Of course, it also means that they are unaware of the need to use protection when undertaking sexual activity.

Stigma and discrimination have been identified as being one of the main prohibitions to effective HIV treatment and prevention for PLWHA (Chen, Choe, Chen & Zhang, 2007; Mahajan et al., 2008; Wu et al., 2008). Extensive research has been undertaken concerning the results of stigma on health outcomes and they are far-reaching and devastating. The UN suggests stigma and discrimination 'discourage people from seeking information and using services that can prevent HIV infection, hinder them from knowing whether they are infected, and impede access to treatment, care and support' (UNAIDS, 2011, p. 131).

For the individual being stigmatised, issues of shame, low self-esteem and isolation may lead to both mental and physical health problems (Su et al., 2013). Discrimination may also result in denial of employment, educational opportunities and, even in some medical settings, denial of services (Burki, 2011; UNAIDS, 2011).

Ultimately, stigma sets people apart from others and leads to the stereotyping of certain individuals as undesirable. Individuals are no longer considered normal but are considered tainted and marked as different. People being stigmatised become a different type of person and are often no longer accepted the community. They become outsiders and are set apart. Stigmatisation of individuals allows collectives of people to band together in mutual contempt for the person being perceived as undesirable. In this manner they collectively identify stereotypes and determine agreed-upon responses for dealing with and discriminating against those considered divergent from the norm. By devaluing the stigmatised individuals and placing them in a context of social undesirability, the collective group is permitted to feel superior.

Reasons for stigma might not be established in fact. A person may be stigmatised simply due to perceived difference. For example, in HIV/AIDS scenarios, individuals may be stigmatised, and relegated to a position of inferior status, if they are perceived as having the disease, regardless of whether they are actually infected or showing symptoms of AIDS. This causes extensive long-term detrimental effects on the individuals being stigmatised. The psychological effects due to the negative feelings associated with their undesirable difference are compounded by very real physical limitations. Social connections are severed, relationships are ended, and resources and support networks are reduced. In situations of HIV/AIDS, this can lead to unemployment, homelessness and, ultimately, sub-optimal health outcomes.

Drawing on research undertaken in psychiatric hospitals and with members of society considered to be socially deviant, such as homosexuals and criminals, Erving Goffman posited a foundational definition of stigma that has informed general understandings of stigma in a HIV/AIDS framework. He defined stigma as 'deeply discrediting' in a manner that differentiates a person from being whole and normal to being tainted or spoiled, discounted and undesirably different (Goffman, 1963). Thus, this binary (whole and normal: spoiled and undesirably different) devalues people due to perceived difference. Unfortunately, this focus on the individual as being undesirably different seems to have led to misconceptions that if HIV/AIDS were understood more, than PLWHA would no longer be stigmatised.

Obviously, this conceptualisation of stigma is limited in scope and does not take into account cultural or social aspects of stigma. Parker and Aggleton (2003) advise that the characterisation of people as being undesirable contextualises stigma as a static attribute that is mapped onto people, rather than a changing and often contested social process. They propose that this understanding of stigma has limited the ways in which stigma and discrimination have been dealt with in HIV/AIDS settings (Parker & Aggleton, 2003). Even though definitions of stigma have been constrained by focusing on the individual as an object of stigma, Goffman (1963) suggested that stigma is also about relationships as well as undesirable difference. Therefore, stigma is best viewed as a societal phenomenon, dependent on the actions of groups of people.

Central to this sociological understanding of stigma is the intersection of power dynamics, whether economic, social or political, that enable individuals to operate as collectives to identify undesirable differences; generate stereotypes; and discriminate against those perceived to exhibit negative stereotypic manifestations divergent from the agreed upon rules governing cultural norms (Mahajan et al., 2008; Parker & Aggleton, 2003). As such, stigma is rooted in the structure of a society and generally intended to shame and discredit certain groups (Zefi, 2013). Goffman (1963) stated: 'By definition, of course, we believe the person with a stigma is not quite human. On this assumption we exercise varieties of discrimination, through which we effectively, if often un-thinkingly, reduce his life chances' (p. 14). The stigmatised person comes to inhabit a space of social inequality that permits one group to feel superior while devaluing another (Parker & Aggleton, 2003).

Due to its concise summation and usefulness, this chapter adopts the following definition of stigma suggested by Hatzenbuehler, Phelan and Link (2013). For these scholars, 'stigma is defined as the co-occurrence of labeling, stereotyping, separation, status loss, and discrimination in a context in which power is exercised' (p. 14). This definition is useful as it highlights the distinction between stigma and discrimination.

While discrimination is a constitutive feature of stigma, it does not adequately encompass all the elements of stigma, such as stereotyping and labelling (Hatzenbuehler et al., 2013). Within a HIV/AIDS context, Herek (2014) defines stigma as:

HIV/AIDS-related stigma (hereinafter HIV stigma) is defined here as the negative regard and inferior status that society collectively accords to people perceived to have HIV, whether or not they are actually infected and whether or not they manifest symptoms of AIDS, and the individuals, groups, and communities with which they are associated.

(p. 123)

Stigma then, has long-term, detrimental effects on the individuals being stigmatised, due to discrimination and the negative feelings associated with their undesirable difference. Hatzenbuehler et al. (2013) suggest: 'Stigma thwarts, undermines, or exacerbates several processes (i.e., availability of resources, social relationships, psychological and behavioral responses, stress) that ultimately lead to adverse health outcomes' (p. 815).

The literature suggests that stigma represents an added encumbrance that impacts individuals beyond any existing impairments or health burden (Hatzenbuehler et al., 2013). Thus, stigma has a very real impact on individuals' efforts to achieve human security. It prevents them from fully engaging in society in a meaningful manner, resulting in them being unable to secure community support, education, employment and health care. Due to the overarching effects of stigma on HIV/AIDS epidemics, there is a range of GBPs aimed at reducing the stigmatisation and discrimination of key populations and PLWHA.

Stigma GBP

In GBP dialogue, stigma reduction has consistently been promulgated as an area needing attention. It does not matter how good programmes are, if people avoid attending them, they are useless. Additionally, research is revealing that it is not enough to just simply apply medical solutions to problems that exist within societal constructs. Numerous studies have indicated that HIV-related stigma has caused individuals to delay testing, decline disclosure of status to partners and have reduced engagement with HIV services (UNAIDS, 2013). For key populations in HIV/AIDS epidemics, there is a double stigma – that of being HIV+ and engagement in socially objectionable practices. It is clear that reducing stigma related to HIV/AIDS is an area of primary concern in attempting to halt and reverse HIV epidemics.

Stigma is enacted and has repercussions for individuals across three different levels. On a macro level, the obvious impacts of stigma in HIV epidemics include lack of treatment and the potential for HIV to spread through continued high-risk sexual practices between individuals. On a mezzo or community level, individuals, particularly PLWHA who are also members of key populations, suffer from extensive human rights violations, such as refutation of health care provision, denial of employment, punitive law enforcement practices and enforced re-education and detention. On the micro level, PLWHA, whether members of key populations or not, suffer stigma-induced feelings of shame and worthlessness, depression and feelings of suicide.

Stigma is a problem that differs according to cultural norms. There is evidence to suggest that when people are correctly educated concerning the ways HIV is transmitted, and they are provided with information on how to prevent themselves being exposed to transmission risks (such as use of condoms and not sharing needles), there is a reduction in the levels of stigma experienced by PLWHA. The imperative is thus to educate people about HIV/AIDS. This is best done in a variety of ways considering that there is no 'one' optimal manner of communicating information.

The media has had a long history of influencing public perceptions in HIV/AIDS epidemics, often negatively. The use of billboards, print media, celebrity advocacy campaigns and films advocating stigmatising messages concerning HIV/AIDS have a negative impact on stigma reduction efforts (Hood, 2011). Understanding that they have the ability to sway audiences, it is rational to conclude that the media have the potential to be used to reverse some of those previously negative stigmatising discourses. The use of media to promote non-stigmatising messages can therefore positively affect the attitudes and behaviours of the general population towards PLWHA.

The issue of double stigmatisation due to affiliation with a key population is more difficult to address, due to entrenched cultural norms. GBP recognises that the language used to describe key populations has had an effect on the way that they are perceived and health care workers recently changed their discourse from a focus on behaviour to their place in HIV epidemics. Micollier (2012) states: 'The label "high-risk groups" reinforces the de facto social stigma and widespread discrimination against the persons concerned and hence their vulnerability in HIV/AIDS infection' (p. 107).

There are structural policy interventions, such as decriminalisation of sex work and MMT and needle syringe programmes (NSPs), which may mitigate the effects of social stigma. The education of police officers in human rights and non-discriminatory practices has also been proven to reduce the impacts of stigma felt by vulnerable populations. Counselling services are also recommended in order to deal with emotional issues and general concerns experienced by PLWHA.

MMT and NSPs

MMT and NSPs are advocated for HIV/AIDS epidemics in PWID key populations. They have proven effective in reducing the number of shared injection practices as well as subsequent criminal activity and high-risk behaviours in these populations. Opioid substitution therapy or MMT is effective because it means that injection heroin users are no longer subject to the ups and downs associated with injection drug use and are therefore less likely to engage in high-risk behaviours, such as exchange of sex for drugs or money (Zandonella, 2006). NSPs provide access to clean injection apparatus negating the need for needle sharing. Together MMT and NSPs are considered to be key interventions necessary for any successful programme to reduce HIV/AIDS transmission associated with PWID (WHO, UNICEF & UNAIDS, 2011).

In 2010, of the 33 countries that provided data to UNAIDS, WHO and UNICEF concerning MMT and NSPs, only three came close to meeting the WHO-recommended NSPs target of 200 syringes per injecting individual be distributed each year (WHO et al., 2011). However, many countries are substantially below that target and, as such, the optimal efficacy of their programmes is not being achieved and there is little change being recorded in the HIV burden in these PWID populations (UNAIDS, 2013). Most recently, WHO advocated for safety-engineered syringes (WHO, 2015). These syringes have a sharps injury prevention feature to prevent accidental needle stick injuries and ensure safe sharps waste management. In addition, they have a re-use prevention feature. When both MMT and NSPs are implemented as programmes according to GBPs' guidelines, they make a substantial contribution towards lessening the HIV/AIDS transmission risk due to high-risk behaviours in PWID communities.

Additionally, PWID are less likely to engage in acts that may be considered criminal, such as selling sex for drugs or money, and are therefore less likely to be arrested and forced into mandatory drug rehabilitation and detention centres. Incarceration is in no way considered an effective response to PWID. WHO, UNAIDS and UNICEF state: 'Drug detention centres have poor records in preventing drug use and high rates of recidivism. In addition, drug detention centres can enhance HIV and related risks, violate human rights and undermine the potential success of proven interventions' (2011, p. 129).

Finally, MMT programmes generally have a counselling component and peer support outreaches. PWID are able to access services that enable them to deal with the issues that may occur in their lives, including stigmatisation and lack of employment. Additionally, for PLWHA, they are able to gain information on HIV/AIDS services, including HIV transmission prevention strategies, behavioural interventions, condoms, advocacy and ART and other social and medical services.

HIV/AIDS is a blood-borne disease and high-risk sharing practices and unsafe injections (including accidental needle-stick injuries) permit the direct introduction of contaminated blood from the vector to the new host. In order to effectively reach PWID, there needs to be a substantial increase in commitment to efficiently and sustainably deliver NSPs and MMT programmes. In order to make any real impact, there must be an optimal coverage of PWID populations; programmes need to reach as many PWID as possible, with sufficient numbers of needles, and in a way that is accessible (Zandonella, 2006).

Condoms

The use of condoms as an effective preventative measure has been well documented and applied extensively in HIV/AIDS epidemics. Globally, condom programming is an essential component of effective prevention strategies, regardless of cultural context. When used correctly and consistently they are one of the best measures for preventing transmission of HIV (UNAIDS, 2013). As earlier discussed, sexual transmission of HIV is relatively inefficient but conditions that exacerbate the infectiousness, such as STIs or pregnancy, can exist. It is intuitively obvious that condoms create a barrier between sexual partners. If the virus cannot breach the epithelium in the vaginal or anal cavities, then transmission cannot occur. It is a solution that is available globally and for little expense.

A number of different types of condoms are available and more are being developed every year. For HIV epidemics, both male and female condoms are advocated. CSW outreach centres generally provide condoms for free and sex workers are able to either collect them personally or arrange for peers to collect a supply that is then distributed. Additionally, most government HIV/AIDS programming attempts to ensure that condom distribution vending machines are available at locations such as bars, karaoke clubs and brothels where sexual activity is likely to be performed or initiated. While these are not free, they are generally low cost and ensure the sustainability of ongoing condom distribution.

Additionally, along with condoms, some outreach services provide lubricants, which aid in sexual intercourse and provide an additional barrier for transmission. During sexual activity, inflammation and tearing of the vaginal or anal wall allow the virus to take advantage of these breaches in the epithelium and gain entry to the host. Generally, this is more likely to occur in the vaginal or anal cavity during dry penetration. Equally, researchers have been working on developing microbicides that will hopefully serve as lubricants and actively destroy viable virus pathogens.

In the CAPRISA 004 microbicide trial undertaken in South Africa, there was a reported overall efficacy of 39 per cent reduction in HIV transmission, which peaked at 50 per cent after 12 months in individuals with good adherence (Karim et al., 2010). Microbicides are compounds that can be formulated as creams, films, suppositories or gels. They are for topical application inside the rectum or vagina to protect against HIV. However, there are some issues concerning microbicides. Microbicides require a high adherence rate to be effective and current sub-optimal adherence remains a challenge for microbicide usage (Gray et al., 2016). While the future of microbicide use in HIV epidemics is promising, there are significant challenges remaining before they move on from the trial phase.

Globally, there are still issues surrounding the use of condoms. This is particularly so for women. Women are often unable to negotiate the use of condoms and, as a result, will undertake sexual activity without them. This is the case for FSWs who may find it difficult to negotiate the use of condoms with clients (especially those operating in the lower hierarchies, such as street walkers), but this is also the situation for many married women or women in non-commercial relationships. Significantly, this is one of the drivers of MTCT. In these circumstances, women, who may have only one sexual partner, become infected by men who engage in sexual intercourse outside of the relationship, particularly with key groups such as PWID, MSM or FSWs, or via other high-risk behaviours. Therefore, while it has been established that condoms remain an essential component of successful HIV/AIDS GBP prevention and treatment programmes, there are still challenges associated with ensuring their optimal usage.

What can China do?

While not every aspect of HIV/AIDS policy in China is discussed in this chapter the major prevention and education programmes for China's HIV/AIDS epidemics are considered. China's main policies for prevention efforts closely follow those of TasP. However, they have been running education programmes and distributing condoms for many years and MMT and syringe programmes since implementing pilot programmes in 2004 (Yin et al., 2010).

World Aids Day has been used as a platform for widespread HIV/AIDS education initiatives in China. Other HIV educational initiatives include the use of billboards and television (albeit mainly in urban areas and in Han Chinese and therefore generally inaccessible to the ethnic minorities speaking different dialects and the uneducated who comprise the majority of internal migrants). Therefore, while China is making some attempts to address the HIV epidemics within its borders, there needs to be an escalation of those efforts and more programming to enable ethnic minorities and marginalised population groups to access these programmes.

As a part of the prevention campaigns, Beijing also provides stigma reduction programmes for PLWHA (Ying-Xia, Golin, Jin, Emrick, Nan & Ming-Qiang, 2014; Yu, 2012). The Confucian worldview and Chinese cultural practices have meant that historically there has been little sympathy for PLWHA. Another difficulty being faced by PLWHA is that of the existing *hukou* system, a household registration system documenting place of birth and rural or urban residency. In the past, PLWHA have been required to attend clinics in the area of their *hukou* registration. This has changed in the past couple of years and now there is provision for PLWHA to access ART and other HIV/AIDS-related services in other areas. Unfortunately, few people know about this and as a result many ART-eligible PLWHA are not accessing services (Chen, pers. comm., November 2013).

Currently, in China, the mainstay for HIV/AIDS prevention and care programming is the 'Four Free and One Care' policy. This policy rests within broader HIV frameworks and future planning targets such as China's five-year action plans (2001–2005, 2006–2010, 2011–2015) and the Regulations on AIDS Prevention and Treatment (2006) (Yu, 2012). It operates at the vanguard of China's commitment to ensure access to ART for all eligible HIV+ persons. The 'Four Free and One Care Policy' states that free ART drugs will be given to all AIDS patients (both urban and rural) in financial difficulty; it will provide free voluntary counselling and testing (VCT) in areas of high prevalence; prevention of mother-to-child transmission (PMCT) and VCT will be provided for all pregnant women; AIDS orphans will be provided with free education; and care will be provided for all AIDS patients with financial difficulties (Zhang et al., 2006, p. 98).

However, the benefits of this programme are not implemented consistently or effectively and the prohibitive associated costs due to multiple fees for extra testing (such as liver function tests), travel costs and loss of income when attending clinics make accessing this programme impossible for some individuals (Yu, 2012). Additionally, those segments of the population engaged in illegal activities such as sex workers, PWID and MSM are reluctant to access government-run medical facilities due to fear of arrest and incarceration. While some NGOs are involved in implementation of HIV/AIDS programmes (such as rapid testing, condom distribution and syringe programmes), at present all ART is administered only at government-run health clinics and hospitals.

China's NGOs: do they have a role to play?

GBP often works hand in hand with NGOs and CBOs in the delivery of HIV/AIDs services. The situation for NGOs and CBOs in China is somewhat restrictive as all NGOs and CBOs are either fully government-operated non-governmental organisations (GONGOs) or partially government-run and government-funded (Yu, 2012). Wang et al. (2016) state: 'Actual NGOs are organizations created at the grassroots level and tend to be small, lack capacity, and lack political and financial resources. GONGOs are government sponsored and tend to be large, with more professional staff, and a bureaucratic structure' (p. 418). Thus, GONGOs are distinct from NGOs in China. While there are GONGOs who are involved in HIV/AIDS programming in Yunnan, they do not have the favoured position and access to marginalised populations that NGOs and CBOs are able to negotiate (Wang et al., 2016).

However, there is little independence in policy decisions and often NGOs are constrained by Beijing's desired outcomes rather than being able to respond to the fluid situation at grassroots levels (Wang, 2012). NGOs are also often constrained by donor expectations (Watkins, Swidler & Hannan, 2012).

In China, NGOs are regulated by Beijing[3] and are sometimes beset by a climate of mistrust due to fears that Beijing will lose control and that NGOs may grow and challenge the state authority (Yu, 2012). Wang et al. (2016) advise: 'Before legally registering with the Ministry of Civil Affairs, an "NGO" must obtain sponsorship from a relevant government ministry or bureau, the leader of which will be personally responsible for any misconduct by the NGO' (p. 420). As a result, many of the HIV/AIDS organisations are comprised of GONGOs and both funding and policy decisions are managed by Beijing (Wang, 2012; Yu, 2012).

The situation in China is slightly better for CBOs (generally run by larger NGOs), such as drop-in centres, which provide a range of services (such as condoms, syringes, rapid testing and counselling) in an anonymous and non-threatening environment (Chen, pers. comm., October 2013). Local governments will often collaborate with them and allow a certain amount of autonomy as they recognise that CBOs have links to communities and key populations that are otherwise not accessible (Chen, pers. comm., November 2013; Yu, 2012).

Therefore, it does seem that Beijing has been making attempts to be more collaborative and outsource many of its services to PLWHA through NGOs and CBOs. It has recognised that, given a certain amount of autonomy, NGOs and CBOs are able to operate in areas that are difficult for governmental bodies. NGOs are still finding their place in China and there are many areas for improvement.

Additionally, the number of permanent NGOs operating is insufficient for the situations they are encountering (Chen, pers. comm., October 2013).

According to Chen, who is a member of one of the few permanent HIV/AIDS NGOs operating in China, there were only five permanent HIV/AIDS NGOs operating in Yunnan and other limited-term NGOs formed spontaneously as funding for projects became available (Chen, pers. comm., November 2013; Wang et al., 2016).[4] While there were larger numbers of permanent NGOs operating as a part of joint programmes with donor agencies (such as the AusAid/China joint HAARP programme which concluded in 2013), considering that China has become a middle-income country and all major international HIV/AIDS donors have now withdrawn, there is now limited funding not only for the permanent HIV/AIDS NGOs but also for the short-term pop-up NGOs offering limited-term programming. As a result, the NGOs operating on a permanent basis are not only short on funding but also short on members with an average of only four core or full-time members (Wang et al., 2016).

Conclusion

In considering the current GBP, it becomes clear that the implementation of these practices is flexible and culturally adaptable. While this is necessary it does allow for inconsistencies in adoption and usage across different HIV epidemics. Countries pick and choose which (if any) GBPs are most suited to the epidemics within their borders. When there is a thorough and comprehensive understanding of the characteristics of a country's differing epidemics (know your epidemic, know your response), then it seems reasonable to assume that GBPs will be used in an optimal manner. Unfortunately this is not always the case and may result in ineffective or insufficient HIV/AIDS programming.

There are a myriad of challenges facing state governments in addressing HIV epidemics, both in attempting to meet the needs of PLWHA and protecting those who have not been infected. As discussed, these challenges become more complicated and perhaps even appear insurmountable when matters of cultural norms or biases and stigma are added. Practices that may appear optimal may be ineffective due to the reluctance of communities to go against accepted cultural norms or attract stigma by openly acknowledging their participation in behaviour that is perceived to be unacceptable by the general population.

While Beijing appears to be increasingly invested in addressing the HIV/AIDS situation funding constraints, lack of scale-up of existing efforts and a reluctance to include 'outsiders', such as NGOs, INGOs and the UN in what is considered a state problem, hamper efforts to move towards a reduction of new infections. The success of GBP initiatives often relies on NGO and CBO participation, both for the dissemination of information but also for the provision of HIV services. China's preferred method for service delivery is through official governmental hospitals and clinics. The implications for this include insufficient attendance by key populations and possible under-reporting of HIV/AIDS cases, due to the fact that most of the almost 2,000 sentinel surveillance sites are located in government-run establishments.

Finally, it is important to realise that GBP changes over time. What was appropriate at the beginning of the pandemic may no longer be appropriate now. As the understandings of the underlying causes and behavioural risks that intensify HIV infectiousness increase and change, so too do the GBPs. As an effective vaccine becomes more likely, the mutability of GBP keeps pace. What does not change is the fact that individuals have HIV/AIDS. They are not abstract entities but real people with real needs. GBP that addresses the needs of PLWHA rather than concentrating on the disease is always appropriate. Understanding the multifarious nature of the problem provides a foundation for the acceptance of human security frameworks as advantageous in HIV/AIDS epidemics.

Case study 4.1 Guoliang's story

Guoliang's case study reveals some of the more pervasive human security threats for PWID. As with many of the case studies presented in this book, health insecurity, food insecurity, community insecurity and economic insecurity are prevalent. Additionally, as with the other case studies presented, Guoliang's exact location remains unidentified but I can reveal that he lives near Ruili in Yunnan Province (which has a population of about 45 million people). Guoliang is an energetic man who is thin, and small in stature with a balding head. He is a former injection drug user but when I met him he was on a methadone maintenance programme and working as a peer worker attached to a PWID drop-in centre. He tried to be in the drop-in centre every day as he felt that he wanted to give back to people and help them in a way that others had helped him. He had such passion for what he was doing that I found myself getting excited about the possibilities. I enjoyed meeting him a great deal.

As with most of the peer workers I met, Guoliang is HIV+. He told me that he had been stupid when he was using drugs because he had shared needles with his friends but he did not know that it could be bad for him. Now he was trying to live his life as healthily as he could. But, he told me he did not really want to talk about himself; instead he wanted to let me know what was happening in the drop-in centre. He told me that it was a bad situation for many people. Then he raised his head, leaned forward and peering into my eyes, he said, 'A lot of people are suffering, especially along the border areas.' I felt pinned down by his intensity like a beetle on an entomologist's tray, and I found myself unable to hold his gaze. I felt uncomfortable and even slightly ashamed that I did not have any solutions to offer him. My life was completely different and for a moment I had found myself wondering what I thought I was doing in China trying to understand a problem, in a context that was so foreign to me on so many levels. But I knew I wanted to try.

I asked him to tell me what kind of services they provided in the drop-in centre. He told me that often the peer workers were just there to be a friend. They listened when people came in and offered them a place to hang out where they did not feel judged. Of course, they also offered other services like needles and syringes and information about why those things were necessary. Guoliang told me that they also tried to do things that would help out the family members of the PWID who came to the centre. When I asked him why, he said that everyone suffers in one way or another, and everyone needs help.

One of the most important things that they offered to those who dropped by was a blood test to ascertain their HIV status. He said it was something that most PWID drop-in centres did because for some people it was the only way they were ever likely to find out. Guoliang said that they were scared to go to the hospital to have any tests done, as they did not know what would happen to them. He told me that at the centre they administered a rapid test, which was a very simple procedure and just required a bit of blood. It is a similar concept to that used by diabetics to test their blood sugar levels. A small pinprick and then blood dropped onto a small opening on the test. The problem was, he sighed, that sometimes they gave a false positive reading so they had to encourage people who tested positive to get further testing. It was difficult to get them to go but peer workers from the centre would go with them if they needed it.

He told me that what they did at the centre was only a small part of the work. The real need was among the homeless PWID who lived without shelter along the China/Myanmar border areas. He said that 85 per cent of all their work was done with these groups and for them it was not about providing somewhere for them to hang out, for them, it was trying to find a way to keep them alive. Most of the people had illegally crossed from Myanmar and so were technically not able to access services in China. Of course, all of the outreach services in places like Ruili offered help when they could. Guoliang said that there were teams of peer workers, who would regularly go out to the areas along the border in order to take them food, rapid tests, medical supplies and other essential needs. He told me that the conditions were rough out there and it was hard even for the peer workers. 'We are dealing with people who are destitute and in the worst way,' he said.

They only had the clothes that they were wearing and often these items were ragged and inadequate for the conditions. He said that people were freezing and that without help they would die. Guoliang told me that this was not the only problem. They had no food either and would often go days without eating. He said they took what they could out to give to them but it was never enough. They were not able to help them with shelter but did take out blankets when they had them in supply. The PWID were often gathered in small groups spread throughout the countryside so they did not always manage to get to everyone. The peer workers just did their best to get to as many people as possible.

Apart from these issues, Guoliang told me that most of the people living rough had significant medical issues. He said that in general for them to get to a point where they were homeless and living in those conditions, they had significant drug habits. 'One of the big problems is that they inject themselves so often that they begin to get really bad sores at the sites of injection,' he informed me. These sores would fester and without medical treatment get worse until they were suppurating, oozing wounds. The peer workers would treat these wounds when they were out in the field, cleaning them and bandaging them but the conditions were unhygienic and the PWID had no way to keep them clean. 'We just do what we can,' Guoliang said, shaking his head.

Apart from the services they offered for food and medicine for those on the border areas, they also offered training and supplies to help prevent overdose. Guoliang told me it was a constant source of concern for PWID. Everyone had seen a friend die of a drug overdose. He told me that to help with that situation they offered training in the use of Naloxone Hydrochloride (Naloxone). They would train special peer workers to administer the drug to their friends. Naloxone reverses the effects of drug overdose by blocking the opioid receptors in the brain. The peer workers had to commit to being available 24 hours a day, every day. They provided their phone number to their peer network and were on call to administer the drug if someone accidently overdosed. Guoliang told me that many lives had already been saved through this programme as people were too scared to call a doctor or take their friends to the hospital in situations of overdose because they are afraid they would be arrested.

I was impressed by Guoliang and could only imagine that the other peer workers involved with drop-in centre were just as passionate about helping other PWID. In many ways, I felt that this was the true face of the HIV/AIDS initiatives in China. The dedicated and very humble individuals who did what they could to support others. They had been there and lived the same life as the people they were supporting. People like Guoliang had managed to turn things around for themselves, perhaps with the help of other individuals, and they were paying it forward in the best way that they could. They offered encouragement and support rather than judgement and discrimination.

Guoliang's story highlights the need for best practice. Outreach services for hard-to-reach populations like PWID are essential. This is not an abstract notion of 'doing something to help' but a boots on the ground, life-saving strategy. Simply put, not only does best practice help mitigate the continued spread of HIV/AIDs, it saves lives. It saves people like Guoliang and those he reaches out to. Best practice reinstates the human security of the populations who need it most. There is a cost for implementing best practice but the cost of not implementing it is even greater. That cost is paid in rampant HIV/AIDS epidemics but also in broken communities, families, and loss of lives, all of which contribute to significant human insecurity, even extending across generations. The high-level theory of global best practice is played out in the lower levels in ad hoc shelters along the border areas of China, in small drop-in centres and in the hands of people administering a drug that will bring a friend back from the brink of death.

Notes

1 This was evidenced at the AIDS 2014 conference where the term PWID was consistently used in place of injection drug user (IDU).
2 MDG Number six calls for extraordinary action to halt and begin to reverse the AIDS epidemic.
3 China NGOs are regulated through the China State Council Order 250, September 1998, regulating the management and registration of social organisations (Wang, 2012).
4 As a primary informant, active and well versed concerning the current information for the situation for NGOs on the ground in China, Chen is considered a reliable source of information. Chen's interview is also supported by discussion contained in Wang et al. (2016).

References

Alvarez-Uria, G., Pakam, R., Midde, M. & Naik, P. K. (2013). Entry, retention, and viro-logical suppression in an HIV cohort study in India: Description of the cascade of care and implications for reducing HIV-related mortality in low- and middle-income countries. *Interdisciplinary Perspectives on Infectious Diseases*, vol. 2013, Article ID 384805, 1–8. http://dx.doi.org/10.1155/2013/384805.

Autran, B., Hamimi, C. & Katlama, C. (2014). One step closer to HIV eradication? *Current Treatment Options in Infectious Diseases, 6*, 171–182. doi:10.1007/s40506-014-0017-1.

Bangsberg, D. (2010). International perspectives of adherence and resistance to HIV antiretroviral therapy. *Journal of the International AIDS Society, 13*(suppl. 4), O2. Retrieved from www.jiasociety.org/content/13/S4/O2

Burki, T. K. (2011). Discrimination against people with HIV persists in China. *The Lancet, 377*(9762), 286–287.

Chen, J., Choe, M. K., Chen, S. & Zhang, S. (2007). The effects of individual- and community-level knowledge, beliefs, and fear on stigmatization of people living with HIV/AIDS in China. *AIDS Care, 19*(5), 666–673. doi:10.1080/09540120600988517.

Cohen, M. S., Chen, Y. Q., McCauley, M., Gamble, T., Hosseinipour, M. C., Kumarasamy, N., … & Fleming, T. R. (2011). Prevention of HIV-1 infection with early antiretroviral therapy. *New England Journal of Medicine, 365*(6), 493–505. doi:10.1056/NEJMoa1105243.

Deeks. S. G., Lewin, S. R. & Havlir, D. V. (2014). The end of AIDS: HIV infection as a chronic disease. *Lancet, 382*(9903), 1525–1533. doi:10.1016/S0140-6736(13)61809-7.

Funnell, S. (1999). An evaluation of the UNAIDS Best Practices Collection: Its strengths and weaknesses, accessibility, use and impact. UNAIDS. Retrieved from: data.unaids. org/topics/m-e/unaids_best-practice_eval_en.doc

Goffman, E. (1963). *Behavior in public place*. Glencoe, IL: The Free Press.

Gray, G. E., Laher, F., Doherty, T., Karim, S. A., Hammer, S., Mascola, J., … & Corey, L. (2016). Which new health technologies do we need to achieve an end to HIV/AIDS? *PLoS Biology, 14*(3), e1002372.

Hallett, T. B. and Eaton, J. W. (2013). A side door into care cascade for HIV-infected patients? *Journal of Acquired Immune Deficiency Syndrome, 63*(S2), S228–S232.

Hankins, C. A. & de Zalduondo, B. O. (2010). Combination prevention: A deeper understanding of effective HIV prevention. *AIDS, 24* (suppl. 4), S70–S80.

Hatzenbuehler, M. L., Phelan, J. C. & Link, B. G. (2013). Stigma as a fundamental cause of population health inequalities. *American Journal of Public Health, 103*(5), 813–821.

Herek, G. (2014). HIV-related stigma. In P. W. Corrigan (Ed.), *The stigma of disease and disability: Understanding causes and overcoming injustices* (pp. 121–138). Washington, DC: American Psychological Association.

Hood, J. (2011). *HIV/AIDS, health and the media in China*. New York, NY: Routledge.

Kalichman, S. C., Hernandez, D., Cherry, C., Kalichman, M. O., Washington, C. & Grebler, T. (2014). Food insecurity and other poverty indicators among people living with HIV/AIDS: Effects on treatment and health outcomes. *Journal of Community Health, 39*(6), 1133–1139. doi:10.1007/s10900-014-9868-0.

Karim, Q. A., Karim, S. S. A., Frohlich, J. A., Grobler, A. C., Baxter, C., Mansoor, L. E., … & Gengiah, T. N. (2010). Effectiveness and safety of tenofovir gel, an antiretroviral microbicide, for the prevention of HIV infection in women. *Science, 329*(5996), 1168–1174.

Kilmarx, P. H. & Mutasa-Apollo, T. (2013). Patching a leaky pipe: The cascade of HIV care. *Current Opinion in HIV AIDS, 8*, 59–64. doi:10.1097/COH.0b013e32835b806e.

Kim, J., Lutz, B., Dhaliwal, M. & O'Malley, J. (2011). The 'AIDS and MDGs' approach: What is it, why does it matter, and how do we take it forward?. *Third World Quarterly, 32*(1), 141–163.

Lourenço, L., Colley, G., Nosyk, B., Shopin, D., Montaner, J. S. G & Lima, V. D. (2014). High levels of heterogeneity in the HIV cascade of care across different population subgroups in British Columbia, Canada. *PLoS ONE, 9*(12): e115277. doi:10.1371/journal.pone.0115277.

Mahajan, A. P., Sayles, J. N., Patel, V. A., Remien, R. H., Ortiz, D., Szekeres, G. & Coates, T. J. (2008). Stigma in the HIV/AIDS epidemic: A review of the literature and recommendations for the way forward. *AIDS, 22*(suppl. 2), S67–S79.

Micollier, E. (2012). Sexualised illness and gendered narratives: The problematic of social science and humanities in China's HIV and AIDS governance. *International Journal of Asia Pacific Studies, 8*(1), 103–124.

Montaner, J. (2014, July, 20–25). Report back from the 2014 treatment as prevention workshop. Paper presented at the meeting of International Aids Society, 20th International AIDS Conference, Melbourne.

Mugavero, M. J., Amico, K. R., Horn, T. & Thompson, M. A. (2013). The state of engagement in HIV care in the United States: From cascade to continuum to control. *Clinical Infectious Diseases;57*(8):1164–71, doi:10.1093/cid/cit420.

Nakagawa, F., May, M. & Phillips, A. (2013). Life expectancy living with HIV: Recent estimates and future implications. *Current Opinion in Infectious Diseases, 26*(1), 17–25.

Nosyk, B., Montaner, J. S., Colley, G., Lima, V. D., Chan, K., Heath, K., … & Gustafson, R. (2014). The cascade of HIV care in British Columbia, Canada, 1996–2011: A population-based retrospective cohort study. *The Lancet, Infectious Diseases, 14*(1), 40–49.

Parker, R. & Aggleton, P. (2003). HIV and AIDS-related stigma and discrimination: A conceptual framework and implications for action. *Social Science & Medicine, 57*(1), 13–24.

Santos, A. F. & Soares, M. A. (2010). HIV genetic diversity and drug resistance. *Viruses, 2*(2), 503–531. doi:10.3390/v2020503.

Slavin, S. (2015). Promoting treatment for HIV prevention. *HIV Australia, 13*(2). Retrieved from www.afao.org.au/library/hiv-australia/volume-13/vol-13-number-2-horizons/promoting-treatment-for-hiv-prevention#.V6P2rWO48dU

Su, X., Lau, J. T., Mak, W. W., Chen, L., Choi, K. C., Song, J., … & Liu, C. (2013). Perceived discrimination, social support, and perceived stress among people living with HIV/AIDS in China. *AIDS Care, 25*(2), 239–248.

UNAIDS. (2000). *Summary booklet of Best Practices in Africa.* Issue 2, summary booklet series. Retrieved from data.unaids.org/Publications/IRC-pub02/jc-summbookl-2_en.pdf

UNAIDS. (2011). *HIV in Asia and the Pacific: Getting to zero.* UNAIDS. Retrieved from www.unaids.org/en/media/unaids/contentassets/documents/unaidspublication/2011/20110826_APGettingToZero_en.pdf

UNAIDS. (2013). *Global report: UNAIDS report on the global AIDS epidemic 2013.* Retrieved from www.unaids.org/sites/default/files/media.../UNAIDS_Global_Report_2013_en_1.pd

Wang, D., Mei, G., Xu, X., Zhao, R., Ma, Y., Chen, R., … & Hu, Z. (2016). Chinese non-governmental organizations involved in HIV/AIDS prevention and control:

Intra-organizational social capital as a new analytical perspective. *BioScience Trends,* *10*(5), 418–423.

Wang, M. L. (2012). Managing HIV/AIDS: Yunnan's government-driven, multi-sector partnership model. *Management and Organization Review, 8*(3), 535–557.

Watkins, S. C., Swidler, A. & Hannan, T. (2012). Outsourcing social transformation: development NGOs as organizations. *Annual Review of Sociology, 38*(1), 285–315.

WHO (World Health Organization). (2015). WHO guideline on the use of safety-engineered syringes for intramuscular, intradermal and subcutaneous injections in health-care settings. Retrieved from http://apps.who.int/iris/bitstream/10665/170470/1/WHO_HIS_SDS_2015.5_eng.pdf

WHO, UNICEF & UNAIDS. (2011). Global HIV/AIDS response: Epidemic update and health sector progress towards Universal Access, Progress Report 2011. Retrieved from: www.who.int/hiv/pub/progress_report2011/en/

Wu, S., Li, L., Wu, Z., Liang, L., Cao, H., Yan, Z. & Li, J. (2008). A brief HIV stigma reduction intervention for service providers in China. *AIDS Patient Care & STDs, 22*(6), 513–520. doi:10.1089/apc.2007.0198.

Yin, W., Hao, Y., Sun, X., Gong, X., Li, F., Li, J., … & Cao, X. (2010). Scaling up the national methadone maintenance treatment program in China: Achievements and challenges. *International Journal of Epidemiology, 39*(suppl. 2), ii29–ii37.

Ying-Xia, Z., Golin, C. E., Jin, B., Emrick, C. B., Nan, Z. & Ming-Qiang, L. (2014). Coping strategies for HIV-related stigma in Liuzhou, China. *AIDS and Behavior, 18*(2), 212–220.

Yu, H. (2012). Governing and representing HIV/AIDS in China: A review and an introduction. *IJAPS, 8*(1), 1–33.

Zandonella, C. (2006). Injection of hope: Needle and syringe programs can lower HIV infection rates and provide important outreach to injection drug users. *IAVI Report, 10*(4). Retrieved from www.iavireport.org/Back-Issues/Pages/IAVI-Report-10(4)-injectionofhope.aspx

Zefi, V. (2013). Stigma toward HIV/AIDS people. *Mediterranean Journal of Social Sciences, 4*(2), 411.

Zhang, F., Hsu, M., Yu, L., Wen, Y. & Pan, J. (2006). Initiation of the national free antiretroviral therapy program in rural China. In J. Kaufman, A. Kleinman & T. Saich (Eds.), *AIDS and social policy in China* (pp. 96–124). Cambridge, MA: Harvard University Asia Center.

5   The 'loving capitalism' disease

The more you try to cover things up, the more exposed they will be.

欲盖弥彰

History of HIV/AIDS in China

China has been dealing with a HIV/AIDS epidemic since 1989 and currently the disease has been identified in all 31 provinces. However, the first actual case of AIDS was discovered in June 1985 in an Argentinian tourist who was reported to have died of severe lung infection and respiratory failure (Settle, 2003; Wu, Sullivan, Wang, Rotheram-Borus & Detels, 2007). The subsequent section provides a brief synopsis of what can be putatively considered the four phases[1] of the HIV epidemic in China (Nutbeam, Padmadas, Maslovskaya & Wu, 2015; Sheng & Cao, 2008).

In understanding the different phases of the disease in China, it is possible to gain an overview of the expansion of the epidemic. The timeline in Figure 5.1 provides a suitable summary of the actions and reactions of the government in Beijing throughout China's HIV epidemic. Beijing's initial contextualisation of the appearance of HIV in China as something from an external source, and the resulting lack of action, contributed significantly to the emergence of the epidemic within China. This was characterised by a period of more than ten years where Beijing fundamentally ignored the emerging epidemic within its borders, resulting in its diffusion throughout the population. Between 1989 and 1995, Beijing refused to publicly acknowledge that China even had a HIV/AIDS epidemic (Nutbeam et al., 2015). This resulted in a continued growth period and eventually to the rampant spread of HIV throughout all provinces of China, particularly in key populations. The four phases of the epidemic in China are considered to be (1) the introduction phase; (2) the diffusion phase; (3) the growth period; and (4) the rampant prevalence of the disease (Hayes, 2005; Wu et al., 2004).

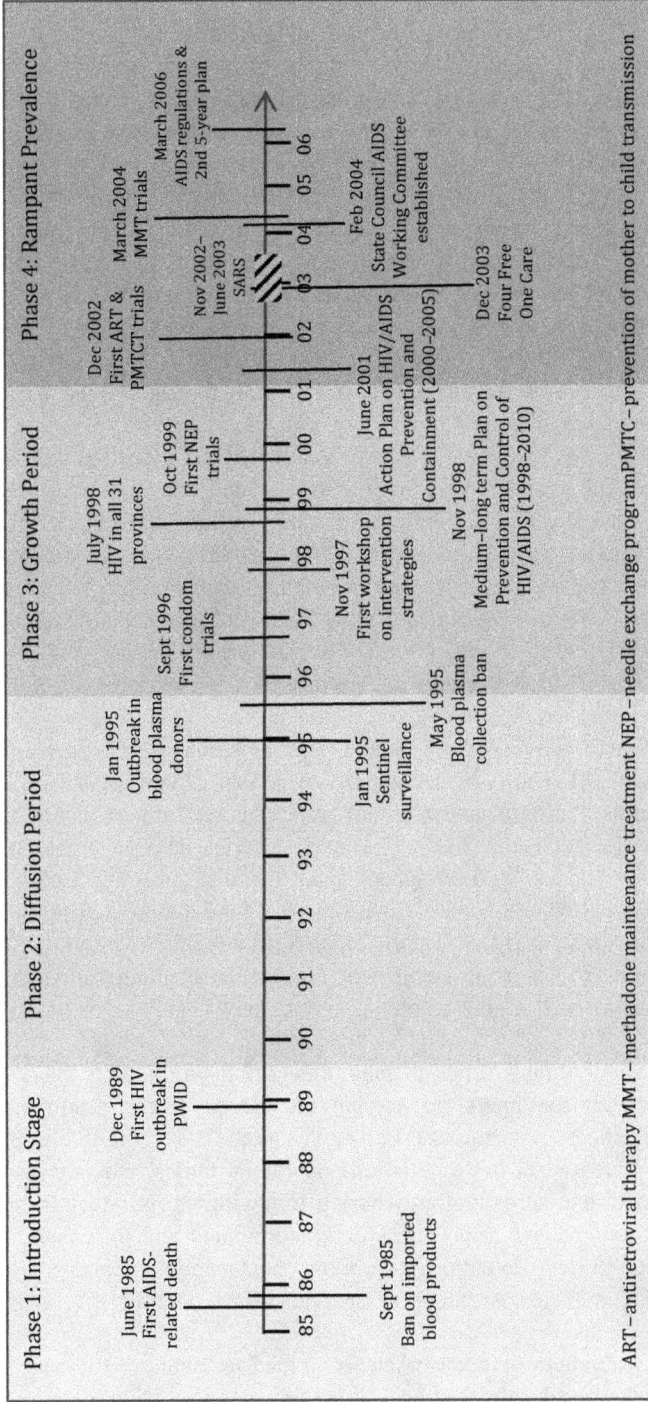

Figure 5.1 Important events in China's HIV/AIDS epidemic.

Phase 1: Introduction Stage

June 1985
First AIDS-
related death

Sept 1985
Ban on imported
blood products

Dec 1989
First HIV
outbreak in
PWID

Phase 2: Diffusion Period

Jan 1995
Outbreak in
blood plasma
donors

Jan 1995
Sentinel
surveillance

May 1995
Blood plasma
collection ban

Phase 3: Growth Period

Sept 1996
First condom
trials

Nov 1997
First workshop
on intervention
strategies

July 1998
HIV in all 31
provinces

Nov 1998
Medium-long term Plan on
Prevention and Control of
HIV/AIDS (1998–2010)

Oct 1999
First NEP
trials

June 2001
Action Plan on HIV/AIDS
Prevention and
Containment (2000–2005)

Phase 4: Rampant Prevalence

Dec 2002
First ART &
PMTCT trials

Nov 2002–
June 2003
SARS

Dec 2003
Four Free
One Care

Feb 2004
State Council AIDS
Working Committee
established

March 2004
MMT trials

March 2006
AIDS regulations &
2nd 5-year plan

85 86 87 88 89 90 91 92 93 94 95 96 97 98 99 00 01 02 03 04 05 06

ART – antiretroviral therapy MMT – methadone maintenance treatment NEP – needle exchange program PMTC – prevention of mother to child transmission

Introduction stage or the 'Western' disease: 1985–1988

The movement of HIV across differing populations has been clearly identified in China. Apart from foreign nationals, the first Chinese citizens to be infected were those returning to China from abroad where they contracted the disease; the second group were haemophiliac patients who contracted the disease through imported contaminated blood (Yu, Xie, Zhang, Lu & Chan, 1996). It is important to understand that in the initial stages of the disease appearing in China, it was considered a Western disease. This categorisation meant that apart from restricting the flow of foreign blood products, testing returning nationals and attempting to crack down on sex workers (who had sex with foreigners), China did very little to halt the spread of HIV in the early stages. As such, it is debatable whether China's focus on prevention in these discrete areas of outbreak contributed positively to a much-needed overall plan to educate the public and potentially halt the epidemic.

In contextualising HIV as a Western disease it was understood that immoral behaviour was the primary driver of the disease and that, by default, Chinese people could not get it due to Confucian morality and racial superiority, resulting in improved immune systems (Dikötter, 2000, p. 1083). Widespread beliefs held that if Chinese simply stayed away from foreigners, they would not contract HIV. Media reports of the time suggested that the West, and America in particular, was the source of all immorality and disease. For example, *The Peking Daily* warned: 'There are social ills that plague the Western world, for instance, drugs, alcoholism, robbery, murder, suicide, divorce, prostitution, homosexuality, venereal disease, AIDS, etc. All these things come from the ideology of capitalism' (cited in Browning, 1987). The inference appears to be that Chinese socialism and the prevailing norms of Confucianism would protect people from becoming infected with HIV. On 25 September 1987, Macartney reported on a government ban on extramarital sex and sex with foreigners, and stated that government officials had proclaimed that AIDS was unlikely to spread in China due to their moral stance against homosexuality and casual sex (*Beijing Review*, cited in Macartney, 1987).

Beijing went so far as to implement legislation, banning foreigners from sexual interactions with Chinese nationals. Macartney (1987) reported:

> Beijing is adopting a series of measures 'strictly forbidding illegal sexual contacts with foreigners' to prevent the spread of the deadly acquired immune deficiency syndrome. Earlier this year [1987], the Public Security Bureau issued a set of 'Regulations on Public Order' making casual sex illegal in China. 'Prostitution, whoring following an introduction, abetting prostitution and whoring are strictly forbidden and offenders face a maximum 15 days detention, a warning, re-education and a maximum fine of 5,000 Yuan,' says Article 30 of the regulations.

However, the numbers of sex workers continued to increase. Previous Maoist crackdowns and re-education and rehabilitation practices including closing the brothels and allegedly stamping out STIs, were no match for emerging markets, changing sexual practices and cross-border trafficking (Hyde, 2000). Incidences of STIs rose at an exponential rate and because sex workers sell sex, and HIV is sexually transmitted, they have been 'perceived as an epidemiological threat the world over' (p. 115). It seems clear that in the early stages of China's epidemic sex workers bore the brunt of censure along with all things Western.

Diffusion period or drug users disease: 1989–1993

The beginning of 1989 revealed that China still had a limited understanding of HIV. Two films dealing with the issue of HIV, and promoted with the characters for 'Super Cancer' and 'AIDS Patients' advertised as 'Pornographic Pestilence' (about three students who had sex with a foreign teacher), were still publicising it as a Western disease contracted through immoral behaviour (Settle, 2003). However, this was soon to change. The first official outbreak of HIV in Chinese nationals appeared in 1989 among 146 infected heroin users in Ruili. In China, the epidemic first manifested in rural areas and spread to urban centres (Cui, Liau & Wu, 2009). It is believed that this group, which lies along a main drug trafficking route from the Golden Triangle, is likely to have been the source of all later transmission of HIV in China (Knutsen, 2012; Settle, 2003). By 1994, having been transmitted to the spouses, sexual partners and children of drug users, the disease was being transmitted by all modes and in all provinces of China (Knutsen, 2012). No longer was the disease one that was exclusive to Westerners, sex workers or drug users.

As a result of this HIV expansion 'The Law of Infectious Diseases Prevention and Control' was passed in 1989, with the methods of implementation passed two years later in 1991. AIDS was declared to be a notifiable disease; AIDS patients required quarantine and cases needed to be reported to local health authorities within 6 hours for urban cases and 12 hours for rural cases (Wu, Rou & Cui, 2004). However, these requirements were unfeasible and inadequate to address the problem, and, as a result, HIV continued to spread throughout China.

This phase also saw the beginnings of an outbreak in former plasma donors (FPDs) and recipients (He & Detels, 2005). From the late 1980s to the early 1990s, thousands of blood and plasma collection points were in operation throughout the country. This was particularly the case in the poorer, least developed regions of central China. They were extremely popular as donors were paid 50 yuan for a unit of plasma and 200 yuan for whole blood (Settle, 2003). A lack of screening for HIV meant that approximately 69,000 FPDs and recipients were infected due to contaminated blood and plasma; resulting in a 10–20 per cent, and in some areas 60 per cent, HIV+ prevalence rate in these cohorts (Cui et al., 2009). For the first time, HIV began to spread throughout significant cohorts of the general population.

It was during this phase, or the diffusion period, that HIV continued expanding into new populations within China. Beijing's lack of attention to the continuing spread meant that there were no existing barriers for expansion or education campaigns to help people understand that HIV was not simply a disease for undesirable elements of the population but rather could be contracted by anyone. The outbreak in FPD was the first time that the general population realised that HIV did not discriminate based on moral behaviour. Throughout this diffusion period, Beijing was still loath to admit that a HIV epidemic was spreading throughout China. Until the publicising of the outbreak in FPDs, Beijing was still reporting on HIV in a limited manner and suggesting that the disease was only manifesting in isolated incidences.

Growth period or anyone's disease: 1994–2000

It was during this growth period that China first acknowledged the epidemic had taken root in the country and that it was no longer being driven by foreigners. For the first time they acknowledged that it was possible for anyone to contract the disease and that it was spreading quickly. In late 1994, the epidemic began its growth period, spreading out from Yunnan. By the mid-1990s, HIV had spread throughout China with all modes of transmission being reported and, by 1998, HIV was reported in all provinces of China (Sheng & Cao, 2008). As a result, the government began to take measures to address the burgeoning epidemic. In 1995, 42 sentinel surveillance sites targeting key populations were introduced in 23 provinces experiencing the highest rates of HIV/AIDS (He & Detels, 2005). These sites sought to identify areas and populations that were experiencing outbreaks in an attempt to come to a more comprehensive understanding about how expansive the epidemic had become.

Also in 1995, China first officially announced the epidemic in FPDs (Wu et al., 2007). By 1996, China began implementing programmes along the international border areas of Yunnan designed to halt the spread of infectious disease and to get the HIV epidemic under control (Settle, 2003). In 1997, Chinese and foreign leaders in HIV/AIDS control met for a workshop which proved to be the turning point in China's efforts and many of the recommendations from that workshop were undertaken (Wu et al., 2004). Rather than addressing the HIV/AIDS epidemic from a strictly public health policy, they began to acknowledge the need to consider the problem from a human perspective.

Regardless of the fact that sex work was illegal in China, in 1997, the CDC implemented programmes promoting condom usage to help limit HIV and other STIs among CSWs (Cui et al., 2009). Even so, figures for 1998 reveal that incidences of STIs had risen alongside numbers of people having multiple sexual partners. He and Detels (2005) state that between 1990 and 1998, the reported incidence of syphilis increased 20-fold while gonorrhoea increased three-fold. However, trials undertaken proved that the interventions were successful and the CDC ramped up the initiatives (Cui et al., 2009). This proved to be the case for interventions targeting PWID and, in 1999, NSPs were initiated in Yunnan and Guangxi Zhuang Autonomous Region (Cui et al., 2009). However, the previous lack of response by Beijing in dealing with the epidemic had taken its toll.

The HIV epidemic had taken hold in these marginalised populations and had begun to move at a rapid rate into other populations. Even though programming had begun, there was still a notable lack of effective HIV education and there was still not enough being done to prevent transmission or treat those who had already been identified as HIV+. Sentinel surveillance was still in its infancy and inadequate coverage resulted in insufficient data to truly grasp the extent of the growth of HIV in China. Moreover, there was still limited understanding concerning the percentages of infection in the different key populations. The response of Beijing to the growing epidemic was lagging behind that required to make any effective advances in halting the spread of the disease.

Rampant prevalence or everyone's disease: 2001–present

Phase four is marked by the implementation of the 'China HIV/AIDS Containment, Prevention and Control Action Plan' covering the period 2001–2005 (He & Detels, 2005) and continues to the present day. This policy paper highlighted effective strategies for dealing with HIV and included condom promotion, needle/syringe exchange and methadone maintenance for PWID (Wu et al., 2004). This phase marks Beijing's acknowledgement that the HIV/AIDS epidemic in China is everyone's problem. In 2002, the National Centre for AIDS implemented pilot methadone replacement and needle/syringe exchange programmes in areas with high proportions of PWID (He & Detels, 2005). Following this, in late December/January 2003, China began trials for antiretroviral therapy (ART) and prevention of mother to child transmission (MTCT) (Wu et al., 2007). However, things did not really improve for PLWHA until issues surrounding the severe acute respiratory syndrome (SARS) epidemic of 2003 brought China's health policies to the forefront.

The SARS epidemic not only focused world attention on China, it also forced the Chinese government to realise that HIV/AIDS could no longer be downplayed and that serious attention needed to be paid to the epidemic. The new administration, led by Hu Jintao, Premier Wen Jiabao and Vice Premier Wu Yi, accelerated the commitment to evidence-based HIV policies (Wu et al., 2007). Attitudes having changed, late in 2003, Premier Wen Jiabao became the first Premier of China to shake hands with AIDS patients in a bid to mitigate stigmatisation ('Handshake highlights fight against AIDS', 2003). That year also saw the implementation of China's 'Four Free and One Care' policy, which is still being enacted.

China has made some important advances in its HIV/AIDS programming since the early days. They have actively initiated programmes that follow GBP and created new programmes allowing for a scale-up of services (Wu et al., 2007). In addition to this, the Chinese government have recognised that economic considerations have to make room for social well-being and public health (Wu et al., 2007). Within key populations in Yunnan, and some other parts of China, the delayed reaction by Beijing in addressing the HIV/AIDS epidemic has resulted in a rampant prevalence, with high infection rate percentages in these populations. It remains to be seen whether China will continue to make ground in halting the epidemic or whether complacency and budget constraints will adversely affect the progress they have already made. Certainly, in Yunnan, HIV/AIDS remains a concern and, when measured against GBP, the initiatives presently in place are not adequate for the current epidemic burden.

The brief overview of the history of the HIV/AIDS epidemic in China reveals Beijing neglected to undertake the necessary steps to halt the spread of the disease in its early stages. There have been ongoing ramifications for that neglect. A prevailing arrogance as to the morality of the Chinese majority population as compared to the perceived lack of morality found in 'others' has also negatively contributed to the diffusion and rampant prevalence of HIV in key populations; and the relatively new, predominant spread of HIV through sexual contact. Beijing has shown itself to still be reluctant to disseminate data; issues of stigma and entrenched ideas that the disease is Western or exclusive to people of low moral status; and a continuing lack of adequate treatment and prevention programmes mean that HIV continues to spread in China.

Limitations of existing data

Gaining a comprehensive understanding of the situation for PLWHA in China can be difficult, due to limitations in available data. As mentioned previously, in order to undertake GBP, it is important to have a thorough understanding of the epidemic in order to create education, treatment and prevention programmes that will be efficient in the area of application. A programme that works well in one area may not be effective in another. China's main data gathering source for estimating numbers of PLWHA is sentinel surveillance in conjunction with a web-based case reporting system.

There are currently over 1,888 sentinel surveillance[2] sites in China, which, in theory, should give an adequate overview of the epidemic. However, there are significant shortfalls in the programme. Surveillance is limited to those who access public clinics and does not account for those accessing private clinics, the many people who are reluctant to be tested for HIV due to issues of stigma or the many undocumented migrants who do not access health services. In addition to these factors, there is also a tendency for local authorities to underestimate figures and a reluctance by Beijing to disseminate the data that it does obtain. Overall, this means that while it is evident that China is dealing with a burgeoning HIV/AIDS epidemic, exact figures cannot be counted on to provide a complete understanding of the situation.

Sentinel surveillance in China is not as effective as it might be for several reasons. First, China's decentralised and fragmented authoritarian political hierarchy means that there is a lack of transparency, accountability, information sharing and cooperation (Zhang, Chow, Zhang, Jing & Wilson, 2012). Currently, all HIV/AIDS surveillance is managed through a central office in China's Centre for Disease Control (CDC) and administered independently at provincial, municipal and county levels (Figure 5.2). This vertical administration of the CDC has

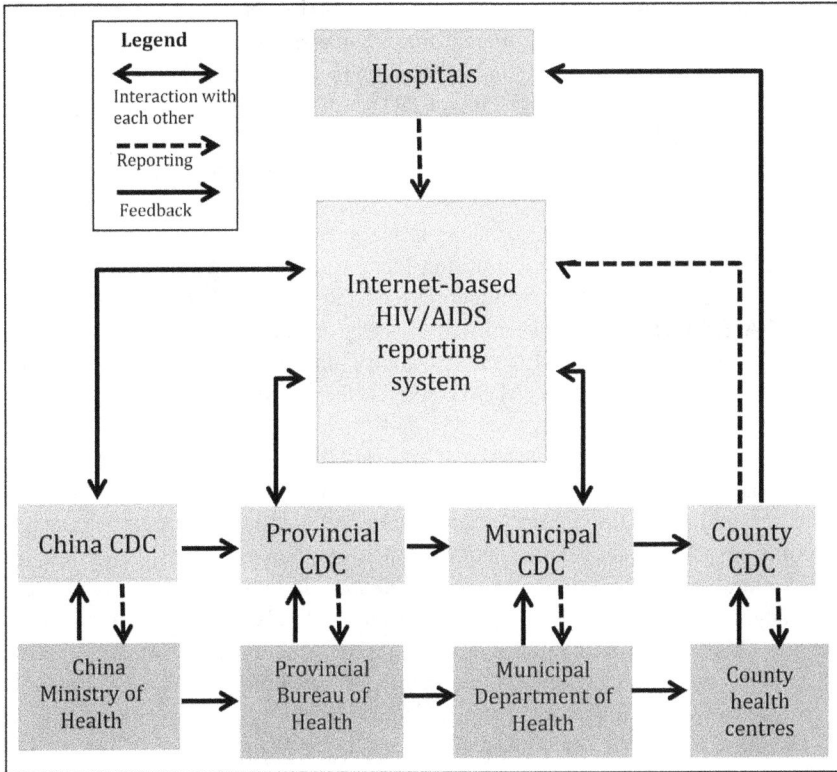

Figure 5.2 Schematic diagram of flow of information for HIV surveillance in China.

implications for research, and the creation and management of HIV pro-grammes. It may lead to backlogs of unanalysed HIV data, large data gaps and lack of quality control (Loo, Saidel, Reddy, Htin, Shwe & Verbruggen, 2012; Mao et al., 2010; Zhang et al., 2012). Significantly, there are few monitoring systems in place to ensure the accuracy of published or reported information (Zhang et al., 2012).

One of the more concerning outcomes of this hierarchy is results-driven policy implementation. Zhang et al. (2012) suggest:

> The absence of genuine engagement of civil society groups, including the media and the scientific communities, and the expectations and pressures from higher-level authorities, often results in a results-oriented policy imple-mentation, such that local officials tend to manipulate nonscientific and arbitrary results to satisfy their superiors perfunctorily.
>
> (p. 167)

Second, there is a shortage of trained personnel and lack of technological capacity and infrastructure, particularly in rural areas (Lin et al., 2012; Zhao et al., 2012). Finally, there is no requirement for public accountability and all decisions about the dissemination of data and openness concerning the HIV situation are at the sole discretion of the central China CDC (under the supervision and approval of the China Ministry of Health). This effectively means that Beijing can withhold information it deems too sensitive or alarming and propagate information that places their efforts in the best light.

While there are obvious challenges in the systems surrounding sentinel surveillance, they are not the only limiting factors in obtaining correct HIV/AIDS data in China. Mobility is a complicating factor in many of China's most at-risk-of-HIV/AIDS populations. In addition to the groups already mentioned (FSW, PWID and floating migrants), there is a high mobility factor for populations of men who have sex with men (MSM). As yet, there appear to be few consistent approaches to sampling highly mobile and hidden people groups who do not routinely access health care facilities (Loo et al., 2012). A research study by Loo et al. (2012) on HIV sentinel surveillance within mobile populations in the Asia Pacific region (including China) states: 'there are insufficient resources to apply rigorous approaches for representative, replicable samples in most countries' (p. 4). Essentially, it is difficult to know the situation in these groups with any real accuracy, as it is impossible to apply the same methods as used for non-mobile people. This is exacerbated in migrant populations due to China's *hukou* system, as many of the floating migrants are unable, or unwilling, to access health services due to their undocumented status (Tuñón, 2006).[3]

There are also difficulties in obtaining surveillance figures for PLWHA, due to a large number of people refusing to be tested. In PWID, FSW, MSM and the floating population, people may refuse to be tested for HIV due to the threat of police crackdowns and enforced incarceration if they are identified as belonging to a key population (Pirkle, Soundardjee & Stella, 2007). Additionally, these population cohorts may feel judged by the cultural bias towards Chinese Confucian philosophy and its stigmatisation of PWID, MSM and sex workers as morally impure members of the community (Ding, Li & Ji, 2011; Qian, Schumacher, Chen & Ruan, 2006; Yang & Kleinman, 2008). Stigmatisation is of particular concern when attempting to form effective policy or collect useable data, due to the fact that the illness is concealed from medical professionals (Dong et al., 2018).

Impacts of stigma in HIV settings in China

In China, the stigmatisation of PLWHA affects not only the individuals themselves but also becomes a shame endured by the entire family (Hong et al., 2008; Ma, Chan & Loke, 2019; Zhou, 2007). Unfortunately, in China there are still misconceptions about how HIV/AIDS is transmitted and this contributes to the discrimination and prejudice against PLWHA being still rampant within the general community (Qian et al., 2007; Yang & Kleinman, 2008; Zhang et al.,

2012). As a result, PLWHA become marginalised and more difficult to interact with, which has significant implications for HIV/AIDS programming and the spread of HIV in general. Without effective surveillance of key populations, there can be little improvement in services and understanding of the epidemiology, or actual HIV/AIDS prevalence in highly marginalised and mobile populations, such as MSM, FSW, PWID and floating migrants (Zhang et al., 2012).

In addition to discouraging PLWHA from accessing services, or often even ascertaining their HIV status, stigma disinclines them from disclosing their HIV+ status to sexual partners or family members (Chen, Choe, Chen & Zhang 2007; Ma et al., 2019). This is due not only to their own feelings of shame and inadequacy but also because they are concerned that their family members will suffer the same discrimination and stigma that they do. This is particularly the case when they have contacted HIV due to practices considered immoral, such as drug use, MSM and sex work (Li et al., 2008). Some literature refers to this as a double stigma, that of HIV and the 'immoral' behaviour, and it impacts both the individual and their family (Li, Wu, Wu, Jia, Lieber & Lu, 2008).

In Chinese society, this is a problem due to the cultural emphasis placed on morals and the family unit because of Chinese Confucianism. This has led to the discrimination of PLWHA, particularly in those groups that might be considered to be morally inferior. Drug use, along with gambling and prostitution, is recorded in official Chinese documents as: 'an ugly social phenomenon' [*Chou'e de shehui xianxiang*] (Tang & Hao, 2007). Interestingly, although these practices are considered to be morally reprehensible, they are also considered to be unofficial requirements within China's governmentality that help to sustain legitimacy and traditional male performance (Uretsky, 2015). This type of business entertaining (*yingchou*), including the solicitation of sex, forms a part of all successful political and economic negotiations (Uretsky, 2015). Even so, it is considered to be contrary to the cultural and moral values of Chinese society as espoused by Confucian philosophy, resulting in a yin/yang type of paradox (Faure & Fang, 2008). For example, Xi Jinping's anti-corruption campaign and the need to appear morally upright and uphold the party values has had the effect of creating juxtaposing discourses; the behaviours are still unofficially required but the evidence of them must be covered up, resulting in serious risks to the men involved in governing China (Uretsky, 2015).

In Chinese culture, treating people who are considered to be of low moral status in a disrespectful or discriminatory manner is considered an acceptable practice (Li, Wu, Wu, Sun, Cui & Jia, 2006). Zhou (2007) suggests: 'Discrimination toward PLWHA is not solely about HIV/AIDS as a disease, but always intersects with existing social prejudices (e.g., homophobia, sexism, racism, and xenophobia) that may have contributed to the social constructions of HIV/AIDS in a society' (p. 815). This is corroborated by societal attitudes towards PLWHA who contracted HIV through blood plasma donation and iatrogenic blood transfusions. These groups of PLWHA were considered innocent and so suffered far less stigmatisation than those who were considered immoral. However, it is interesting to note that this group of PLWHA were themselves discriminatory and stigmatised PLWHA who contracted the infection through other means (Zhou, 2007).

As mentioned, this stigmatisation results in PLWHA being very cautious about disclosing their HIV+ status. However, in a Chinese context, this is not always an option as there have been numerous incidences when medical professionals have disclosed patients' status without their permission (Li et al., 2008). In addition to creating problems within the family, this disclosure has led to loss of employment, isolation by other community members and withdrawal of the PLWHA from the community through feelings of shame (Burki, 2011; Yang & Kleinman, 2008; Zhou, 2007, 2009). In China, such unauthorised disclosure has been made illegal and as such it does not occur with the same frequency as in the past, but it does still occur (Burki, 2011; Zhou, 2007).

This is a particular concern for HIV+ pregnant women. In China, routine HIV testing is available for all pregnant women; and voluntary counselling, information on treatment options for themselves, and information concerning vertical transmission of the virus to their babies are available for those women who test HIV+. In general, women are presented with two options – terminating the pregnancy or receiving free clinical interventions to reduce the risk of spreading the disease to the baby (Liang, Meyers, Zeng & Gui, 2013). Unfortunately, there is some possibility that ongoing HIV/AIDS stigma among medical practitioners might induce them to allow their personal beliefs to influence their advice and willingness to care for patients (Cai, Moji, Honda, Wu & Zhang, 2007; Gill & Okie, 2007; Liang et al., 2013). Women who learn their HIV status during pregnancy are more likely to undergo and abortion due to fear and stigma (Liang et al., 2013). Overall they found that the rates of abortion for HIV+ women were higher than those of the general population.

Upon disclosure of their status, PLWHA are often treated as highly contagious and required to be separate in their living arrangements within a household, including having separate eating utensils, bedding and laundry arrangements (Qian et al., 2007; Zhou, 2007). They are cautious about interacting with people and carry internalised shame and profound feelings of hurt (Zhou, 2013). They become convinced that they deserve to have contracted this disease due to their bad or immoral behaviour and therefore deserve to be treated discriminatorily (Zhou, 2007).

In China, this moralising discourse concerning HIV/AIDS has been exacerbated by media portrayals of PLWHA (Hong et al., 2008; Hood, 2005). Although this situation has changed somewhat over time, the portrayal of PLWHA as being a danger and immoral has increased attitudes of stigma and done little to advance HIV education and prevention efforts within the general community. The public stigmatisation of PLWHA has also led to misconceptions regarding methods of contracting HIV, with many people believing they are safe and that only those participating in unsafe behaviour are susceptible (Burki, 2011; Hong et al., 2008).

While Beijing has implemented policies to stop the stigmatisation of PLWHA, there are still significant challenges to be overcome. Community attitudes concerning the moral standing of key populations are entrenched within the cultural consciousness and fear and lack of education on HIV/AIDS still contribute to stigmatising behaviours. In general, PLWHA still suffer stigmatisation and marginalisation, which is impacting on their willingness to be forthcoming about their HIV+ status or to be tested for fear of a positive result. The consequence is that many individuals are not being identified as PLWHA; they are also not receiving the care and education that they need to manage their infections. Therefore, the lack of human security and failure to identify and alleviate the wants and fears inherent in situations of stigma are having detrimental effects on current efforts to confront the HIV/AIDS epidemics.

For PLWHA, issues of stigma and discrimination in combination with cultural sensitivities, marginalisation and high mobility (both across international and provincial borders) create an environment where receiving adequate and appropriate health care becomes problematic. This is important because not only does it directly impact upon the human security of the individual, it also has far-reaching security implications for China. This is a non-traditional security threat that not only impacts PLWHA but also has the potential to weaken China's military forces (through high rates of infection); generate a significant financial burden for the state, due to increasing medical expenses; and, finally, result in a greater divide between the educated and un-educated as a result of children being unable to attend school. Finally, without effectively addressing the needs of PLWHA, the epidemic will continue to spread.

Additionally, the loss of income, resulting in decreased gross domestic product (GDP) due to unemployment, the breakdown in societal structures and the financial burden of increasing numbers of PLWHA, will weaken the security and financial health of the nation-state. There are challenges inherent in affecting populations that are marginalised and essentially closed off from the general population. In attempting to understand how some of those ongoing challenges affect current HIV/AIDS prevention programmes, it is important to consider the successes and shortfalls in current treatment and prevention efforts being implemented in China.

Shortfalls and challenges of current treatment and prevention efforts

Although China has increased its attempts to deal with HIV in the last ten years, there are still significant gaps in population coverage and resources. China relies on HIV sentinel surveillance sites, concentrating mainly on key populations. These were implemented in 1986 and by 2009 there were 1,029 sites throughout the country, with the greatest number in Yunnan (Pirkle et al., 2007; Qin et al., 2005). This increased to 1,888 sites in 2010 (Lin et al., 2012). Unfortunately, China was slow to deal with the emerging HIV epidemic when it was first reported in PWID in Ruili in Yunnan, and it was not until after an outbreak among plasma donors in Henan Province, and the SARS outbreak, that Beijing began serious efforts to deal with the growing epidemic. The SARS outbreak not only highlighted deficiencies in China's public health care system it also highlighted the need for concerted political will and improved resources for dealing with health emergencies in China (Liu & Kaufman, 2006).

Sustained political will is particularly important in China's decentralised fiscal health care system and must encompass both central and local government political commitment (Liu & Kaufman, 2006). In 2013, China became a middle-income country,[4] according to world classifications, and thus became ineligible to continue to receive funding from INGOs such as AusAID and the Global Fund to Fight AIDS, Tuberculosis and Malaria. The Global Fund has a threshold of $2,000 gross national income per capita, after which funding is substantially reduced in order to encourage governments to take responsibility for the health and well-being of their own populations (Stuart, Lief, Donald, Wilson & Wilson, 2015). In June 2014, the Global Fund stopped its funding support for HIV/AIDS programmes in China, resulting in China establishing the 'Fund for Social Organizations Participating in HIV/AIDS Prevention and Control' (Wang et al., 2016).

Since the withdrawal of funding, China now bears 80 per cent of the cost of its HIV/AIDS programmes and seems to be genuinely making every effort to address the expansion of HIV (Zhao, Poundstone, Montaner & Wu, 2012). In addition to the 'Four Free and One Care' programme, Beijing is also actively involved in providing methadone maintenance programmes and harm reduction programmes, including needle exchange programmes (NEP) for PWID. They have also provided HIV education, counselling and testing, and condom and lubricant distribution among MSM. However, there are still ongoing shortfalls in the policies that Beijing has implemented and effective coverage requires them to exceed the current parameters to meet the challenges identified.

Therefore, while there have been various attempts to improve the current HIV health sector, there is an ongoing deficiency both in political will and resources in HIV/AIDS healthcare policies. Hood (2012) suggests, 'Many of China's HIV positive, and those who lobby for them, negotiate and navigate the condition of being left behind economically, socially and medically' (p. 132). Globally, HIV/AIDS intervention programmes must be targeted at the local situation and populations of concern (Meyer-Rath et al., 2018). Chu and Liu (2011) state: 'The classic treatment of AIDS is highly active antiretroviral therapy, but most people living with HIV/AIDS – especially those in developing countries – have little or no access to the treatment because of the high cost of the therapy' (p. 67). In China, as a still developing country, low annual incomes and limited disposable income after expenses (Table 5.1) mean that in the HIV scenario, user fees and out-of-pocket expenses are quite often prohibitive. This is due to the fact that the free ART package does not cover formal fees, diagnostics (such as regular liver functions tests for those on ART), or informal fees such as travel expenses and accommodation when travelling to and from clinics (Li et al., 2009; Yu, Souteyrand, Banda, Kaufman & Perriëns, 2008; Zhou et al., 2011). For some PLWHA, the cost of annual ART medical fees is almost equivalent to heir annual income (Moon et al., 2008). With a daily disposable income (after expenditures) of 33.19 yuan for

Table 5.1 Average Chinese per capita income for 2017

	Urban	Rural
Per capita disposable income (CNY/yuan)	36,396.19	13,432.43
Average monthly income	3,033.01	1,119.36
Average daily Income	101.10	37.31
US$ per day equivalent	14.99	5.53
(Exchange rate US$1 = 6.74 CNY on 5 January 2019)		
Per capita annual expenditures (yuan)	24,444.95	10,954.53
Total annual income remaining after expenditure (yuan)	11,951.24	2,477.90
Average monthly remaining	995.93	206.49
Average daily remaining	33.19	6.88
US$ per day equivalent	4.92	1.02

Source: income/expenditure figures: National Bureau of Statistics China: Retrieved 5/01/2019 from http://data.stats.gov.cn/english/easyquery.htm?cn=C01.

urban dwellers and 6.88 yuan for rural dwellers, there is little remaining to cover the cost of the additional tests, travel and accommodation.

This is particularly relevant considering the limited public health infrastructure in rural areas (necessitating travel to urban centres for medical assistance at government-run clinics) where more than 80 per cent of all PLWHA are residents (Gill, 2006; Yip, 2006). Additionally, compared to other households, PLWHA households have been found to have significantly lower incomes (Zhang et al., 2012). A further complication for PLWHA lies in China's 'massive restructuring of its social systems into profit-making institutions and its subsequent attempt at health system reform (*yigai*) have made healthcare a luxury many can no longer afford' (Hood, 2011, p. 10). Therefore, in reflecting upon the narrow window of opportunity to mitigate the spread of HIV in China, strategies need to be implemented to ensure that HIV health care is accessible to everyone (Yip, 2006).

However, presently, and increasingly, this is not the case even with the 'Four Free and One Care' policy in place. Naiqun (2006) suggests that the spread of HIV/AIDS in China 'implies specific political-economic inequalities and socio-cultural institutions' (p. 194). Hyde (2007) suggests, '[D]iseases map onto certain places and people more readily than onto others and … HIV/AIDS becomes embedded in political and economic relations, embodied practices, and cultural imaginations' (p. 2). In China, HIV cases have been reported in every province but the vast majority (over 80 per cent) of the HIV epidemic is located in six prefectures; with Yunnan reporting the highest rates of infection (Jia et al., 2010; UNAIDS 2011). In addition, many of the PLWHA in these provinces live in rural areas and are members of key population groups.

FSWs, PWID and floating migrants are by no means the only significant contributors to China's HIV/AIDS epidemic. China is also attempting to manage HIV/AIDS outbreaks in FPD, MSM, MTCT groups and in the general population not belonging to any of the specific groups mentioned. Although the epidemic first began in PWID populations, it is now primarily driven through sexual contact. As such, the role of the CSW and MSM populations has increased in importance. This does not diminish the need for continued research and programming for PWID and other migrant populations. It does mean, however, that the HIV situation in Yunnan is still of high importance. This is still the province with the highest numbers of HIV+ in key populations, such as PWID, migrant and ethnic populations and FSWs, and Yunnan still has the highest percentage rates of PLWHA.

HIV/AIDS in Yunnan

As mentioned, Yunnan is the province with the highest rates of HIV infection in China. The location of Yunnan near the drug production area of the Golden Triangle makes southern Yunnan particularly important, not only in China's HIV/AIDS epidemic and how it is responding to it, but also regionally in the countries that make up the Golden Triangle, namely, Myanmar, Thailand, Cambodia and Laos. There are significant security challenges in dealing with issues crossing national borders. Particularly considering the vast distances encountered along the China-Myanmar boundary line at 2,185 km, and the overall border including Myanmar, Laos and Vietnam at 4,060 km (HIV/AIDS Asia Regional Program (HAARP), 2012). The transmission of HIV in Yunnan is increasing and the epidemic has spread not only across national borders but also from China's rural border areas to urban areas. It has also increasingly spread from the marginalised, rural ethnic minorities to the urbanised Han majority (Xiao, Kristensen, Sun, Lu & Vermund, 2007).

Programmes dealing with HIV in border cities require complex solutions to issues such as:

- a highly mobile migrant population;
- extensive poverty;
- difficult geographical obstacles;
- an extensive trade system both cross-border and internally.

Due to these challenging environments, traditional health care approaches targeting specific groups through a formal system, although seemingly practical, have been found to be ineffective (Du Guerny, Hsu & Hong, 2003). Collaboration between nation-states does not always produce effective resolutions as threats to national security and apportioning accountability (and ultimately financial responsibility) for issues that evolve often result in stalemates and lack of action (Chen, pers. comm., December 2013).

Population mobility impacts upon the spread of HIV/AIDS. Population movement is complex and raises issues concerning not only the populations who are mobile, but also their interactions on the stable populations through which they pass and with whom they interact. Skeldon (2000), for example, describes the problematic nature of accounting for population movement and suggests: '[It is] not often a simple movement from an origin to a destination but a complex system of multiple movements which are extremely difficult and time-consuming to map out' (p. 2). Thus, the difficulty of researching population movement has implications for the research of mobility in the spread of HIV/AIDS in Yunnan.

Often people who cross borders are undocumented and, therefore, there is no information on their health status and it is difficult to obtain accurate numbers of people moving (Beyrer, Razak, Lisam, Chen, Lui & Yu, 2000). Ruxrungtham et al. (2004) discuss the problem of obtaining accurate figures when dealing with the issue of HIV/AIDS and the state:

> Unfortunately, despite the high rankings generally accorded Asian surveil-
> lance systems, significant gaps in coverage of key populations and quality
> problems remain, and few Asian countries have translated these data into
> effective prevention programmes, as can be seen by the continuing growth
> of epidemics throughout the region.
>
> (p. 75)

Presently a large number of China's HIV/AIDS sentinel surveillance sites are located in Yunnan and, thus, there is a great deal of knowledge about the epidemiology of HIV/AIDS in this region. Jia et al. (2010) suggest that Yunnan's HIV/AIDS situation can act as a useful case study for understanding the epidemiology of HIV in other regions and therefore can inform future intervention programmes. However, there are still gaps in research concerning the transmission of HIV throughout mobile, ethnic and cross-border populations.

Similar to the challenges of population movement for established health care approaches is that of cultural diversity. Yunnan's population is diverse, and in addition to the Han ethnic group, there are more than 25 minor ethnic groups accounting for more than one-third of the entire population (Xu et al., 2013). Before 1996, the majority of all HIV cases in the area were concentrated in minority populations. While this situation has changed, pockets of high-risk minority groups still demonstrate increased incidence rates. Ethnic minorities are likely to be poor, less educated, unemployed and marginalised, which leads them into risk-taking behaviour (Hammett et al., 2006). Therefore, it is essential that HIV/AIDS treatment and prevention programmes consider the challenges faced in these populations and address current shortfalls in HIV education programming and accessibility.

Drug use among rural minorities is also disproportionately high due to their proximity to the Golden Triangle (Xiao et al., 2007). In addition, they are more likely to live in rural areas with limited access to health care and remote from many of the more established HIV/AIDS programmes (Du Guerny et al., 2003; Saich, 2006; UNAIDS China, 2011). The geographical location of the rural farmlands means that many of the rural minorities overlap international borders and cross-border (international) marriage is common as is cross-border trade (HAARP, 2012).

In Yunnan, the highest percentages of HIV/AIDS cases overall are now in the Han ethnicity. This is due to the spread of HIV from rural minority areas into the urban areas, such as Kunming, where there are higher numbers of individuals in this Han majority population. Modes of transmission for the Han majority encompass many of those encountered by minority populations. In rural areas, PWID are more likely to be male minority residents whereas in urban environments the highest percentage of PWID are Han Chinese, with females thought to be between one-third and almost one-half of all PWID (McCoy, McCoy, Shenghan, Zhinuan, Xue-ren & Jie, 2001; Xiao et al., 2007). This is particularly significant when recognising that high numbers of PWID are believed to provide sex in exchange for drugs or money (Li, He, Wang & Williams, 2009). Additionally, in Yunnan, it is estimated that 70 per cent of FSWs are poorly educated Han Chinese (Xiao et al., 2007). While injection drug use is still a driver, sexual interaction is now the main transmission mode for HIV among the Han population. However, drug use often plays a role in high-risk sexual behaviours.

Currently there are a number of government organisations, NGOs and local CBOs working in Yunnan. The HIV/AIDS Asia Regional Program (HAARP), which ended in November 2013, was an AusAid collaboration with the Yunnan CDC and various local NGOs and CBOs, along the Yunnan/Myanmar border areas. A particular concern for this programme is providing PWID harm reduction both to users and their extended networks (partners, wives, girlfriends). They suggest that some of the most difficult-to-reach populations implicated in the expansion of HIV comprise Chinese and foreign nationals crossing borders from Myanmar, Thailand and Vietnam. Key ethnic population groups in the transmission of HIV and other blood-borne infections include: Vietnamese fishermen, cross-border mobile construction workers, long-haul truck drivers traversing national boundaries, and FSWs, PWID and their partners passing between borders (HAARP, 2012).

Cross-border prevention and education programmes have shown they can be effective in accessing these populations. However, there are a number of inhibiting factors that reduce the efficacy of cross-border health initiatives between China and its neighbouring states. There are very few programmes actually running and those that are running vary in quality and impact (UNAIDS China, 2011). As well as these issues, many national programmes do not cover key populations from the ethnic minority populations in Yunnan's border and rural areas. This produces a gap in the dissemination of HIV/AIDS services and prevention education (UNAIDS China, 2011). There is also a lack of political commitment by Beijing to the improvement of health and development in the ethnic minority areas, due to complex historical contexts between the Han Chinese and ethnic minority groups (UNAIDS China, 2011). In the main, this is due to the Han Chinese belief in their pre-eminence as the culturally superior rulers of China. In general, the ethnic minorities are considered backward and uncivilised (Hansen, 1999). Regardless of ongoing difficulties, recently Beijing has been making some attempts to include cross-border PLWHA in their available HIV/AIDS initiatives.

However, even when services are available, there are issues for non-Chinese citizens attempting to access harm reduction facilities. At this time, only those with Chinese national identity cards can be admitted into existing HIV/AIDS programmes (HAARP, 2012; UNAIDS China, 2011). The cultural diversity and non-Chinese citizenship of many of those crossing borders, combined with the lack of adequate programme, challenging operational environments, and the reluctance of Beijing to finance programmes for these highly mobile groups create an environment that facilitates the spread of HIV. For example, this is particularly problematic when considering the significant number of Myanmar nationals, including students, at a number of universities in Kunming, who are newly identified as being HIV+ in Yunnan (UNAIDS China, 2011; Xu et al., 2013).

With millions of people crossing the border between Myanmar and Yunnan every year, this poses a significant security risk (as porous national borders are unable to regulate the flow of people or goods) for the expansion of HIV within China and the border areas (UNAIDS China, 2011). Unfortunately, as noted earlier, Beijing is generally hesitant (or unable) to accept the burden of HIV prevention and education for non-citizens, even when there is some evidence to suggest prevention and treatment for Yunnan-based non-Chinese will benefit their own HIV/AIDS prevention efforts (UNAIDS China, 2011). Many of the non-Chinese based in Yunnan are sexually active in the region and, without adequate education and health care, they have a great potential for transmitting the disease within both their own ethnic groups and in the Han population. In Yunnan, as with the rest of China, HIV is currently being driven through sexual transmission. Of the 54,000 newly estimated cases in 2011, heterosexual transmission accounted for 42.2 per cent and homosexual transmission accounted for 32.5 per cent of cases (Wu et al., 2013).

Despite the increasing rates of infection, in the years since Beijing first began dealing with the HIV epidemic, important steps have been made to halt the expansion of the disease. This has mainly been done through the implementation of various education and prevention programmes and, in recent years, TasP. However, while in some areas Beijing has been actively running some programmes (including pilot programmes) that conform to GBP, there is room for improvement in outreach efforts to rural minorities, and within highly mobile Chinese and non-Chinese populations. This is particularly the case in rural and international border areas where the NGO presence is limited.

Conclusion

In the initial stages of the epidemic, the Chinese government was disinclined to accept the possibility of HIV becoming a problem for Chinese citizens. Due to Confucian ideas of morality, a negative portrayal of the West and initial outbreaks being confined to foreign nationals, HIV was considered a 'Western' disease confined to foreigners and those of low moral standing. In the subsequent years, the Chinese government has attempted to address the ensuing stigma and misunderstandings of earlier years and many of the initiatives implemented by China have proven to be effective but are somewhat mitigated by the difficulties of the operational environment, lack of funding and existing punitive laws faced by key populations.

As shown, out-of-pocket treatment costs are prohibitive for most PLWHA. While there are some positive changes in the requirements for migrants to be able to access ART (although many migrants remain unaware of these changes), the financial burden of tests and counselling, travel to and from clinics, and ongoing need for stability and regular attendance at government-run hospitals and clinics do create issues for those needing to access therapy. Unless Beijing implements cost-cutting initiatives for these groups, issues concerning adherence to ART regimes and voluntary testing and treatment will be further complicated. This is particularly so given the epidemic has now become sexually driven due to unsafe sexual practices and therefore has the capability to make debilitating inroads into the general population.

These conflicting initiatives must be reconciled if any substantial progress is to be made in halting the HIV epidemic in these groups. Especially when considering that such practices drive these marginalised populations underground, making them even more difficult to access. The hidden nature of these groups means that current prevention and treatment programmes may not be as effective due to lack of substantial data informing decision-making processes. This is particularly the case in Yunnan where the highly porous international borders allow the cross-border transmission of HIV. Finally, it is essential for Beijing to adequately address issues of stigma and discrimination in high-risk, marginalised populations. The shame and fear that accompany attendance at medical treatment facilities, particularly those that are government-run, mean that many high-risk individuals refuse to be tested and, when tested, are reluctant to reveal their HIV+ status.

Case study 5.1 Ming-Hua's story

Ming-Hua's story is important, as it highlights the fact that human insecurity not only affects the vulnerable individual but also has direct impacts on family members. In circumstances of food insecurity, community insecurity and health insecurity, individuals are often forced to make decisions and undertake behaviours that can exacerbate HIV epidemics. In that moment, they are not concerned with the macro-level analysis of a situation or whether their behaviours may have a detrimental effect. In fact, most individuals that I met wanted to contribute positively and not harm others. They would love to be a part of the solution but they are unable to do so when they using all of their energy to simply live each day. Often they no longer think about the future. Ming-Hua had stopped worrying about the future for herself. The circumstances that she found herself in meant that she simply had to turn her attention to survival, not only for herself but also for her son. Although she had little expectation for herself, she hoped that she might be able to give him a future. This is her story.

I had been in China for some time when I met Ming-Hua. It was the coldest winter that Yunnan had seen in decades. With great excitement, I had joined many of the Kunming locals gathering on the streets to take photos and stare in wonder at the unusual sight of heavy snow falling in the city. While it seemed magical at the time, the results were less so and thousands of tourists were stranded at Kunming airport as it closed due to thick ice on the runways. Traffic on the roads between Lijiang and Dali had come to a standstill and almost 2,000 people had been trapped in their cars without food because rescue vehicles could not get through the mountain passes. A week later as I drove out of Kunming to the village where Ming-Hua lived, much of the snow had melted but it was still bitterly cold and I was bundled in a thick coat, gloves and had a warm hat jammed on my head.

I had already met a number of different PLWHA and heard quite a few stories about the struggles that people were encountering on a daily basis. I knew that circumstances could be dire for some people, while others seemed to be coping well and as I walked from the car to Ming-Hua's home, I was hopeful that she would be one of the luckier ones. I went to meet her with a friend of mine from Kunming and I was glad of the company as Ming-Hua lived in a run-down area of the town. After walking for some time, I had turned down a small street that was filled with potholes, ragged edges and no gutters. The directions that had been provided indicated that I needed to enter a small alleyway and I hesitated as I looked at the rough buildings that overshadowed the uneven path.

Nevertheless I pressed on, and the alleyway soon flowed into what seemed to be some kind of open courtyard that I had to cross before heading down another small alley. It seemed to me that Ming-Hua must live in some kind of community arrangement but after crossing the courtyard the conditions deteriorated. The sides of the small buildings either side of the path were littered with rubbish and small patches of black ice. As I approached the building she lived in, I had stepped over a dead rat decomposing in the open gutter and I had been glad of the cold as it was preventing it from smelling as it slowly rotted. The place where Ming-Hua's home was located was very dark even though the day had been bathed in sunshine; and to me it seemed quite oppressive.

Very little light penetrated the spaces between the water stained walls of the buildings pressing at it from all angles. They were made with brick, wood and concrete and seemed dilapidated and uncared for. Her place was not really a house but rather a small room that had a decaying wooden door and a small window near the corrugated roofline. It haphazardly joined one of the buildings but I learned later that Ming-Hua rented the room as a separate dwelling. As I knocked, the door opened and Ming-Hua came outside to greet us.

Ming-Hua was a very thin, petite woman with stringy, long black hair. She had an air of deep weariness that hung around her like a shadow. Her face was lined and she looked care-worn but I could still see a beauty that had not been completely eroded. She was bundled up against the cold and as we stood chatting, she would reach a thin arm up every now and then to tuck her hair behind her ears as the wind stirring between the buildings caught hold of it. We both had red noses and cheeks and found ourselves stamping on the ground periodically to warm our muscles. Eventually, we went inside and while I had hoped that we would find it warm and snug, the reality was far different. The air inside was only marginally warmer than the chilly conditions we had been enduring outside.

The room was just a bit larger than a walk-in wardrobe. The only furniture it contained was a double bed, which was shoved up in a corner of the room to make space for the buckets used for the toilet and water and the dozens of plastic tubs, baskets and boxes that filled the rest of the room. There seemed to be a big mound of grimy blankets and sweat-stained sheets piled up on the bed but as I looked closer the dark tousled head of a teenage boy emerged from the heap. Ming-Hua told us her son lived there with her and that he was still in bed at such a late hour because it was the only way that he could stay warm. They had electricity but they did not have the money to pay for heating. There were no kitchen or bathroom facilities. Ming-Hua kept her food and a few bowls and other crockery in a plastic tub. Another tub held a few food items and Ming-Hua reached into this to find something to offer us. There was nowhere for us to sit since the bed was occupied so we stood in the cluttered space and Ming-Hua told me her story.

She told me that she used to run a mobile noodle shop when her husband was still alive. The shop had operated from a small cart that Ming-Hua used to move from place to place in the town. They had not been wealthy but they had been doing ok. Even before her husband had died, things had begun to change. He had started to inject heroin and the money began to decrease. It had gotten worse when they found that he had contracted HIV. He had been sharing needles and one of those shared needles had delivered the virus into his blood. Once that had happened, no one would employ him any more and fewer and fewer people had come to the noodle shop. The situation had deteriorated further when Ming-Hua had contracted the disease from her husband. He had died soon after, leaving her to care for their son. Since Ming-Hua had been HIV+, she had not been able to sell noodles, instead she had been forced to sell sex.

She said people did not blame her for having HIV, as they knew that her husband had given it to her, but they were scared. She told me that people were afraid to buy her noodles as they thought they would get HIV from eating the noodles that she had touched. She said most people had never learned anything about how the disease worked and so they believed it was easy to catch. She hardly knew much about it herself, she told me. She had only learned a few things after she had found out that she had the disease. Ming-Hua did not use words like stigmatisation or discrimination, she just knew that people who had been her friends and neighbours were now too afraid to be around her or eat a meal with her, let alone buy her noodles.

Ming-Hua told me that she did not want to be a sex worker, but what choice did she have? Sometimes she had to bring clients back to her home and when that happened she had to make her son wait outside until she was done. She hated having to do this, but she had to take care of him and this was the only way that she could make money. She worried that she could not make much as she could only have clients who did not know, or did not care, that she was HIV+. 'We make enough to survive,' she told me. She had dreams to try and open another noodle shop and thought that if she could just get enough money together, then maybe she could give it a chance. Perhaps people who did not know about her status would buy from her or perhaps people would come to understand more about how the disease was transmitted and be less afraid. 'I was very good at selling noodles,' she said wistfully. 'People used to like them very much.'

Ming-Hua's story highlights some of the challenges that have been discussed in this chapter. China's HIV/AIDS epidemics have changed from being driven through high-risk drug injection practices to being sexually driven. The overview of the history of HIV/AIDS in China reveals the delayed responses in term of public policy to combat the spread of the disease, but also the lack of education that resulted from this delay. When it was thought that only immoral individuals and westerners were susceptible, it was less concerning; the revelation that anyone could get it caused panic and extreme stigmatisation of those infected. While that has changed dramatically in the last number of years, the wheels of belief and understanding turn slowly. Stigmatisation is still a major problem for PLWHA. The resulting human insecurity, food insecurity, health insecurity, and economic insecurity exacerbate this as people like Ming-Hua appear to have no other options but to sell sex for survival, due to a lack of a social security safety net, which further increases her human insecurity.

Notes

1 Scholars such as Huang (2006) and Zhang and Ma (2002) suggest three stages, as they combine significant events into an overarching final time period, but in doing so they detract somewhat from the significance of Beijing's actions of the time.
2 This type of surveillance annually measures the HIV seroprevalence of selected at-risk populations. Data are sourced from selected sites/locations that are repeated in subsequent rounds. Some of the sampling may include sequential sampling among facility-based populations, convenience sampling in community settings and cluster sampling or respondent-driven sampling (Loo et al., 2012).
3 For populations identified as HIV+, this is no longer the case. They are able to access services in any province. However, the caveat is that they must first be officially identified as being HIV+.
4 A middle-income country is a nation with a per capita income (as of 2012) of between $1,036 and $12,615. See www.worldbank.org/en/country/mic/overview

References

Beyrer, C., Razak, M. H., Lisam, K., Chen, J., Lui, W. & Yu, X. F. (2000). Overland heroin trafficking routes and HIV-1 spread in south and south-east Asia. *AIDS, 14*(1), 75–83.
Browning, M. (1987). U.S. freedoms would open China to AIDS, other ills, paper warns. *Philadelphia Inquirer* [Philadelphia, PA]. 5 February 1987, A.22.
Burki, T. K. (2011). Discrimination against people with HIV persists in China. *The Lancet, 377*(9762), 286–287.
Cai, G., Moji, K., Honda, S., Wu, X. & Zhang, K. (2007). Inequality and unwillingness to care for people living with HIV/AIDS: A survey of medical professionals in southeast China. *AIDS Patient Care & STDs, 21*(8), 593–601. doi:10.1089/apc.2006.0162.
Chen, J., Choe, M. K., Chen, S. & Zhang, S. (2007). The effects of individual- and community-level knowledge, beliefs, and fear on stigmatization of people living with HIV/AIDS in China. *AIDS Care, 19*(5), 666–673. doi:10.1080/09540120600988517.
Chu, Y. & Liu, H. (2011). Advances of research on anti-HIV agents from traditional Chinese herbs. *Advances in Dental Research, 23*(1), 67–75.
Cui, Y., Liau, A. & Wu, Z. (2009). An overview of the history of epidemic of and response to HIV/AIDS in China: Achievements and challenges. *Chinese Medical Journal (English Edition), 122*(19), 2251–2257.
Dikötter, F. (2000). Racial discourse in China: continuities and permutations. In J. Hutchinson & A. D. Smith (Eds.), *Nationalism: Critical concepts in political science*, vol. 3. London, UK: Routledge.

Ding, Y., Li, L. & Ji, G. (2011). HIV disclosure in rural China: Predictors and relationship to access to care. *AIDS Care, 23*(9), 1059–1066. doi:10.1080/09540121.2011.554524.

Dong, X., Yang, J., Peng, L., Pang, M., Zhang, J., Zhang, Z., … & Chen, X. (2018). HIV-related stigma and discrimination amongst healthcare providers in Guangzhou, China. *BMC Public Health, 18*(1), 738.

Du Guerny, J., Hsu, L. N. & Hong, C. (2003). Population movement and HIV/AIDS: The case of Ruili, Yunnan, China. UNDP South East Asia HIV and Development Programme. Retrieved from www.hivdevelopment.org/Publications_english/The%20 case%20of%20Ruili.htm

Faure, G. O. & Fang, T. (2008). Changing Chinese values: Keeping up with paradoxes. *International Business Review, 17*(2), 194–207.

Gill, B. (2006). China's health care and pension challenges. Testimony before the US-China Security and Economic Review Commission hearing on major internal challenges facing the Chinese Leadership, February 2, Washington, DC. Retrieved from www.uscc.gov/hearings/2006hearings/written_testimonies/06_02_02_bates.pdf

Gill, B. & Okie, S. (2007). China and HIV: A window of opportunity. *The New England Journal of Medicine, 356*(18), 1801–1805. doi:10.1056/NEJMp078010.

HAARP (HIV/AIDS Asia Regional Program). (2012). *Yunnan Cross Border Transition Project. Annual progress report 2011.7–2012*. AusAid, 64–22.

Hammett, T. M., Kling, R., Johnston, P., Liu, W., Ngu, D., Friedmann, P., … & Des Jarlais, D. C. (2006). Patterns of HIV prevalence and HIV risk behaviors among injection drug users prior to and 24 months following implementation of cross-border HIV prevention interventions in northern Vietnam and southern China. *AIDS Education & Prevention, 18*(2), 97–115.

Hansen, M. H. (1999). The call of Mao or money? Han Chinese settlers on China's south-western borders. *The China Quarterly, 158*, 394–413.

Hayes, A. (2005). AIDS, bloodheads & cover-ups: The 'ABC' of Henan's AIDS epidemic. *AQ: Australian Quarterly, 77*(3), 12–40.

He, N. & Detels, R. (2005). The HIV epidemic in China: History, response, and challenge. *Cell Research, 15*(11), 825–832.

Hong, Y., Li, X., Stanton, B., Fang, X., Lin, D., Wang, J., … & Yang, H. (2008). Expressions of HIV-related stigma among rural-to-urban migrants in China. *AIDS Patient Care & STDs, 22*(10), 823–831. doi:10.1089/apc.2008.0001.

Hood, J. (2005). *Narrating HIV/AIDS in the PRC media: Imagined immunity, distracting others, and the configuration of race, place and disease*. Canberra, Australia: Australian National University.

Hood, J. (2011). *HIV/AIDS, health and the media in China*. London, UK: Routledge.

Hood, J. (2012). HIV/AIDS and shifting urban China's socio-moral landscape: Engendering bio-activism and resistance through stories of suffering. *IJAPS, 8*(1), 125–144.

Hyde, S. T. (2000). Selling sex and sidestepping the state: Prostitutes, condoms, and HIV/AIDS prevention in Southwest China. *East Asia, 18*(4), 108–136.

Hyde, S. T. (2007). *Eating spring rice: The cultural politics of AIDS in Southwest China*. Berkeley, CA: University of California Press.

Huang, Y. (2006). The politics of HIV/AIDS in China. *Asian Perspective, 30*(1), 95–125.

Jia, M., Luo, H., Ma, Y., Wang, N., Smith, K., Mei, J., … & Zhang, Q. (2010). The HIV epidemic in Yunnan Province, China, 1989–2007. *JAIDS: Journal of Acquired Immune Deficiency Syndromes, 53*, S34.

Knutsen, W. L. U. (2012). An institutional account of China's HIV/AIDS policy process from 1985 to 2010. *Politics & Policy, 40*(1), 161–192.

Li, L., Wu, Z., Wu, S., Jia, M., Lieber, E. & Lu, Y. (2008). Impacts of HIV/AIDS stigma on family identity and interactions in China. *Families, Systems & Health, 26*(4), 431.

Li, L., Wu, S., Wu, Z., Sun, S., Cui, H. & Jia, M. (2006). Understanding family support for people living with HIV/AIDS in Yunnan, China. *AIDS and Behavior, 10*(5), 509–517. doi:10.1007/s10461-006-9071-0.

Li, X., He, G., Wang, H. & Williams, A. B. (2009). Consequences of drug abuse and HIV/AIDS in China: Recommendations for integrated care of HIV-infected drug users. *AIDS Patient Care & STDs, 23*(10), 877–884. doi:10.1089/apc.2009.0015.

Liang, K., Meyers, K., Zeng, W. & Gui, X. (2013). Predictors of elective pregnancy termination among women diagnosed with HIV during pregnancy in two regions of China, 2004–2010. *BJOG: An International Journal of Obstetrics & Gynaecology, 120*(10), 1207–1214.

Lin, W., Chen, S., Seguy, N., Chen, Z., Sabin, K., Calleja, J. G. & Bulterys, M. (2012). Is the HIV sentinel surveillance system adequate in China? Findings from an evaluation of the national HIV sentinel surveillance system. *Western Pacific Surveillance and Response Journal, 3*(4), 76–85.

Liu, Y. & Kaufman, J. (2006). Controlling HIV/AIDS in China: Health system challenges. In J. Kaufman, A. Kleinman & T. Saich (Eds.), *AIDS and social policy in China* (pp. 75–95). Cambridge, MA: Harvard University Asia Center.

Loo, V., Saidel, T., Reddy, A., Htin, K. C. W., Shwe, Y. Y. & Verbruggen, B. (2012). HIV surveillance systems in the Asia Pacific region. *Western Pacific Surveillance and Response, 3*(3).

Ma, P. H., Chan, Z. C. & Loke, A. Y. (2019). Self-stigma reduction interventions for people living with HIV/AIDS and their families: A systematic review. *AIDS and Behavior, 23*(3), 707–741.

Macartney, J. (1987). Chinese authorities ban sex with foreigners to stop AIDS. Beijing: United Press International. Retrieved from www.upi.com/Archives/1987/09/29/Chinese-authorities-ban-sex-with-foreigners-to-stop-AIDS/2564559886400/

Mao, Y., Wu, Z., Poundstone, K., Wang, C., Qin, Q., Ma, Y. & Ma, W. (2010). Development of a unified web-based national HIV/AIDS information system in China. *International Journal of Epidemiology, 39*(suppl. 2), ii79–ii89.

McCoy, C. B., McCoy, H. V., Shenghan, L., Zhinuan, Y., Xue-ren, W. & Jie, M. (2001). Reawakening the dragon: Changing patterns of opiate use in Asia, with particular emphasis on China's Yunnan Province. *Substance Abuse & Misuse, 36*(1 & 2), 49–69.

Meyer-Rath, G., McGillen, J. B., Cuadros, D. F., Hallett, T. B., Bhatt, S., Wabiri, N., … & Rehle, T. (2018). Targeting the right interventions to the right people and places: The role of geospatial analysis in HIV program planning. *AIDS (London, England), 32*(8), 957.

Moon, S., Van Leemput, L., Durier, N., Jambert, E., Dahmane, A., Jie, Y., … & Saranchuk, P. (2008). Out-of-pocket costs of AIDS care in China: Are free antiretroviral drugs enough? *AIDS Care, 20*(8), 984–994.

Naiqun, W. (2006). Flows of heroin, people, capital, imagination, and the spread of HIV in southwest China. In T. Oakes & L. Schein (Eds.), *Translocal China: Linkages, identities, and the reimagining of space* (pp. 193–212). New York, NY: Routledge.

Nutbeam, D., Padmadas, S. S., Maslovskaya, O. & Wu, Z. (2015). A health promotion logic model to review progress in HIV prevention in China. *Health Promotion International, 30*(2), 270–280.

Pirkle, C., Soundardjee, R. & Stella, A. (2007). Female sex workers in China: Vectors of disease? *Sexually Transmitted Diseases, 34*(9), 695–703.

Qian, H., Schumacher, J. E., Chen, H. T. & Ruan, Y. H. (2006). Injection drug use and HIV/AIDS in China: Review of current situation, prevention and policy implications. *Harm Reduction Journal, 3*(1), 4. doi:10.1186/1477-7517-3-4.

Qian, H., Wang, N., Dong, S., Chen, H., Zhang, Y., Chamot, E., ... & Shao, Y. (2007). Association of misconceptions about HIV transmission and discriminatory attitudes in rural China. *AIDS Care, 19*(10), 1283–1287. doi:10.1080/09540120701402814.

Qin, L., Yoda, T., Suzuki, C., Yamamoto, T., Cai, G., Rakue, Y. & Mizota, T. (2005). Combating HIV/AIDS in mainland China: An epidemiological review of prevention and control measures. *Southeast Asian Journal of Tropical Medicine and Public Health, 36*(6), 1479–1486.

Ruxrungtham, K., Brown, T. & Phanuphak, P. (2004). HIV/AIDS in Asia. *The Lancet, 364*(9428), 69–82.

Saich, T. (2006). Social policy development in the era of economic reform. In J. Kaufman, A. Kleinman & T. Saich (Eds.), *AIDS and social policy in China* (pp. 15–46). Cambridge, MA: Harvard University Asia Center.

Settle, E. (2003). *AIDS in China: An annotated chronology 1985–2003*. Monterey, CA: China AIDS Survey.

Sheng, L. & Cao, W. K. (2008). HIV/AIDS epidemiology and prevention in China. *Chinese Medical Journal, 121*, 1230–1236.

Skeldon, R. (2000). *Population mobility and HIV vulnerability in South East Asia: An assessment and analysis*. Bangkok: UNDP South East Asia HIV and Development Project.

Stuart, R. M., Lief, E., Donald, B., Wilson, D. & Wilson, D. P. (2015). The funding landscape for HIV in Asia and the Pacific. *Journal of the International AIDS Society, 18*. https://doi.org/10.7448/IAS.18.1.20004.

Tang, Y. & Hao, W. (2007). Improving drug addiction treatment in China. *Addiction, 102*(7), 1057–1063. doi:10.1111/j.1360-0443.2007.01849.x.

Tuñón, M. (2006). Internal labour migration in China: Features and responses. Beijing, ILO, April 1–51. Retrieved from www.ilo.org/wcmsp5/groups/public/--asia/--ro-bangkok/--ilo-beijing/documents/publication/wcms_158634.pdf

UNAIDS. (2011). *HIV in Asia and the Pacific: Getting to zero*. UNAIDS. Retrieved from www.unaids.org/en/media/unaids/contentassets/documents/unaidspublication/2011/20110826_APGettingToZero_en.pdf

UNAIDS China. (2011). Background paper Cross-border programming to strengthen integrated HIV response in China. UNAIDS, July.

Uretsky, E. (2015) 'Sex' – it's not only women's work: A case for refocusing on the functional role that sex plays in work for both women and men, *Critical Public Health, 25*(1), 78–88, doi:10.1080/09581596.2014.883067.

Wang, D., Mei, G., Xu, X., Zhao, R., Ma, Y., Chen, R., ... & Hu, Z. (2016). Chinese non-governmental organizations involved in HIV/AIDS prevention and control: Intra-organizational social capital as a new analytical perspective. *BioScience Trends, 10*(5), 418–423.

Wu, J., Meng, Z., Xu, J., Lei, Y., Jin, L., Zhong, P., ... & Su, B. (2013). New emerging recombinant HIV-1 strains and close transmission linkage of HIV-1 strains in the Chinese MSM population indicate a new epidemic risk. *PLoS ONE, 8*(1), e54322. doi:10.1371/journal.pone.0054322.

Wu, Z., Rou, K. & Cui, H. (2004). The HIV/AIDS epidemic in China: History, current strategies and future challenges. *AIDS Education and Prevention, 16*(suppl. A), 7–17.

Wu, Z., Sullivan, S. G., Wang, Y., Rotheram-Borus, M. J. & Detels, R. (2007). Evolution of China's response to HIV/AIDS. *The Lancet, 369*(9562), 679–690.

Xiao, Y., Kristensen, S., Sun, J., Lu, L. & Vermund, S. H. (2007). Expansion of HIV/ AIDS in China: Lessons from Yunnan Province. *Social Science & Medicine, 64*(3), 665–675.

Xu, J., An, M., Han, X., Jia, M., Ma, Y., Zhang, M., ... & Geng, W. (2013). Prospective cohort study of HIV incidence and molecular characteristics of HIV among men who have sex with men (MSM) in Yunnan Province, China. *BMC Infectious Diseases, 13*(1), 1.

Yang, L. H. & Kleinman, A. (2008). 'Face' and the embodiment of stigma in China: The cases of schizophrenia and AIDS. *Social Science & Medicine, 67*(3), 398–408. doi:10.1016/j.socscimed.2008.03.011.

Yip, R. (2006). Opportunity for effective prevention of AIDS in China: the strategy of preventing secondary transmission of HIV. In J. Kaufman, A. Kleinman & T. Saich (Eds.), *AIDS and social policy in China* (pp. 96–124). Cambridge, MA: Harvard University Asia Center.

Yu, D., Souteyrand, Y., Banda, M. A., Kaufman, J. & Perriëns, J. H. (2008). Investment in HIV/AIDS programs: Does it help strengthen health systems in developing countries? *Globalization and Health, 4*(1), 8.

Yu, E. S., Xie, Q., Zhang, K., Lu, P. & Chan, L. L. (1996). HIV infection and AIDS in China, 1985 through 1994. *American Journal of Public Health, 86*(8), 1116–1122.

Zhang, K. L. & Ma, S. J. (2002). Epidemiology of HIV in China: Intravenous drug users, sex workers, and large mobile populations are high risk groups. *BMJ, 324*. Retrieved from https://doi.org/10.1136/bmj.324.7341.803.

Zhang, L., Chow, E. P. F., Zhang, J., Jing, J. & Wilson, D. P. (2012). Describing the Chinese HIV surveillance system and the influences of political structures and social stigma. *The Open AIDS Journal, 6*(suppl. 1), 163.

Zhao, Y., Poundstone, K. E., Montaner, J. & Wu, Z. (2012). New policies and strategies to tackle HIV/AIDS in China. *Chinese Medical Journal, 125*(7), 1331–1337.

Zhou, F., Kominski, G. F., Qian, H. Z., Wang, J., Duan, S., Guo, Z. & Zhao, X. (2011). Expenditures for the care of HIV-infected patients in rural areas in China's antiretroviral therapy programs. *BMC Medicine, 9*(6), 1–10. doi:10.1186/1741-7015-9-6.

Zhou, Y. R. (2007). "If you get AIDS... you have to endure it alone": Understanding the social constructions of HIV/AIDS in China. *Social Science & Medicine, 65*(2), 284–295. doi:10.1016/j.socscimed.2007.03.031.

Zhou, Y. R. (2009). Help-seeking in a context of AIDS stigma: Understanding the healthcare needs of people with HIV/AIDS in China. *Health & Social Care in the Community, 17*(2), 202–208. doi:10.1111/j.1365-2524.2008.00820.x.

Zhou, Y. R. (2013). Morality, discrimination, and silence: Understanding HIV stigma in the sociocultural context of China. In P. Liamputtong (Ed.), *Stigma, discrimination and living with HIV/AIDS* (pp. 117–132). Dordrecht, the Netherlands: Springer.

6   HIV/AIDS-affected populations

One justice can overpower a hundred evils.

正压百邪

Female sex workers (FSWs), people who inject drugs (PWID) and floating migrants, are by no means the only significant contributors to China's HIV/ AIDS epidemic. China is also attempting to manage HIV/AIDS outbreaks in former blood plasma donors (FPD), men who have sex with men (MSM), transgender (TG) sex workers, mother-to-child transmission (MTCT) and in the general population not belonging to any of the specific groups mentioned. They have significant impacts on the continuing transmission of HIV/AIDS in China and, along with FSW, PWID and migrants, are briefly considered in this chapter. Although the epidemic first began in PWID populations, it is now primarily driven through sexual contact. As such, the role of CSW and MSM populations has increased in importance. This does not diminish the need for continued research and programming for PWID and other migrant populations, who still act as primary drivers in the epidemic. These groups interact on several levels and all of them to differing degrees are engaged in sexual risk behaviours.

MSM populations

The situation for men who have sex with men (MSM) populations in China is nascent as one of the areas of greatest concern for the spread of HIV. Globally, there is a lack of reliable data on this key population and evidence suggests that HIV/AIDS programmes are lacking. UNAIDS reports:

> Where data exist on HIV in these populations, they show that our collective responses are failing far more often than they are reaching scale or succeed- ing. Just as disconcerting, in many parts of the world, is the fact that few reliable data exist at all.

(2009, p. 2)

China is one of those countries where very limited data exist at all. MSM are a hidden population and yet are thought to be significantly contributing to the spread of HIV/AIDS in China. In almost all provinces of China, these groups have increasingly high percentages of HIV infection.

The term MSM is an overall designation representing the different communities of men who have same sex intercourse, including bisexual, homosexual, transgender (TG) and predominantly heterosexual men. China's current MSM population is estimated to be between 5 and 10 million, with 47,000 of them estimated to be living with HIV/AIDS (Ma et al., 2012; Peng et al., 2012). Some researchers comment that unless the HIV epidemic in MSM populations is brought under control, China will become the global centre for MSM transmission (Ma et al., 2012). Not only have the percentages of people living with HIV (PLWHIV) significantly increased within this group over the course of China's HIV epidemic, there are also reports of new recombinant, more virulent, forms of the disease circulating within MSM populations.[1]

Research recommends that 60 per cent of at-risk MSM populations need to engage in safer behaviours to generate any significant impact on the spread of HIV/AIDS. To achieve that, programmes need to cover 80 per cent of the population (Commission on AIDS in Asia, 2008). China currently falls far short of this figure (Ma et al., 2012). MSM populations did not form a primary target for HIV prevention and education policy in China until 2004 (Ma et al., 2012). While Beijing has increased research and programmes to connect with this cohort, increased efforts are needed before a complete understanding of the situation emerges.

The MSM communities in China have been highly stigmatised and thus operate as a hidden community (Chen et al., 2012). This means that delivering HIV/AIDS treatment and prevention programmes within these communities is extremely challenging. This is even more so due to the migrant status of many MSM. Research has found that HIV and STI infection rates among migrant MSM are higher than those among non-migrant MSM (Guo, Li, Song & Liu, 2012). Additionally, many of these migrants are from rural areas and return to their hometowns for traditional Chinese holidays, potentially worsening the spread of HIV from urban to rural areas. This constant mobility, coupled with a reluctance to be identified as *homosexual*, makes it difficult to gain access to these vulnerable MSM populations (Chen et al., 2012; Jie, Ciyong, Xueqing, Hui & Lingyao, 2012).

This suggests that there is a combination of events or circumstances occurring among MSM cohorts, creating a worse situation than would transpire if each happened separately (UNAIDS, 2009). It might be labelled a *syndemic*, a term coined by medical anthropologist Merrill Singer, and it suggests that a collection of interacting social and psychosocial circumstances can lead to increased risks of HIV within a population (Jie et al., 2012). Research has also indicated that people infected with HIV who experience these types of psychosocial problems may have decreased CD4 T-lymphocytes, increased viral loads, a faster clinical decline and higher AIDS-related mortality (Jie et al., 2012).

In China, conditions for a syndemic occur in homosexual and bisexual MSM cohorts, as they are likely to encounter intimate partner violence, high-risk sexual behaviour and depression, which can lead to a higher risk of contracting HIV (Jie et al., 2012). These issues are compounded by alcohol and drug use among MSM populations with both recreational synthetic drugs (which may cause a two-fold increase in the chances of HIV transmission) such as 'poppers' (inhaled alkyl nitrites), and drugs such as heroin (Luo, Hong, Wang, McGoogan, Rou & Wu, 2018). This is exacerbated by events such as stigma and discrimination, leading to psychosocial circumstances, such as expectations of rejection, internalised homophobia, anxiety, depression and thoughts of suicide, which then interact with HIV to magnify its impact both on the individual and their family lives (Jie et al., 2012; Peng et al., 2012). In addition to the psychological pain, the discrimination encountered by MSM causes them to fear accessing prevention services or being tested for HIV. The main reasons for this were concerns for confidentiality, fear of people learning their sexual orientation and fear of test results being positive (Ma et al., 2012). This is particularly concerning because if they are in stage one or two of the HIV infection, they may incorrectly dismiss the symptoms and spread the disease to others. Overall, the combination of psychosocial issues and lack of knowledge concerning HIV status may lead to MSM cohorts engaging in high-risk sexual activities.

High-risk behaviour in MSM populations therefore specifically includes not being routinely tested for HIV, unprotected anal sex, multiple partners, group sex, commercial gay sex and sex with male strangers (Chen et al., 2012; Ma et al., 2012; Peng et al., 2012). Also condom usage levels still remain below acceptable prevention levels to be effective. Research findings suggest that only 39.2 per cent of MSM used condoms each time and only 62.5 per cent used condoms in their last same-sex encounter (Peng et al., 2012). MSM in high-risk groups mistakenly believe that male homosexual activity would not increase the likelihood for contracting HIV and that no venereal diseases could be contracted if the sexual organs looked normal (Chen et al., 2012). They also report that, within these high-risk MSMs, there was also a greater diversity in sexual behaviours and condom malfunction (such as slippage or breakage).

This becomes more troubling when considering that many of the MSM in China are involved in heterosexual relationships in addition to their homosexual encounters. Studies show that 44 per cent of all MSMs are either married or cohabitating with women (Peng et al., 2012). One of the main reasons why MSM cohorts engage in marriage and partner relationships with women is to hide their sexual preferences (Guo et al., 2012; Peng et al., 2012). Chinese culture disapproves of homosexuality and, as a result, MSM are highly stigmatised and suffer high levels of emotional and psychological stress.

In studies undertaken among MSM populations, it was found that some 50 per cent of those involved had suffered abuse or discrimination due to their sexual orientation (Chen et al., 2012). It was also found that 50 per cent of MSM do not use condoms with their spouses (Chen et al., 2012). As such, there is concern that MSM may act as bridging populations for the expansion of self-sustaining HIV epidemics within the general population. While MSM are a key population in China, it is very difficult to obtain data on their current situation due to the hidden nature of their activities and their reluctance to be identified as belonging to this cohort.

While the situation is changing, and more researchers are venturing into this area, certainly more research needs to be undertaken. However, this book does not focus on this group due to the decision to target PWID populations as the epicentre of the outbreak; FSWs due to sexual interaction as an emerging transmission route into the general population; and undocumented migrants as an under-researched cohort with the potential to exacerbate the spread of HIV/AIDS throughout China, due to their high mobility between urban areas and location of origin.

TG sex workers

The situation for transgender (TG) women in China is unclear, beyond being able to state that it is troublesome. They are referred to as ghost people (*ren yao*). This is because they are rarely seen in public. They are neither men nor women in the eyes of most people and inhabit a world somewhere between the two (Chen, pers. comm., November 2013). They are highly stigmatised and not accepted in society. Their very name in Chinese is an indication of how difficult they are to reach. Obtaining medical assistance is difficult due to discrimination and other legal barriers (such as needing to use male gendered birth identity when presenting for treatment) (UNAIDS, 2009). To fully understand the HIV/AIDS risks in TG populations, it is important not to simply look at the biological transmission routes but also their psycho-sexual and social determinants (Guadamuz et al., 2011). Clearly, they are particularly under-researched and little is known about their access to appropriate treatment or HIV/AIDS information but anecdotally it is considered to be inadequate.

Although TG sex workers face many of the same issues as MSM populations, and are generally included in the statistics for MSM, it is worth discussing them as a separate sub-group. They are often exposed to unique challenges associated with their activities as sex workers. Additionally, most TG women do not identify as male and therefore do not consider they are men engaging in sex with other men.[2] When incarcerated, TG women are processed as males and therefore exposed to brutality and forced sexual encounters on a level that MSM and most FSWs do not endure.[3] There is no legal recourse for them to be treated as women regardless of whether they have had gender reassignment surgery (Emerton, 2006).

Additionally, there appears to be limited HIV/AIDS information, or government will, targeted towards this key population. In order to address this situation, UNAIDS suggested that:

> Based on local epidemiological and social realities, enhanced responses must combine efforts focused specifically on men who have sex with men

and transgender people, attention to their needs in broader HIV responses, and bridge-building with broader efforts to achieve gender equality, promote human rights and protect public health.

(2009, p. 3)

Unlike MSM in general, TG people may have additional high-risk behaviours derived from inadequate availability of health services. The lack of availability of products routinely used for gender changes, such as liquid silicon for breast augmentation and hormones (which do not have government approval for the purposes of body augmentation) may result in their injection without medical supervision (Guadamuz et al., 2011). Apart from individuals using products that are not medically sound for the purpose, these back alley procedures result in high-risk behaviours, such as needle sharing and the potential for HIV, hepatitis B and C and other infectious diseases – in addition to injection drug use and sexual risk behaviours (Guadamuz et al., 2011).

Mother-To-Child-Transmission (MTCT)

MTCT transmission of HIV is an increasing problem in China. While percentage rates overall are low, especially when compared to other key populations, there is still a slowly expanding epidemic in this cohort. Transmission of HIV from mother to child occurs during pregnancy, labour, delivery or breastfeeding. Yunnan not only had the first outbreak of HIV in China, in 1995, it also reported the first outbreak of MTCT transmission of HIV in China (Chen & Qian, 2005). Since that time, transmission rates have continued to increase at a low percentage rate and of the 780,000 PLWHA in China, 1.1 per cent of those individuals were affected through MTCT (Qian, Vermund & Wang, 2005; UNAIDS and China's Ministry of Health (CMOH), 2012). However, prevalence rates differ significantly in different geographical regions (Liang, Meyers, Zeng & Gui, 2013). Regardless of MTCT transmission being a very low risk in China, there are some concerns that infection rates are on the increase. Moreover, Beijing has continued to scale up efforts to reach pregnant women with HIV prevention measures.

Beijing has been offering MTCT services for HIV+ pregnant women since implementing pilot programmes in 2002. In China, screening for HIV during pregnancy has become a routine health initiative. Women who are confirmed to be HIV+ are presented with options, including termination of their pregnancy or clinical interventions to reduce the risk of vertical transmission from mother to child (Liang et al., 2013). China is committed to following GBP in this area and currently offers counselling, the option of an abortion or antiretroviral therapy (for women with CD4 T-cell counts below 350) and other assistance during the pregnancy, including caesarean delivery when available (Liang et al., 2013; Wu, Sullivan, Wang, Rotheram-Borus & Detels, 2007).

In addition to these initiatives during pregnancy, they are also offered infant formula for 12 months to reduce the risks of transmission via breast milk

(Coovadia et al., 2007; Wu et al., 2007). In the latter half of 2010, Beijing implemented a new combination programme that combines HIV prevention with syphilis and hepatitis B prevention (UNAIDS & CMOH, 2012). By the end of 2011, the CMOH stated that these service programmes had achieved 100 per cent coverage in provinces with more serious epidemics[4] (including Yunnan) and 39 per cent nationwide (UNAIDS & CMOH, 2012). WHO suggests that, without these interventions, the transmission of HIV from mother to child would range from 15–45 per cent (WHO, 2014). With the interventions, the rate is reduced to levels below 5 per cent.

Beijing has facilitated, and thereby increased, the coverage of HIV+ pregnant women by integrating these programmes into routine mother and child health care networks (UNAIDS & CMOH, 2012). However, cases of MTCT have continued to increase. The CMOH (UNAIDS & CMOH, 2012) reported that in 2011 the number of reported cases of MTCT transmission in China had increased to 5,315 (an increase of 1,169) from 2010 figures of 4,146. Of significant note are the high rates of abortion among HIV+ pregnant women as these figures are not included in prevalence percentages. As such, it is highly probable that the actual rates of transmission may be higher than those reported (Liang et al., 2013).

The figures point to an increasing problem and with rates of 1.1 per cent of new HIV infections overall, there are indications that HIV has crossed into the general population in China. This is particularly problematic because MTCT rates of infections of 1 per cent or higher are used as a baseline indicator that the epidemic has progressed into the general population (Chen & Qian, 2005; UNAIDS, 2011a). In Dehong prefecture in Yunnan, the rate of HIV prevalence in pregnant women exceeded 1.3 per cent in 2003, suggesting that the prefecture has been undergoing a generalised epidemic for a number of years (Shan et al., 2014; Xiao, Kristensen, Sun, Lu & Vermund, 2007). Jia et al. (2010) state:

> Increasing prevalence among blood donors and pregnant women indicate HIV has begun to spread among the general low-risk population. HIV prevalence rates amongst these groups in Yunnan are above the national average and are increasing annually. In eight counties, prevalence rates reported by antenatal clinics already reached or passed 1%.
>
> (p. 39)

Therefore, although HIV/AIDS is still concentrated in high-risk groups, in some areas it has become generalised (Sun et al., 2010). MTCT transmission of HIV is also an important vector for the spread of the disease in China. Generally the other key populations are either implicated in the transmission of HIV to mothers or the mothers themselves belong to one of the key populations. Therefore, while they are recognised as an important indication of the expansion of HIV into a generalised epidemic and an increasing route for transmission in China this group. is not a main focus.

FPDs and blood transfusion recipients

Two significant groups of PLWHA are former plasma donors (FPDs) and iatrogenic blood transfusion recipients. Globally China is unique for the large numbers of FPDs who became infected through commercial plasma donation (Dou et al., 2010). This was largely due to the unregulated collection practices and the reinjection of pooled red blood cells (Dou et al., 2010; Hayes, 2005). Additionally, most infections occurred over a small timeframe in the early to mid-1990s. The cohort was rural, generally poor and generally engaged in high-risk practices, such as injection drug use or sex work. The infection became a self-sustaining epidemic after infected individuals passed on HIV to their spouses and children but virtually no new infections occurred after the population reached infection saturation point (Dou et al., 2010).

China does have a financial and HIV/AIDS percentage burden due to the large numbers of HIV+ FPD. Financial costs continue to increase as large numbers of HIV+ FPD are currently receiving ART. There is also the risk of HIV being spread through unprotected sex between serodiscordant couples (L. Wang et al., 2010). Serodiscordant couples are those where one person in the relationship is HIV+ and the other is HIV negative. Significantly, the seroconversion rate between these couples is showing an upward trend (L. Wang et al., 2010). Possible reasons for this increase include: the patients advancing to AIDS and higher viral loads, leading to increased transmission; riskier sexual behaviours (such as lack of condom use) and a decrease in knowledge and self-protection; and finally, a desire to have children, regardless of the risks (L. Wang et al., 2010). Overall, the research highlights the need to strengthen education and prevention services, condom promotion and counselling and support services.

While there have been few new cases of HIV infection through blood collection practices due to PRC regulations concerning blood donation, the unregulated practice of blood collection still exists to some extent (Reynolds & McKee, 2009). This has obvious implications for the renewed spread of HIV though these collection sites should these practices increase. There is very limited information concerning this area and their contribution to percentages of HIV infection. However, recently (reported in February 2019), China's second largest supplier of blood products was forced to recall 12,000 units due to fears of a HIV contamination after the discovery of HIV antibodies in its intravenous immunoglobin product (Needham, 2019). In addition to this, blood heads have changed their black market operations from purchasing blood to purchasing blood donor certificates. In China, in order to receive blood from state-run blood banks, it is necessary to supply the medical facility with a donor certificate (family members and friends are expected to donate blood). Blood heads now recruit individuals off the street to donate blood and sell their donor certificates; these are then sold to individuals needing blood and blood plasma transfusions (Harney, 2015).

While these new contaminations and blood head practices are concerning, overall within China new infections due to blood collection practices are very low (Qian, Vermund & Wang, 2005). Therefore, the main concern with this cohort of

PLWHA lies with the ongoing treatment of HIV+ individuals and the protection of serodiscordant partners and children. While this group is important to mention for its historical and ongoing contribution to issues surrounding HIV in China, they are no longer a main source of transmission. This cohort are generally geographically stable and do not currently pose a significant threat to the spread of HIV.

Marginalised and mobile populations

PWID, FSWs and floating migrants are highly mobile, generally engage in illegal activities and are highly stigmatised due to nature of their activities, resulting in a high risk for the spread of HIV in China in general and Yunnan Province specifically. Each cohort operates individually, and poses unique challenges for HIV prevention and education but tends to intersect with each other at some level, and all three groups can act as HIV conduits to the general population.

For example, FSWs might be both migrants and injecting drug users or a combination of all three; the clients of FSWs may be migrants and may or may not be injecting drug users; and injecting drug users may be migrants and may or may not be clients of FSWs (Figure 6.1). There are also other key populations

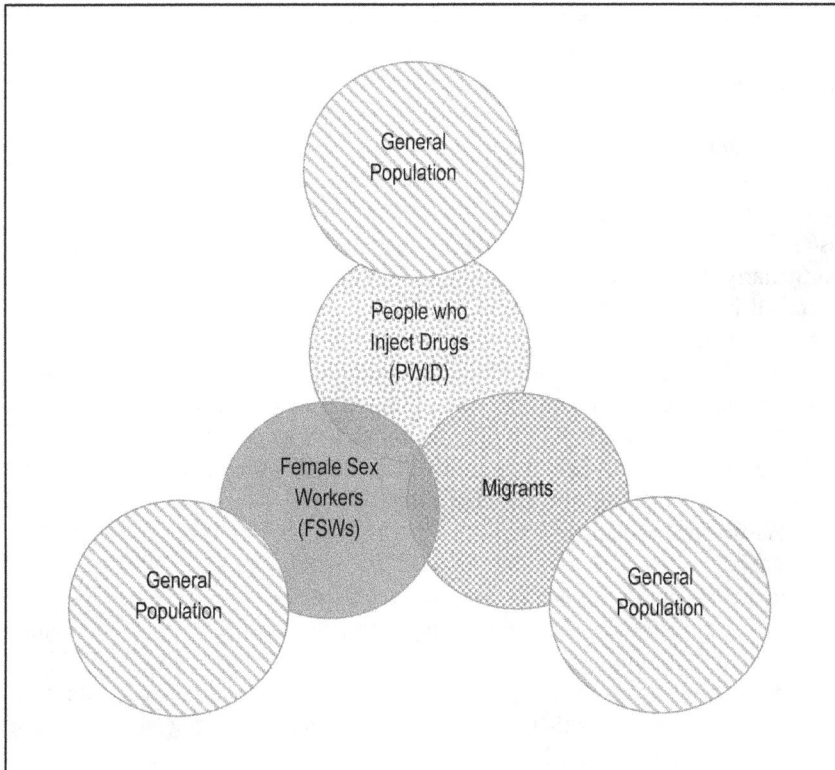

Figure 6.1 Possible interactions between cohorts.

(such as MSM) that they may intersect with on some level but this chapter concentrates on the three being researched as the most pertinent for understanding past and future HIV/AIDS epidemic trends in China.

PWID

Injecting drug use (IDU) and the cross-border passage of illicit drugs are implicated in the spread of HIV/AIDS in the region surrounding Yunnan and in the province itself (Beyrer et al., 2006). Wang et al. (2009), undertaking research in Yunnan, found although low condom usage rates increased the risk of commercial sex worker-to-client transmission, injection drug use was 'the single largest risk factor for HIV acquisition among FSWs, much larger than any risk factor traditionally associated with sex work, such as condom use rates, numbers of partners, and STIs' (p. 168). In China, PWID who are HIV+ are stigmatised and marginalised for engaging in immoral practices and suffer the additional ignominy of infection with an incurable disease. Coinciding with the stigmatisation involved with drug use, it is an illegal activity that may lead to incarceration and compulsory rehabilitation programmes.

Regardless of the contraindications for drug use in China, there was an estimated increase from 70,000 PWID in 1990 to over 1.16 million registered PWID in 2005 (Li, Ha, Zhang & Liu, 2010), which is an astonishing 1,557 per cent increase. However, the 2005 figures are out of date, and are potentially and most likely now considerably higher, but there is extreme difficulty in obtaining more precise numbers due to under-reporting and a general lack of dissemination of current figures by Beijing. While these figures are not specific to Yunnan, it does show that China is experiencing a continued increase in the numbers of drug users. Increases in drug use can be intuitively applied to the situation in Yunnan particularly due to their proximity to the Golden Triangle and drug trafficking routes. It is clear that a cumulative number of users and public perceptions, and subsequent stigmatisation, exacerbate the situation for drug users in China.

The main drug of choice for PWID in China is heroin (this is possibly owing to the extensive cross-border flow of opiates from Myanmar) (Qian et al., 2006). Due to increases in illicit drug prices, many users changed from inhaling heroin (chasing the dragon) to injecting heroin as it provides greater cost effectiveness to the user in achieving the required effect at lower doses (Bao & Liu, 2009; Che, Assanangkornchai, McNeil, Li, You & Chongsuvivatwong, 2011; Qian, Schumacher, Chen & Ruan, 2006). Intravenous drug use (IDU) has been well documented as being responsible for efficient transmission of HIV due to unsafe injecting practices, such as needle sharing, and other high-risk behaviours within the drug-using community (Hammett, Des Jarlais et al., 2007; Qian et al., 2006). It seems clear then that the high-risk behaviours involved with injecting drug use mean that those areas with the highest rates of injection drug abuse are also likely to be the areas where HIV is most prevalent.

The severity of the HIV epidemic in China is currently most prevalent in PWID, varies extensively and as of 2007, 78.2 per cent of all drug cases in

Yunnan were reported in Dehong, Honghe, Dali, Lincang, Wenshan and Kunming municipality (Jia, Luo et al., 2010). Significantly, in China, injecting drug use is more prevalent among unemployed, poor ethnic minority populations already marginalised by society (Hammett, Des Jarlais et al., 2007). This makes the delivery of HIV/AIDS programmes problematic as these groups of people are already disengaged from society and often in difficult-to-reach areas.

Delivering good HIV clinical care for PWID is complicated by a range of challenges related to drug dependency, such as social problems including marginalisation, and medical and psychological issues (Li, He, Wang & Williams, 2009; Liu, Lian & Zhao, 2006). Some estimates, such as those suggested by Philbin and Zhang (2010), advise that as of October 2007 there were between 40,000 and 50,000 PLWHA in Yunnan being serviced by 11 methadone clinics, government-run needle exchange programmes and a small number of NGOs. According to Tsai et al. (2010), Chinese authorities have made efforts to provide harm reduction facilities and education as: 'Compelling evidence suggests that availability of clean injecting equipments for injection drug users is a cost-effective and cost-saving strategy for reducing HIV/AIDS' (p. 546). Added to these issues are difficulties involved with HIV+ PWID not being able to afford methadone treatment with many PWID having no stable job and less access to basic needs, such as housing, food and medication (Li, He et al., 2009). Their high mobility and marginalisation also make it difficult for PWID to access methadone drug programmes and regular medical care (Zhang, Hsu, Yu, Wen & Pan, 2006).

The illegality of drug use in China can also pose access difficulties for the effective implementation of harm reduction and HIV treatment and prevention, as there is a fear of arrest and detention (Philbin & Zhang, 2010). In China, campaigns of law enforcement are categorised by long periods of weak or lax enforcement and short periods of intense and coercive enforcement (Van Rooij, 2016). These periods of intense enforcement are known as *strike hard (Yanda)* campaigns. In effect, they are intense police campaigns targeting illegal activities. They have been strongly condemned for their brutality, human rights abuses and neglect of criminal procedural laws, with different campaigns resulting in deaths (in the 2001 *strike hard* campaign, 2,960 people were sentenced to death and 1,781 were executed within the first three months) (Van Rooij, 2016).

These crackdowns are problematic in HIV/AIDS scenarios as they create a climate of fear of police and pressure PWID and CSWs to become even more hidden, marginalised and harder to reach. *Strike hard* campaigns often focus on specific areas known to be frequented by CSWs and drug users in an attempt to arrest and/or detain them for re-education. Hammett, Wu et al. (2007) confirm:

crackdowns, mass arrest, forced detoxification and incarceration of drug users … and in many places crackdowns on drug users have become almost continuous. Strategies include arrest quotas, use of paid informants and bounties for turning in dealers and users, and further expansion of compulsory detoxification centers and re-education through labor camps.

(p. 138)

Initially PWID may be offered a voluntary detention in detoxification centres but if they are caught using drugs again, they may be sent to compulsory centres or labour camps for up to 12 months (Li, Ha et al., 2010; Qian et al., 2006).

Additionally, law enforcement crackdowns have contributed to the changing nature of drug use from nasal inhalation *chasing the dragon*, to injection use. This is due to increased prices and the need for compact, refined drugs that are easier to distribute (McCoy, McCoy, Shenghan, Zhinuan, Xue-ren & Jie, 2001). The result is that users turn from inhalation to injection as it provides a less expensive, more satisfying, quicker result as well as being more portable as syringes are relatively easy to dispose of and hide from police (McCoy et al., 2001; Qian et al., 2006).[5] This is particularly important when simply carrying a syringe can raise police suspicions, resulting in them demanding a urine test which can then be used against them as evidence (Chen, pers. comm., November 2013). In 2007, one anti-narcotics campaign called 'Wind and Thunder Sweeping Narcotics' not only strengthened random urine testing permissions but also offered monetary incentives for neighbours, family and friends to report drug users to authorities (Cohen & Amon, 2008). Another result of police law enforcement has been to cause users to pool together in areas they consider safe from police but where sharing of needles is more likely to occur (McCoy et al., 2001).

There is also strong evidence to suggest that in Yunnan, male PWID who frequent FSWs, and FSWs who are themselves PWID, may have played a crucial role in the transition of the HIV epidemic from being IDU-driven to being sexually driven (Jia, Luo et al., 2010). Molecular genetic evidence in Yunnan, as discussed on p, 84, points to the HIV strains which are spreading through sexual transmission as likely to have originated in the PWID population (Hammett, Wu et al., 2007). One possible reason for this is indicated in research which has demonstrated that PWID engaging in sexual contact were less likely to use condoms, more likely to have multiple sex partners and have a PWID sex partner and engage in unsafe injecting practices (Li, He et al., 2009).

There is an increasing overlap between drug use and sex work, particularly among female sex worker populations, which may be providing a growing bridge between these high-risk groups and the general population thereby exacerbating the rapid spread of the epidemic in China (Jin et al., 2010; Jun et al., 2008; Yang, Latkin, Luan & Nelson, 2005). This is a common pattern with HIV epidemics globally. Although local and national HIV treatment and harm prevention programmes for PWID generally focus on reduction of drug use, studies suggest there is a need to expand programmes to deal with promoting safer sex and reductions in the number of sexual partners (Hu et al., 2011). Thus, a need for further understanding of the connections between drug use and sexual activity is of continuing concern to researchers. Without implementation of these types of programmes, it is possible that the local and global human security risks intrinsic to a HIV epidemic in China may evolve from concept to reality.

FSW populations

The highly permeable international borders in Yunnan mean that in addition to drug trafficking, there is a cross-border trade in other goods and services (Tagliacozzo, 2001). Women are subject to both internal and cross-border trafficking and this has been shown to directly contribute to mutations of the HIV virus and the global dispersions of HIV sub-types through sex trafficking (Huda, 2006). Additionally, rapid industrialisation has created unprecedented migration flows in China (Long, Zou & Liu, 2009). Rural workers are flocking to urban centres in search of higher-paying jobs with which they may support family members in their home communities.

Generally, FSWs have a very high rate of mobility, increasing the potential for them to facilitate the spread of HIV, and other STIs implicated in the increased risk of infection with HIV, between rural and urban areas (Ding et al., 2005; Knutsen, 2012; Wang, Li, Stanton, Fang, Lin & Mao, 2007). One reason for FSWs' forced mobility is the need to maintain an income in an environment where brothels are pressured by clients to continually provide a line-up of new faces (Wong & Yilin, 2003). Migrants are thus absent from their usual support networks and community and family constraints, causing them to indulge in high-risk behaviours. such as paid sex and drug use (Zhao et al., 2005).

This situation creates both a supply and demand for sex workers. While there are both male and female commercial sex workers (CSWs), FSWs represent the highest number of individuals working in the sex industry. As migrant women appear to have increased sexual risk and higher rates of STIs than their male counterparts, coupled with a low socio-economic status, it has been suggested that a high proportion of them may be engaging in sex work (Knutsen, 2012; Wang, Li et al., 2007). This has implications for the expansion of HIV/AIDS in China and poses a significant human security risk as transmission is now predominantly taking place through sexual contact.

The prevalence of sex work in China has increased rapidly since the beginning of China's reform and opening period and the relaxing of constraints with the West from 1978 (Pirkle et al., 2007). CSWs can be found in a myriad of locations in China from remote rural villages to large urban cities and number in the region of between 4–6 million (Kaufman & Meyers, 2006; Pirkle, Soundardjee & Stella, 2007). However, depending on how sex work is categorised and including those who occasionally accept gifts and money for sex, that figure might be as high as 20 million sex workers (Jeffreys, 2015). Significantly, the highest rates of FSWs who are HIV+ are found in Yunnan and particularly in the border areas near Thailand, Myanmar and Vietnam (Wang et al., 2009). Programmes dealing with FSWs in Yunnan face challenges for accessibility as rather than congregating in a specific red light area, FSWs are distributed throughout the village or city (Chen, pers. comm., November 2013). As such, it is impossible to reach them other than on an individual level with peer educators known to individual FSWs or referred to them by trusted friends.

The high numbers of HIV+ FSWs in Yunnan may be attributed to injecting drug use and infrequent use of condoms with clients and regular sexual partners (Wang et al., 2009). Jun et al. (2008) suggest: 'It is possible that drug users who also engage in unsafe sex with both high-risk populations (sex workers) and low-risk populations (regular partners or spouses) may be fueling the current epidemic, especially in the high-IDU area of Yunnan' (p. 564). The large number of mobile FSWs in Yunnan is largely due to the key role played by drug abuse and the pull-factors caused by servicing the overall demographics of the rural population who are young, male, and suffering from high unemployment (Jia, Wang et al., 2010).

With the majority of sex workers being female, an additional driver thought to be responsible for the increased rate of sex workers is the Chinese one-child policy and China's cultural preference for sons (Chi, Dong, Lei, Jun, Lu & Hesketh, 2013).[6] Women traditionally leave home to become a member of their husband's family (Hesketh & Xing, 2006; Tucker et al., 2005) while culturally the son is tasked with taking care of the parents in their old age and carrying on the family line (Xiaolei et al., 2013). As a result, there has been a tendency for women to abort their child if an ultrasound reveals it to be female. While female infanticide is forbidden by Beijing, sex-selective abortions are still relatively easy to obtain (Xiaolei et al., 2013). The imbalance in sex ratios, resulting in about 118 males born to every 100 females in China (in 2010), has left many single men unable to find partners (Tucker et al. 2005; Xiaolei et al., 2013; C. Yang et al., 2010; Zhou, Yan & Hesketh, 2013). As a result of being unable to find a partner, they are more inclined to frequent FSWs, which adds to the demand for sexual services.

While research has been undertaken on the role of FSWs in the spread of HIV in China, far less research is being undertaken on the role of commercial sex clients, in particular, male migrants as bridging populations (Zhao et al., 2005). Therefore, more research needs to be done on the formation of effective HIV education programmes targeting the clients of FSWs. It must be noted that the onus for prevention efforts (through attendance at treatment and prevention programmes) and the spread of HIV (due to the need to demand condom usage) must not be placed on sex workers alone, as they are often the least powerful partners in sexual negotiations, but also upon the clients of sex workers as bridging populations to the general community (Yang et al., 2010; Yi et al., 2010).

Prevention programmes in FSW communities have had some limited success but still many FSWs and their clients are engaging in high-risk behaviours. This may be partially due to the high turnover rates of FSWs (Ding et al., 2005; Wong & Yilin, 2003). Additionally, intervention workers are faced with challenges due to the varied types of sex workers (Parish & Pan, 2006). UNAIDS comment: 'Sex work is continually evolving. Many interventions are missing new categories of mobile and informal sex workers. Critically, prevention programmes seldom reach out to clients of sex workers' (2011, p. 20). Commercial sex is generally venue-based with a ranking system from that of hotel courtesans through to massage girls and, finally, streetwalkers, all of whom display a considerable variation of sexual practice and HIV risk (Parish & Pan, 2006; Yang et al., 2010).

There is often little room for FSWs to negotiate condom use and often the male clients feel little concern for the girls' welfare, particularly in the lower hierarchies (Burris & Xia, 2009; Parish & Pan, 2006). The level of risk exposure is reported to vary, depending on which rank of the sex industry a worker is employed in, with FSWs in the lower ranks having a HIV prevalence of 17.9 per cent as compared with the 5.7 per cent prevalence rate of those higher up in the industry (Yang et al., 2010). Added to which:

> Sex work is a fluid occupation influenced by economic conditions. Due to the illegal nature of sex work and FSWs' geographical mobility, it is difficult to sustain outreach, education, and counselling programs targeted at the individual level among these mobile populations.
>
> (Yi et al., 2010, p. 8)

Irrespective of the illegality of commercial sex work in China, the government has implemented programmes aimed at reducing rates of HIV infection such as condom distribution, education programmes, and free HIV treatment programmes for those infected (Wang et al., 2009). However, FSWs are obliged to negotiate double risks and stigmatisation, that of STI/HIV and of arrest and mandatory detention due to the *strike hard* campaign. Under the terms of this campaign, they may be confined from three months to six years and be tested for HIV and other STIs without consent and simply carrying a condom may be grounds for arrest (Burris & Xia, 2009; Pirkle et al., 2007; Sharma & Chatterjee, 2012). This adds to the increasing prevalence of HIV as the perpetual movement of FSWs contributes to the expansion of their sexual networks and refusal to be tested and treated for STIs and HIV for fear of police crackdowns and arrest (Pirkle et al., 2007).

The constant mobility of FSWs not only causes dilemmas in accessing health services, it also means that FSWs potentially spread HIV to new regions through an expanded client base. FSWs' combination of high mobility, drug use, early first sexual encounters, low education levels, youth and low rates of condom use create a perfect synergy for the expansion of HIV infection into lower-risk populations through their clients and casual boyfriends (Chen et al., 2005; Merli & Hertog, 2010). When this is combined with a disinclination to be tested for HIV, resulting in ignorance as to HIV status, the potential ramifications for the spread of HIV increase exponentially.

The floating migrant population

China has an extensive number of internal labour immigrants moving throughout the country in search of work (Hyde, 2007). Many of them are registered in accordance with the existing *hukou* system of household registration but a large number are not and make up what has been termed China's floating population.

In China's current *hukou* system, every person is allocated a permanent household registration with an official agricultural or non-agricultural status.

According to China's National Bureau of Statistics, at the end of 2011, there were an estimated 252.78 million migrant workers in China. Of which, an estimated 73 per cent had come from poorer regions of China (Li, Huang, Cai, Xu, Huang & Shen, 2009). Economic migrants are those who have left their place of household registration to take up employment in general professions, such as factory workers or labourers, in urban centres (Li, Huang et al., 2009). To legally make such a move, residents are required to obtain official approval and obtain a temporary or permanent residency permit. However, many do not do so (Tuñón, 2006).

The fact that these migrants are outside of official channels not only makes them difficult to document, but it also means that they may find it extremely difficult to access health care and education and prevention programmes (Tucker et al., 2011). Indubitably, having an undocumented status complicates the situation for both cross-border and internal labour migrants. Tuñón (2006) states:

> [O]btaining a precise representation of the scale of migration is further complicated by its clandestine nature: only an estimated 40% of migrants obtain either a temporary or permanent resident permit. The remainder, who have lived without local authorization for at least six months, are known as the 'floating population' and migrate, reside and work through informal and unregulated channels.
>
> (p. 7)

Mobile populations in the region have already been identified as important vectors of HIV transmission (Kaufman, Kleinman & Saich, 2006). Piot, Greener and Russell (2007) suggest that rapid economic development has increased the mobility of people both within and across borders and that this mobility correlates with higher rates of HIV infection. This increase in mobility has also aided the cross-border trade in illicit drugs between Myanmar and Yunnan, further facilitating the expansion of HIV/AIDS in the region (Beyrer et al., 2006). The most affected states in the context of HIV/AIDS are the Myanmar border zones with Yunnan (Beyrer & Lee, 2008). The migration of people for labour is a factor that worldwide has been found to increase HIV risk as it separates spouses, families and individuals from their kinship and support networks for extended periods of time (Lin et al., 2011; Skeldon, 2000).

Studies have found that labour migrants face considerably greater risks of contracting HIV due to increased risk-taking behaviours (Su et al., 2018). Approximately 11 per cent of male migrants had engaged the services of sex workers and in Shanxi and Shandong Provinces, almost 70 per cent of all PLWHA were migrants (Jun et al., 2008). Wang et al. (2007) state: 'The separation from family, lack of social control, relative affluence, and anonymity of living in a city make male migrants particularly vulnerable to commercial sex and HIV risk behaviors' (p. 2). Many of these labour migrants are surplus young men stemming from the sex ratio imbalance inherent in the one-child policy and a cultural bias against female children (Merli & Hertog, 2010; C. Yang et al., 2010).

In addition to this, their relative youth, lower socio-economic status, frequent migration and loosening of community restraints have been found to increase risk-taking behaviours and social and sexual mixing (Knutsen, 2012; Li, Huang, Cai, Xu, Huang & Shen, 2009). Xiao et al. (2007), examining the spread of the HIV/AIDS problem in Yunnan, submit that the migration of young men may be fuelling the sex industry. There appears to be a higher likelihood that migrant men will indulge in casual sex or use sex workers, and in doing so they may increase their exposure to HIV through multiple partners, high rates of unprotected sex and drug use (Knutsen, 2012; B. Wang et al., 2007; C. Yang et al., 2010).

Migrants have a low knowledge of HIV and the risk behaviours to be avoided and limited access to information that may help them understand those risks (Huda, 2006; Liao et al., 2011; Zhao et al., 2005). As stated by Tuñón (2006, pp. 14–15): '[M]igrants are faced with a dearth of information and limited services in the area of sexual and reproductive health ... HIV/AIDS also looms over the large, young and mobile population free of traditional constraints.' There is also some concern that rural labour migrants may be uninformed and ill-prepared for the situations that they may face when arriving in urban areas. This seems to be particularly the case with girls and young women who may be forced into situations of exploitation, such as debt bondage, sexual exploitation and forced labour (Tuñón, 2006).

However, it would be incorrect to assume that Beijing is doing nothing to help facilitate access to prevention and education services for labour migrants, as they have introduced a number of different interventions addressing migrants' vulnerabilities, but they are still well short of what is needed, and these efforts are limited by the complexities of the current *hukou* system and urban biases (Hu, Cook & Salazar, 2008; Tuñón, 2006). As a result, there continues to be many migrants who are unable to access even the most basic of education and health care. Generally the cost of health care is prohibitive for people who are not covered by their employer's health insurance schemes, and China's insurance system mostly excludes migrants, as even public clinics and hospitals require payment (S. Li et al., 2009). Conversely, even though migrants may find accessing basic health care needs easier in their home communities, the health care systems for sexual health may be poorly established (Yi, Mantell, Wu, Lu, Zeng & Wan, 2010).

In the past, it was necessary to get drugs from an appointed health care site according to the *hukou* system in order to be eligible for the 'Four Free and One Care' policy (X. Li et al., 2009). As a result of this requirement, many migrant workers were excluded from accessing health services. This was no longer entirely correct as requirements for free ART are simply a range of tests and counselling to determine status and CD4 count (now increased from below 200 to below 350), regardless of registration status (Chen, pers. comm., November

2013). Unfortunately, information regarding these new regulations is poorly disseminated which, when added to the high cost of health care and low annual incomes, leaves an estimated 80 per cent of the rural population without health insurance. As HIV/AIDS services are exclusively administered in government treatment facilities, migrants remain reluctant to access health care services outside of their *hukou* registrations (Tuñón, 2006).

Migrant populations, especially those who are outside the *hukou* system, may act as links between FSWs and PWID as they can belong to, or interact with, both cohorts, and the general population when returning to their home communities. When considering that male migrants indulge in high-risk behaviours and represent an important subgroup of CSW clients, some researchers believe that these population groups may represent the tipping point for the transmission of HIV in China (Jun et al., 2008; S. Li et al., 2009; B. Wang et al., 2007; Zhao et al., 2005). This is particularly due to their high mobility and regular return to rural home communities.

Conclusion

The situation for HIV/AIDS in China is one of continuing concern. The epidemic is dynamic and there are new cases of HIV reported regularly. Although this chapter provides a brief overview of a number of vectors for the transmission of HIV in China, such as MSM, MTCT, FPDs, FSWs, PWID and floating migrants, they do not equally contribute to high-risk factors for the spread of HIV. As shown, with the exception of MSM, the PWID, FSW and floating migrants engage in the highest risk behaviours of populations implicated in the spread of HIV/AIDS in China. In addition to all of them being the main transmission routes for HIV in Yunnan, with high rates of infection in selected pockets, they are all key populations that are highly mobile and marginalised by society.

A case has also been made for the epidemiological evidence, suggesting that the initial spread of HIV in China started in PWID populations in Yunnan. While the overall percentages for China as a whole do remain low, the cohorts mentioned in this chapter all engage in high-risk behaviours and have ongoing HIV epidemics. This is particularly the case in Yunnan where proximity to the Golden Triangle and porous borders with Myanmar, Vietnam and Laos create an environment that is particularly conducive to drug use, sexual trafficking and high mobility. Subsequently, they continue to require resources and treatment and prevention initiatives that keep pace with the changing nature of infection in China.

The epidemic is still active in more long-standing groups of PLWHA, both within Yunnan and the rest of China, and vigilance is required within these cohorts to improve upon current levels of infection. As an example of this, even though blood collection practices have changed and the epidemic has generally halted in cohorts of FPDs, there is increasing concern that individuals are becoming more blasé about how they are managing their prevention efforts and, therefore, numbers of infections have increased in some areas. This is even more so in key populations, such as PWID, CSWs, MSM and the floating population, as they are less likely to seek medical intervention or be tested for HIV than other population groups due to the illegal nature of their practices, high mobility and stigma.

In Yunnan and other areas within China, HIV/AIDS interventions within these cohorts becomes even more difficult when issues such as arrest and detention hamper treatment and prevention programmes. The illegal nature of sex work and drug use, coupled with the current *strike hard* campaigns, is deleterious to the work being undertaken in the promotion of safe injection practices and condom usage. As long as carrying a condom can lead to suspicion of sex work and possible arrest, it will not be seen as an attractive option for FSWs.

Case study 6.1 highlights the problems associated with forced incarceration for PWID, economic insecurity, food insecurity, community insecurity and health insecurity. PWID have unique needs within the HIV/AIDS epidemics due to the nature of their addictions. While Beijing follows GBP in supplying MMT programmes, they are not always accessible to individuals. Ruili is well known as a drug trafficking transit and destination location for drugs entering from the Golden Triangle.

Case study 6.1 Yong's story

Ruili is a beautiful town in Yunnan Province in Southern China. The city itself is dotted with golden temples and has a stunning backdrop of mountains that fade off into the distance. It sits on the edge of a river (the Irrawaddy) that borders China and Myanmar. It is not a large city, in fact, hardly more than a large town but it has a bustling energy that makes it seem far larger than it really is. It is a holiday playground for Chinese citizens from Kunming and the surrounding area. While not every person who arrives in Ruili is interested in sex tourism, it is one of the main attractions. The main reason for this is its proximity to the area of the Golden Triangle. The sex trade and the drug trade are travel companions on the Silk Roads that criss-cross Southern Yunnan.

The morning after my arrival in Ruili, I travelled to an area close to the middle of town. I spent the morning meeting with two peer workers involved with a drop-in centre for PWID. The centre itself was a small shopfront with a few wooden stools and a desk. It was coated in green paint that was lazily peeling itself from the walls and the floor was stained, unsealed concrete but as this is quite common in China, it does not denote a lack of care. The peer workers I met were both HIV+ and on methadone maintenance regimes. I asked them if the police knew of the centre and whether they supported its operation. One of the workers told me that they did know of it and that although drug use is not legal, and the police were not actively supportive, they did not usually raid the place and in general left them alone.

We were there for some hours chatting about the clientele and the different ways that individuals would use the service. They provided counselling services and HIV rapid tests so that PWID did not have to go to a clinic to ascertain their status (rapid tests are small blood tests that give an immediate result. While they are generally accurate, they have been known to produce false positive results so most people were encouraged to confirm the result through further testing.) They said that most people were afraid to go to the clinic, as they feared that they would be arrested for being drug users. They told me that as well as running the drop-in centre, they would go to the area along the border to take supplies to the PWID who lived in the bush. These people had no access to health services and very little in the way of food and shelter. As a result of this conversation, they offered to take me to visit some injection drug users in the area.

There was no public transport available to where the PWID were squatting, so I had to go by motorbike. It is a common form of transport in Yunnan, so I was not surprised when they wheeled out two decrepit-looking bikes and told my interpreter and me to climb on the back. I use the word motorbike very generously; it was actually a little scooter, like a Vespa. With some trepidation I swung my leg over and perched myself on the back of the bike behind one of the peer workers. As we sped through Ruili, swerving in and out of the traffic and hordes of other bikers, I found myself clinging to him like a barnacle. I was helmetless and as I am much bigger than the average Chinese, I feared that I might topple us as we leaned into the corners. After what seemed an inordinately long time, we arrived at the edge of nowhere. The road simply ceased. I slid from the back of the bike and stood at the edge of a rocky slope overlooking rice fields surrounded by areas of thick vegetation.

The place we were heading for was out past the field and I had to scramble down the incline, cross the rice paddies, and cross a shaky bamboo bridge over a small creek to get there. The trail on the other side was narrow and as we approached a small, ad hoc shelter. the peer workers went ahead with long sticks, using them to flick aside human excrement from where we were walking. There were no toilets or running water and the people sheltering in the small hut simply squatted outside. The hut itself was little more than rusting corrugated iron and blue and white tarpaulin stretched over sticks. There were no windows but there was a small entrance space that was draped in a brightly patterned fabric. One of the peer workers hammered on the tin and stood back waiting.

A short time later the curtain moved, revealing a dishevelled young man named Yong. Behind him we could see a man and a woman sleeping on a grass mat on the mud floor of the hut. Yong is an injection drug user who had just been released from a mandatory detention centre where he was supposed to be rehabilitated. He had been incarcerated there for two years, which is the normal period given for repeat drug offenders. He had been living in the hut for some weeks at the time we met. He did not have anywhere else to go. He told me that the first thing that he did when he was released was find a heroin supplier. He knew that he was better off not taking drugs but said that he now had no choice because his body needed it. The two other people living with him had also recently been released from a detention centre. He said they all did whatever they needed to in order to survive.

In addition to living in a space that was barely adequate to provide shelter from the rain and entirely inadequate for the cold winter nights that were common during the time of year that I was there, Yong and his companions had no other support. They were all unemployed and had no money to buy even the most basic of essentials. Yong told me that they barely had enough to eat each day and that they could not afford to seek medical attention. Apart from which, they were afraid that if they did, they would be returned to detention. He told me that whatever money they were able to get was mostly spent on drugs, and that after taking them they just spent the day sleeping. He also told me that the woman was working as a sex worker in order to bring in some income. I did not ask him how he and the other man made the money to buy drugs and purchase the small amounts of food that they were able to eat. I did ask him if he was HIV+ and he responded that all three of them were.

While mandatory rehabilitation in detention centres is standard policy for repeat drug offenders in China, there is much debate about its efficacy and whether it constitutes a violation of an individual's human rights (Knutsen, 2012). China's record for human rights is not good. In cases where they deem public safety to be paramount, the rights of the individual are superseded by the need to minimise the perceived risk for the general public. Mandatory incarceration for drug users is not a viable solution. This is the stance that is supported by WHO, UNAIDS and UNICEF who state: 'Drug detention centres have poor records in preventing drug use and high rates of recidivism. In addition, drug detention centres can enhance HIV and related risks, violate human rights and undermine the potential success of proven interventions' (WHO, UNICEF & UNAIDS, 2011b, p. 129). This seems to be graphically highlighted by the three people living in a shanty hut in an area outside Ruili.

The story of Yong and his companions is not an isolated tale of hardship. Often PWID who enter rehabilitation centres clean of HIV will exit with a positive status (Cohen & Amon, 2008). In addition, some drug users advance to more high-risk drug-taking practices while undertaking mandatory re-education. Considering that PWID are one of the key populations in HIV/AIDS epidemics it is essential that they receive effective education about the risks of injection drug use and the steps they can take to minimise harm. The conditions and circumstances in which Yong and his shanty companions are living demonstrate that the current practices are insufficient. Upon being released from incarceration in a mandatory re-education and rehabilitation centre, Yong told me that one of the first things he did was to source heroin and get high.

While China is continually improving its responses to HIV/AIDS, they remain insufficient. MMT programmes are available for injection heroin users but the risk of incarceration makes applying for them an unattractive option for many. Additionally, PWID face stigmatisation and are marginalised from their communities. They are often unable to get employment and, therefore, may live in conditions of poverty and despair. Without some form of support, PWID return to what they know best. For some, it may be a coping mechanism to deal with the shortfalls characteristic of their lives in situations of poverty and human insecurity, for others, it is a way to forget and chemically simulate an alternate existence.

Notes

1 New 01B recombinant strains have emerged in MSM populations in Anhui Province from circulating CRF01_AE and US-derived B strains. This reveals transmission links among different epidemic region-derived strains. These new recombinants appear to have increased pathogenesis. Studies show that even patients under the age of 25 (who should be adept at forming immune responses against invading pathogens) are

progressing to AIDS with low CD4+ counts and obvious AIDS-like symptoms (J. Wu et al., 2013).
2 The AIDS 2014 conference provided a platform for TG sex workers to share their experiences through public discussions. At the conference, this was one of the points repeatedly made by TG women, regardless of their nationality.
3 At the AIDS 2014 conference many TG women shared stories of having their heads shaved (and being put in the male prison population); being raped in prison; and being forced to perform oral sex on entire groups of prison populations. When removed from the general population, to prevent such violations from occurring, they were put in the segregated paedophile prison population. This reinforced feelings of despair as it accorded them a proxy status with those generally considered sexually perverted.
4 The national Prevention of Mother-To-Child-Transmission (PMTCT) Work Management Information System showed that in 2011, HIV counselling and testing services were provided to over 8 million pregnant women, and testing coverage increased to 92.9 per cent. The percentage of HIV positive pregnant women receiving ART for PMTCT stood at 74.1 per cent (UNAIDS & CMOH, 2012, p. 9).
5 This situation is similar to that which occurred in Xinjiang. *Strike hard* campaigns resulted in a change in drug-taking practices from smoking heroin to IDU (Hayes, 2012).
6 The one-child policy was revised in 2015 and, on 1 January 2016, a two-child policy law became effective.

References

Bao, Y. & Liu, Z. (2009). Systematic review of HIV and HCV infection among drug users in China. *International Journal of STD & AIDS, 20*(6), 399–405.

Beyrer, C. & Lee, T. J. (2008). Responding to infectious diseases in Burma and her border regions. *Conflict and Health, 2*(2). Retrieved from www.biomedcentral.com/content/pdf/1752-1505-2-2.pdf

Beyrer, C., Suwanvanichkij, V., Mullany, L. C., Richards, A. K., Franck, N., Samuels, A. & Lee, T. J. (2006). Responding to AIDS, tuberculosis, malaria, and emerging infectious diseases in Burma: Dilemmas of policy and practice. *PLoS Medicine, 3*(10), e393.

Burris, S. & Xia, G. (2009). The 'risk environment' for commercial sex work in China: Considering the role of law and law enforcement practices. In J. Tucker, D. L. Poston Jr., Q. Ren, B. Gu, X. Zheng, S. Wang & C. Russell (Eds.), *Gender Policy and HIV in China* (pp. 179–188). Dordrecht, the Netherlands: Springer.

Che, Y., Assanangkornchai, S., McNeil, E., Li, J., You, J. & Chongsuvivatwong, V. (2011). Patterns of attendance in methadone maintenance treatment programs in Yunnan province, China. *The American Journal of Drug and Alcohol Abuse, 37*(3), 148–154.

Chen, G., Li, Y., Zhang, B., Yu, Z., Li, X., Wang, L. & Yu, Z. (2012). Psychological characteristics in high-risk MSM in China. *BMC Public Health, 12*(1), 1.

Chen, K. T. & Qian, H. (2005). Mother to child transmission of HIV in China. *BMJ, 330*, 1282–1283.

Chen, X., Yin, Y. P., Liang, G. J., Gong, X. D., Li, H. S., Poumerol, G., ... & Yu, Y. H. (2005). Sexually transmitted infections among female sex workers in Yunnan, China. *AIDS Patient Care & STDs, 19*(12), 853–860.

Chi, Z., Dong, Z. X., Lei, W. X., Jun, Z. W., Lu, L. & Hesketh, T. (2013). Changing gender preference in China today: Implications for the sex ratio. *Indian Journal of Gender Studies, 20*(1), 51–68.

Cohen, J. E. & Amon, J. J. (2008). Health and human rights concerns of drug users in detention in Guangxi Province, China. *PLoS Medicine, 5*(12), e234.

Commission on AIDS in Asia. (2008). *Redefining AIDS in Asia: Crafting an effective response.* Oxford, UK: Oxford University Press. Retrieved from http://data.unaids.org/pub/report/2008/20080326_report_commission_aids_en.pdf

Coovadia, H. M., Rollins, N. C., Bland, R. M., Little, K., Coutsoudis, A., Bennish, M. L. & Newell, M. L. (2007). Mother-to-child transmission of HIV-1 infection during exclusive breastfeeding in the first 6 months of life: An intervention cohort study. *The Lancet, 369*(9567), 1107–1116.

Ding, Y., Detels, R., Zhao, Z., Zhu, Y., Zhu, G., Zhang, B., ... & Xue, X. (2005). HIV infection and sexually transmitted diseases in female commercial sex workers in China. *Journal of Acquired Immune Deficiency Syndromes, 38*(3), 314–319.

Dou, Z., Chen, R. Y., Xu, J., Ma, Y., Jiao, J. H., Durako, S., ... & Zhang, F. (2010). Changing baseline characteristics among patients in the China national free antiretroviral treatment program, 2002–09. *International Journal of Epidemiology, 39*(suppl. 2), ii56–ii64.

Emerton, R. (2006). Finding a voice, fighting for rights: The emergence of the transgender movement in Hong Kong 1. *Inter-Asia Cultural Studies, 7*(2), 243–269.

Guadamuz, T. E., Wimonsate, W., Varangrat, A., Phanuphak, P., Jommaroeng, R., McNicholl, J. M., ... & van Griensven, F. (2011). HIV prevalence, risk behavior, hormone use and surgical history among transgender persons in Thailand. *AIDS and Behavior, 15*(3), 650–658.

Guo, Y., Li, X., Song, Y. & Liu, Y. (2012). Bisexual behavior among Chinese young migrant men who have sex with men: Implications for HIV prevention and intervention. *AIDS Care, 24*(4), 451–458.

Hammett, T. M., Des Jarlais, D., Johnston, P., Kling, R., Ngu, D., Liu, W., ... & Donghua, M. (2007). HIV prevention for injection drug users in China and Vietnam: Policy and research considerations. *Global Public Health, 2*(2), 125–139. doi:10.1080/17441690600981806.

Hammett, T. M., Wu, Z., Tran, T. D., Stephens, D., Sullivan, S., Liu, W., ... & Des Jarlais, D. C. (2007). 'Social evils' and harm reduction: The evolving policy environment for human immunodeficiency virus prevention among injection drug users in China and Vietnam. *Addiction, 103*(1), 137–145. doi:10.1111/j.1360–0443.2007.02053.x.

Harney, A. (2015). China's 'blood famine' drives patients to the black market. *Reuters Health News*, February 16. Retrieved from www.reuters.com/article/us-china-health-blood/chinas-blood-famine-drives-patients-to-the-black-market-idUSKBN0LI0W920150216

Hayes, A. (2005). AIDS, bloodheads & cover-ups: The 'ABC' of Henan's AIDS epidemic. *AQ: Australian Quarterly, 77*(3), 12–40.

Hayes, A. (2012). HIV/AIDS in Xinjiang: A serious 'ill' in an 'autonomous' region. *IJAPS, 8*(1), January, 77–102.

Hesketh, T. & Xing, Z. W. (2006). Abnormal sex ratios in human populations: Causes and consequences. *Proceedings of the National Academy of Sciences, 103*(36), 13271–13275.

Hu, X., Cook, S. & Salazar, M. A. (2008). Internal migration and health in China. *The Lancet, 372*(9651), 1717–1719.

Hu, Y., Liang, S., Zhu, J., Qin, G., Liu, Q., Song, B. ... & Qian, H. (2011). Factors associated with recent risky drug use and sexual behaviors among drug users in southwestern China. *Journal of AIDS Clinical Research, 2*(120), 3. Retrieved from www.omicsonline.org/2155-6113/2155-6113-2-120.php

Huda, S. (2006). Sex trafficking in south Asia. *International Journal of Gynecology & Obstetrics, 94*(3), 374–381.

Hyde, S. T. (2007). *Eating spring rice: The cultural politics of AIDS in southwest China.* Berkeley, CA: University of California Press.

Jeffreys, E. (2015). *Sex in China.* Chichester, UK: John Wiley & Sons, Ltd.

Jia, M., Luo, H., Ma, Y., Wang, N., Smith, K., Mei, J., ... & Zhang, Q. (2010). The HIV epidemic in Yunnan province, China, 1989–2007. *JAIDS: Journal of Acquired Immune Deficiency Syndromes, 53*, S34.

Jia, Z., Wang, W., Dye, C., Bao, Y., Liu, Z. & Lu, L. (2010). Exploratory analysis of the association between new-type drug use and sexual transmission of HIV in China. *American Journal of Drug & Alcohol Abuse, 36*(2), 130–133. doi:10.3109/00952991003734269.

Jie, W., Ciyong, L., Xueqing, D., Hui, W. & Lingyao, H. (2012). A syndemic of psychosocial problems places the MSM (men who have sex with men) population at greater risk of HIV infection. *PloS ONE, 7*(3), e32312.

Jin, X., Smith, K., Chen, R. Y., Ding, G., Yao, Y., Wang, H., ... & Wang, N. (2010). HIV prevalence and risk behaviors among male clients of female sex workers in Yunnan, China. *Journal of Acquired Immune Deficiency Syndromes, 53*(1), 131–135.

Jun, J., Ning, W., Lin, L., Yi, P., Guo, L., Wong, M., Zheng, L. & Xi, W. (2008). HIV and STIs in clients and female sex workers in mining regions of Gejiu City, China. *Sexually Transmitted Diseases, 35*(6), 558–556. doi:10.1097/OLQ.0b013e318165926b.

Kaufman, J., Kleinman, A. & Saich, T. (2006). Introduction: Social policy and HIV/AIDS in China. In J. Kaufman, A. Kleinman & T. Saich (Eds.), *AIDS and social policy in China* (pp. 3–14). Cambridge, MA: Harvard University Asia Center.

Kaufman, J. & Meyers, K. (2006). AIDS surveillance in China: Data gaps and research. In J. Kaufman, A. Kleinman & T. Saich (Eds.), *AIDS and social policy in China* (pp. 47–71). Cambridge, MA: Harvard University Asia Center.

Knutsen, W. L. U. (2012). An institutional account of China's HIV/AIDS policy process from 1985 to 2010. *Politics & Policy, 40*(1), 161–192

Li, J., Ha, T. H., Zhang, C. & Liu, H. (2010). The Chinese government's response to drug use and HIV/AIDS: A review of policies and programs. *Harm Reduction Journal, 7*, 1–6. doi:10.1186/1477-7517-7-4.

Li, S., Huang, H., Cai, Y., Xu, G., Huang, F. & Shen, X. (2009). Characteristics and determinants of sexual behavior among adolescents of migrant workers in Shangai (China). *BMC Public Health, 9*(1), 195.

Li, X., He, G., Wang, H. & Williams, A. B. (2009). Consequences of drug abuse and HIV/AIDS in China: Recommendations for integrated care of HIV-infected drug users. *AIDS Patient Care & STDs, 23*(10), 877–884. doi:10.1089/apc.2009.0015.

Liang, K., Meyers, K., Zeng, W. & Gui, X. (2013). Predictors of elective pregnancy termination among women diagnosed with HIV during pregnancy in two regions of China, 2004–2010. *BJOG: An International Journal of Obstetrics & Gynaecology, 120*(10), 1207–1214.

Liao, S., Weeks, M. R., Wang, Y., Li, F., Jiang, J., Li, J., ... & Dunn, J. (2011). Female condom use in the rural sex industry in China: Analysis of users and non-users at post-intervention surveys. *AIDS Care, 23*, 66–74. doi:10.1080/09540121.2011.555742.

Lin, D., Li, X., Wang, B., Hong, Y., Fang, X., Qin, X. & Stanton, B. (2011). Discrimination, perceived social inequity, and mental health among rural-to-urban migrants in China. *Community Mental Health Journal, 47*(2), 171–180. doi:10.1007/s10597-009-9278-4.

Liu, Z., Lian, Z. & Zhao, C. (2006). Drug use and HIV/AIDS in China. *Drug & Alcohol Review, 25*(2), 173–175. doi:10.1080/09595230500538835.

Long, H., Zou, J. & Liu, Y. (2009). Differentiation of rural development driven by industrialization and urbanization in eastern coastal China. *Habitat International, 33*(4), 454–462.

Luo, W., Hong, H., Wang, X., McGoogan, J. M., Rou, K. & Wu, Z. (2018). Synthetic drug use and HIV infection among men who have sex with men in China: A sixteen-city, cross-sectional survey. *PloS ONE, 13*(7), e0200816.

Ma, W., Raymond, H. F., Wilson, E. C., McFarland, W., Lu, H., Ding, X., ... & He, X. (2012). Participation of HIV prevention programs among men who have sex with men in two cities of China – a mixed method study. *BMC Public Health, 12*(1), 1.

McCoy, C. B., McCoy, H. V., Shenghan, L., Zhinuan, Y., Xue-ren, W. & Jie, M. (2001). Reawakening the dragon: Changing patterns of opiate use in Asia, with particular emphasis on China's Yunnan Province. *Substance Abuse & Misuse, 36*(1 & 2), 49–69.

Merli, M. G. & Hertog, S. (2010). Masculine sex ratios, population age structure and the potential spread of HIV in China. *Demographic Research, 22*, 63–94.

Needham, K. (2019). Blood plasma scandal latest stain on China's medical products image. *The Sydney Morning Herald*, February 7. Retrieved from https://tinyurl.com/y3ydceu8

Parish, W. L. & Pan, S. (2006). Sexual partners in China: Risk pattern for infection by HIV and possible interventions. In J. Kaufman, A. Kleinman & T. Saich (Eds.), *AIDS and social policy in China* (pp. 190–213). Cambridge, MA: Harvard University Asia Center.

Peng, Z., Yang, H., Norris, J., Chen, X., Huan, X., Yu, R. ... & Chen, F. (2012). HIV incidence and predictors associated with retention in a cohort of men who have sex with men in Yangzhou, Jiangsu Province, China. *PloS ONE, 7*(12), e52731.

Philbin, M. M. & Zhang, F. (2010). Exploring stakeholder perceptions of facilitators and barriers to accessing methadone maintenance clinics in Yunnan province, China. *AIDS Care, 22*(5), 623–629. doi:10.1080/09540120903311490.

Piot, P., Greener, R. & Russell, S. (2007). Squaring the circle: AIDS, poverty, and human development. *PLoS Medicine, 4*(10), e314.

Pirkle, C., Soundardjee, R. & Stella, A. (2007). Female sex workers in China: Vectors of disease? *Sexually Transmitted Diseases, 34*(9), 695–703.

Qian, H. Z., Schumacher, J. E., Chen, H. T. & Ruan, Y. H. (2006). Injection drug use and HIV/AIDS in China: Review of current situation, prevention and policy implications. *Harm Reduction Journal, 3*(1), 4. doi:10.1186/1477-7517-3-4.

Qian, Z., Vermund, S. & Wang, N. (2005). Risk of HIV/AIDS in China: Subpopulations of special importance. *Sexually Transmitted Infections, 81*(6), 442–447.

Reynolds, L. & McKee, M. (2009). Matching supply and demand for blood in Guizhou province, China: An unresolved challenge. *Journal of Public Health, 90*(1), 32–36. doi:10.1016/j.healthpol.2008.09.002.

Shan, D., Sun, J., Khoshnood, K., Fu, J., Duan, S., Jiang, C., ... & Liu, H. (2014). The impact of comprehensive prevention of mother-to-child HIV transmission in Dehong prefecture, Yunnan province, 2005–2010: A hard-hit area by HIV in Southern China. *International Journal of STD & AIDS, 25*(4), 253–260.

Sharma, M.,& Chatterjee, A. (2012). Partnering with law enforcement to deliver good public health: The experience of the HIV/AIDS Asia regional program. *Harm Reduction Journal, 9*(1), 24–29.

Skeldon, R. (2000). *Population mobility and HIV vulnerability in South East Asia: An assessment and analysis*. Bangkok, Thailand: UNDP South East Asia HIV and Development Project.

Su, L., Liang, S., Hou, X., Zhong, P., Wei, D., Fu, Y., … & Yang, H. (2018). Impact of worker emigration on HIV epidemics in labour export areas: A molecular epidemiology investigation in Guangyuan, China. *Scientific Reports, 8*(1), 16046.

Sun, X., Lu, F., Wu, Z., Poundstone, K., Zeng, G., Xu, P., … & Liau, A. (2010). Evolution of information-driven HIV/AIDS policies in China. *International Journal of Epidemiology, 39*(suppl. 2), ii4–ii13.

Tagliacozzo, E. (2001). Border permeability and the state in Southeast Asia: Contraband and regional security. *Contemporary Southeast Asia, 23*(2), 254–274. Retrieved from http://search.proquest.com/docview/205217465?accountid=26503

Tsai, T., Morisky, D. E. & Chen, Y. A. (2010). Role of service providers of needle syringe program in preventing HIV/AIDS. *AIDS Education & Prevention, 22*(6), 546–557. doi:10.1521/aeap. 2010.22.6.546.

Tucker, J. D., Henderson, G. E., Wang, T. F., Huang, Y. Y., Parish, W., Pan, S. M., … & Cohen, M. S. (2005). Surplus men, sex work, and the spread of HIV in China. *AIDS, 19*(6), 539–547.

Tucker, J. D., Peng, H., Wang, K., Chang, H., Zhang, S. M., Yang, L. G. & Yang, B. (2011). Female sex worker social networks and STI/HIV prevention in South China. *PLoS ONE, 6*(9), e24816.

Tuñón, M. (2006). Internal labour migration in China: Features and responses. Beijing, ILO, April, 1–51. Retrieved from www.ilo.org/wcmsp5/groups/public/--asia/--ro-bangkok/--ilo-beijing/documents/publication/wcms_158634.pdf

UNAIDS. (2009). *UNAIDS action framework: Universal access for men who have sex with men and transgender people*. Geneva, Switzerland: World Health Organization.

UNAIDS. (2011a). UNAIDS terminology guideline 2011. Retrieved from: www.unaids. org/sites/default/files/media_asset/JC2118_terminology-guidelines_en_1.pdf?fbclid=I wAR0qRc8BT5i6VNMDzLTW7R6wb05gyAROHYsJLCfgwHKCLIF-2FlCJRQeiN8

UNAIDS. (2011b). *HIV in Asia and the Pacific: Getting to zero*. UNAIDS. Retrieved from www.unaids.org/en/media/unaids/contentassets/documents/unaidspublication/2011/20110826_APGettingToZero_en.pdf

UNAIDS & CMOH (China's Ministry of Health). (2012). *2012 China AIDS response progress report. Ministry of Health of the People's Republic of China. 31 March.* Retrieved from www.unaids.org/sites/default/files/country/documents//file,68497,es..pdf

Van Rooij, B. (2016). The campaign enforcement style: Chinese practice in context and comparison. In F. Bignami & D. Zaring (Eds.), *Comparative law and regulation: Understanding the global regulatory process* (pp. 217–237). Cheltenham, UK: Edward Elgar Publishing.

Wang, B., Li, X., Stanton, B., Fang, X., Lin, D. & Mao, R. (2007). HIV-related risk behaviors and history of sexually transmitted diseases among male migrants who patronize commercial sex in China. *Sexually Transmitted Diseases, 34*(1), 1.

Wang, H., Chen, R. Y., Ding, G., Ma, Y., Ma, J., Jiao, J. H., … & Wang, N. (2009). Prevalence and predictors of HIV infection among female sex workers in Kaiyuan city, Yunnan province, China. *International Journal of Infectious Diseases, 13*(2), 162–169.

Wang, L., Zeng, G., Luo, J., Duo, S., Xing, G., Guo-wei, D., … & Ning, W. (2010). HIV transmission risk among serodiscordant couples: A retrospective study of former plasma donors in Henan, China. *Journal of Acquired Immune Deficiency Syndromes, 55*(2), 232.

WHO (World Health Organization). (2014). *HIV prevention, diagnosis, treatment and care for key populations: Consolidated guidelines*. Geneva, Switzerland: World Health Organization.

WHO, UNICEF & UNAIDS. (2011). Global HIV/AIDS response: Epidemic update and health sector progress towards Universal Access, Progress Report 2011. Retrieved from: www.who.int/hiv/pub/progress_report2011/en

Wong, W. C. W. & Yilin, W. (2003). A qualitative study on HIV risk behaviors and medical needs of sex workers in a China/Myanmar border town. *AIDS Patient Care and STDs, 17*(8), 417–422.

Wu, J., Meng, Z., Xu, J., Lei, Y., Jin, L., Zhong, P., ... & Su, B. (2013). New emerging recombinant HIV-1 strains and close transmission linkage of HIV-1 strains in the Chinese MSM population indicate a new epidemic risk. *PLoS ONE, 8*(1), e54322. doi:10.1371/journal.pone.0054322.

Wu, Z., Sullivan, S. G., Wang, Y., Rotheram-Borus, M. J. & Detels, R. (2007). Evolution of China's response to HIV/AIDS. *The Lancet, 369*(9562), 679–90.

Xiao, Y., Kristensen, S., Sun, J., Lu, L. & Vermund, S. H. (2007). Expansion of HIV/AIDS in China: Lessons from Yunnan province. *Social Science & Medicine, 64*(3), 665–675.

Xiaolei, W., Lu, L., Dong, Z. X., Chi, Z., Wei, L., Jun, Z. W. & Hesketh, T. (2013). Rising women's status, modernisation and persisting son preference in China. *Indian Journal of Gender Studies, 20*(1), 85–109.

Yang, C., Latkin, C., Luan, R. & Nelson, K. (2010). Condom use with female sex workers among male clients in Sichuan Province, China: The role of interpersonal and venue-level factors. *Journal of Urban Health, 87*(2), 292–303.

Yang, H., Li, X., Stanton, B., Liu, H., Liu, H., Wang, N., ... & Chen, X. (2005). Heterosexual transmission of HIV in China: A systematic review of behavioral studies in the past two decades. *Sexually Transmitted Diseases, 32*(5), 270–280.

Yi, H., Mantell, J. E., Wu, R., Lu, Z., Zeng, J. & Wan, Y. (2010). A profile of HIV risk factors in the context of sex work environments among migrant female sex workers in Beijing, China. *Psychology, Health & Medicine, 15*(2), 172–187.

Zhang, F., Hsu, M., Yu, L., Wen, Y. & Pan, J. (2006). Initiation of the national free antiretroviral therapy program in rural China. In J. Kaufman, A. Kleinman & T. Saich (Eds.), *AIDS and social policy in China* (pp. 96–124). Cambridge, MA: Harvard University Asia Center.

Zhao, R., Gao, H., Shi, X., Tucker, J. D., Yang, Z., Min, X., ... & Wang, N. (2005). Sexually transmitted disease/HIV and heterosexual risk among miners in townships of Yunnan province, China. *AIDS Patient Care & STDs, 19*(12), 848–852.

Zhou, X., Yan, Z. & Hesketh, T. (2013). Depression and aggression in never-married men in China: A growing problem. *Social Psychiatry and Psychiatric Epidemiology, 48*(7), 1087–1093.

7 The situation in Yunnan

Coming events cast their shadows before them.

山雨欲来风满楼

Current operational environment

NGOs interviewed at the time of writing were taking a very pragmatic approach to the use of current funds in the hopes of continuing their programmes until the government funding was released. China had just been elevated to being a middle-income country and there was still a lot of uncertainty about what this would mean for HIV/AIDS programming. In the past, China had received funding from external donors and the Global Fund but Beijing would have to carry the responsibility for continued funding from this point onwards. Wang (pers. comm., October 2013) stated that, in his opinion, quite a number of community-based organisations (CBOs) and non-governmental organisations (NGOs) would be unable to survive the transition from receiving international non-governmental organisation (INGO) funds to being mainly government-funded. However, there was no real unanimity on whether this was a totally negative course of events. Wu (pers. comm., November 2013) commented:

> The question about NGOs and CBOs should not be about whether there are enough of them or if they have enough money but rather whether they are valuable and if not they should close down and make the money they have available to others that are making an impact.

It seems clear that a complete overhaul of the organisations currently working on HIV/AIDS in China is underway. Whether this ultimately translates into a more streamlined but efficient NGO/CBOs engagement, or whether it opens up the door to greater shortfalls and lack of programming, remains to be seen.

Consideration of the current NGO/CBOs; participation reveals that the majority are working in the area of policy implementation and overarching programmes such as methadone maintenance therapy (MMT) and needle exchange, antiretroviral therapy (ART) and condom distribution to female sex workers

(FSWs) and migrant workers. Of the organisations where it was possible to undertake research, none of them were extensively involved in assisting clients with employment, training, housing or advocacy. They did provide some food, clothing and shelter particularly for homeless injection drug users (IDUs) and FSWs. While free programmes, such as MMT, ART and condom distribution, do uphold some of the human security needs of people living with HIV/AIDS (PLWHA), they fall short of addressing many of their essential requirements.

This is particularly so in the public health model of treatment as prevention (TasP) currently preferred in China. TasP is focused more on protecting the general population by getting HIV+ individuals on ART than meeting the societal needs of key populations. Policy occurs as a top-down initiative and Beijing has little control about how this is implemented at ground level. Therefore, these initiatives often face problems in community settings. For example, Beijing is committed to initiatives, such as MMT and needle exchange, but at the local level they are often unwanted and communities react negatively. These problems in a community setting only exacerbate issues of stigma and marginalisation.

This partially stems from China's division of labour allocation and current conceptualisation of HIV/AIDS as mainly occurring in key populations comprising the more undesirable segments of the community (Ding, Li & Ji, 2011; Yang & Kleinman, 2008). Understandably, the police are concerned with protecting the public from criminal elements within the community. Thus, for many of these officers, the main focus of their interactions with PWID and FSWs is to remove them from public spaces. With police being responsible for issues concerning FSWs and PWID, these cohorts often find out their HIV status through compulsory testing upon arrest and incarceration in detention centres (R. Li et al., 2018; Wu, pers. comm., November 2013). However, this has the knock-on effect of reducing the efficacy of HIV/AIDS prevention efforts, as key populations are reluctant to attend clinics or other programmes for fear of the police.

One NGO reported that there were still problems with the operating environment and that on the day following outreach events FSWs in attendance had been arrested by police (Wu, pers. comm., November 2013). Wu commented, 'it creates a lack of trust between FSWs and the organisations trying to provide assistance'. As such, interviews with organisations on the ground have confirmed the need for education of law enforcement agencies to better deal with high-risk individuals engaging in illegal activities (Philbin & Zhang, 2010).

During interviews in both Ruili and Kunming, participants commented that they did not routinely attend outreach services and drop-in centres due to fear of arrest. The fear of arrest and incarceration still acts as a deterrent for those wishing to access service organisations and medical interventions. Wang (pers. comm., December 2013) stated: 'Sometimes police need to meet targets and so will arrest PWID and FSWs to meet those targets.' Interestingly, this scenario does not appear to be applied everywhere as one CBO working with PWID commented that the police were aware of their drop-in centre and, while not actually supporting their efforts, did nothing to hinder their activities.

The effect of hard-line policing of key populations has proven to be detrimental in addressing HIV/AIDS epidemics. Without addressing the fundamental needs and human security threats of these populations, a sustainable response to HIV/AIDS will be impossible. Punitive legislation and policing practices should be revised where practicable, to allow meaningful engagement of key populations (WHO, 2014). Not only does hard-line policing create a climate of fear but it also adds to the stigma experienced by key populations, as it reinforces the stereotype that they are bad people. In short, while some policing is, of course, necessary, the types of results stemming from *strike hard* campaigns are of little help.

Significantly, Beijing has made some very encouraging steps towards addressing the needs of highly mobile PLWHA and there are now some services addressing their mobility and their reluctance to publicise their HIV+ status. In Yunnan, they have begun using a new rapid test. Whereas the time from testing to notification of HIV status formerly took weeks, individuals are now able to find out their status almost immediately. In Dehong prefecture, the period of time from testing to treatment can now be completed in 10 days (Wu, pers. comm., November 2013). This is having a positive impact on drop-out rates as individuals are able to receive their results before moving on. In saying that, some issues still have to be resolved concerning the rapid tests returning false positives (Wu, pers. comm., November, 2013). However, regardless of temporary technical issues, this is a positive contribution to the existing interventions.

Another positive policy change for highly mobile populations concerns universal access to treatment for PLWHA. Whereas for most individuals the *hukou* system requires them to obtain medical treatment in their registered *hukou*, the situation has recently changed for PLWHA. HIV+ individuals are now able to access services such as ART in any *hukou* in China. This is an extremely important initiative when considering the high mobility of high-risk individuals, such as migrants, FSWs and PWID, who are often outside their *hukou* and therefore previously needed to return home for treatment. It is a relatively new initiative by Beijing to address the expanding HIV/AIDS epidemic and does make a positive contribution to the human security of PLWHA.

Already in Yunnan, PLWHA are able to access a range of free services but now, if they are HIV+, they are able to access these services anywhere in China. Moreover, they are able to access this treatment without the need to identify as FSW, PWID or MSM. This is an initiative that covers all provinces. Wu (pers. comm., November 2013) commented that HIV+ individuals are given a type of universal medical code, or for the purposes of this book unicode, that allows them to access ART treatment in any province. However, this is only available for people who have already tested as HIV+. Their status must be established through the usual testing methods.

The old policy of only being able to access treatment within an individual's *hukou* made it extremely difficult for highly mobile PLWHA to maintain ART regimes. In spite of this positive progress, there was no mention of the unicode being applicable in cases of opportunistic infections (OI). In Yunnan, treatment for OI is free, as is the testing, but Chen (pers. comm., November 2013) stated that this was only accessible in Yunnan. As such, it seems that this is not covered by the unicode in other provinces. Whether this is a detrimental oversight in the policy is unknown and further research would be beneficial in understanding the full ramifications of the unicode and any current shortfalls in the policy.

While this new policy will undoubtedly prove to be extremely beneficial to China's continuing efforts to manage HIV/AIDS, many of those who need the unicode do not know that it exists. The information regarding these new rules has not successfully been disseminated and, as a result, many highly mobile PLWHA are still unaware that they can access treatment in any province. As such, if they are unable to access services through their *hukou*, many people, particularly those who are highly mobile and/or involved in illegal activity, do not access services at all. One of requirements of the ART is the need for PLWHA to attend clinics to receive their drug regimens; as already stated, this has proven difficult for highly mobile populations. The unicode addresses this issue and has the potential to significantly assist mobile PLWHA in China.

In order to successfully address the needs of highly mobile PLWHA in accessing ART regimes outside of their *hukou*, Beijing must increase their efforts to make the information regarding the unicode more widely available. This represents a shortfall in an otherwise positive contribution to the current situation for PLWHA in China. Although ART regimes must still be administered in government-run facilities (with the inherent fear of stigmatisation, as already discussed), the considerable financial benefits to vulnerable populations able to use the unicode make undergoing ART a more affordable proposition.

In addition to the problems of the unicode for individuals within the *hukou* system, there are significant problems with cross-border migration from Myanmar. Foreign nationals are not eligible for free HIV/AIDS services and yet they make a significant contribution to the ongoing HIV/AIDS epidemics in Yunnan. In a research project testing 1 in every 500 individuals crossing the borders between Yunnan and the neighbouring countries, it was found that 0.85 per cent of the 280,961 individuals tested were HIV+. The rate increased dramatically for the borders in Dehong prefecture with 5.12 per cent or 1,163/22,699 individuals testing HIV+ (Wang et al., 2015; Xuan et al., 2018). This represents a significant area for concern for HIV/AIDS programmes in Yunnan.

TasP in China: challenges and shortfalls

Information provided by Chen (pers. comm., December 2013) confirms that, for Chinese citizens, ART is available to everyone who is HIV+ after they have gone through testing and compulsory counselling (F. Zhang et al., 2006). This counselling takes the form of three to four visits to a doctor approved to administer ART. The first session is generally used in dealing with the shock an individual feels upon learning of the HIV+ status. The next few sessions are spent in discussion as patients struggle to come to terms with the fact that they will need to take this medication at 11a.m., every day, for the rest of their lives. However, there are many PLWHA who are still afraid to obtain health care. While Beijing has adopted a 'zero discrimination' policy, there are still problems surrounding health care as almost 50 per cent of PLWHA are afraid to disclose their status and 80 per cent are afraid of being blamed or refused services (R. Li et al., 2018). This means that while ART is available, not everyone eligible is on an ART regimen.

In addition to this, the margin for non-compliance in their daily drug-taking programme is very small. Chen (pers. comm., December 2013) conveyed that if a PLWHA misses three doses, their entire ART regime may be rendered useless and they may develop drug resistance. In order to maintain viral suppression strict patient adherence levels of greater than 95 per cent are required (Smith, 2005). However, 40–60 per cent of PLWHA are less than 90 per cent adherent and this has a tendency to decrease over time (Smith, 2005). This is a serious and ongoing problem for PWID as they often forget to take medications due to being under the influence of drugs, or simply not getting out of bed on time to take it when scheduled (Chen, pers. comm., December, 2013). As a result of this, PWID have a high drop-off rate and currently less than 30 per cent of all HIV+ PWID are on ART and there is a high drug resistance in this group of PLWHA (Chen, pers. comm., July 2014).

The first three to six months on ART are extremely difficult for patients due to brutal drug side effects (Garcia-Prats, McMeans, Ferry & Klish, 2010; Gill, 2006). Chen (pers. comm., November 2013) commented that there are a great many of them and that a large number of people stop therapy because they are unable to cope with the side effects. Of those undertaking ART, a number get sick and actually die from taking the drug cocktail. Although side effects generally diminish within the three-to-six-month time period, this initial phase, coupled with the knowledge that this is a lifetime commitment. is often overwhelming for many. Chen (pers. comm., November 2013) states, 'For some, it is too much.'

This becomes very problematic within the national Chinese TasP policy paradigm. As such, doctors are encouraged or even pressured to get people on ART and maintain this for their lifetimes. This means that doctors are invested in ensuring that PLWHA begin and then continue therapy and, as a result, doctors continue to encourage and counsel patients towards an ART regime (Chen, pers. comm., December 2013). Additionally, the majority of PRC funding is channelled into this policy rather than other prevention programmes. Chen (pers. comm., December 2013) who, in addition to working for a HIV/AIDS NGO, is also a medical doctor commented: '[T]he medicine itself is not enough. If they have poor nutrition in the first three to six months, they can actually get sick and die from taking the therapy.'

Chen went on to comment that while the blood tests to ascertain HIV status are free, the requisite kidney and liver function tests are not. These tests are required regularly (every 6–12 months) for the remainder of the patient's life. However, in Chen's opinion, one of the greatest barriers to PLWHA receiving treatment is transportation costs:

[T]reatment and testing are free. The worst problem is transportation – each county has only one hospital that will distribute ARV meds. Not only that but if the hospital is far away, they may need to stay overnight. This is complicated as they lose one or two days of income as well as having to pay for transport and accommodation – too expensive for many.

Unfortunately, problems due to lack of willingness to participate made it difficult to establish whether any NGOs exclusively addressed these needs or the full extent towards which the human security of PLWHA is considered at a grass-roots level. However, one interviewee mentioned some programmes that assisted in the distribution of food and clothing; the re-training of PWID; the provision of small micro-finance type loans in order to set up small business; and organisations involved in teaching handicrafts.

Thus, it is safe to assume that such programmes do exist but it is not possible to comment on the extent or efficacy of these programmes. However, when asked, Chen (pers. comm., July 2014) commented that these were smaller organisations that were mostly urban-based and that, while they were making a positive contribution, they were limited in scope. Unfortunately, other programmes that are in operation such as MMT, PWID and FSW outreach and drop-in services or condom distribution are plagued by difficulties, such as lack of funding, community opposition and issues with law enforcement agencies. As such, this could be one area where HIV/AIDS programming in China could be improved, particularly the case in highly mobile at-risk populations whose members may be unemployed and living in conditions of poverty.

To date, Ruili remains at the epicentre of the HIV/AIDS epidemic in China (Chen, pers. comm., December 2013). Much of the HIV/AIDS programming, however, is run from Kunming, which is home to the larger NGOs engaged in assisting CBOs working with the highly mobile and marginalised populations.in the border areas. One of the reasons for this is that Kunming is a destination city for illegal migrants, whether internal economic migrants or those who have crossed international borders. It also has large, highly mobile FSW, PWID and MSM populations.

Marginalised and mobile populations

FSWs

In Yunnan, there is no one particular red light area where sex workers congregate. Instead, they are spread throughout the city. Wang (pers. comm., October 2013) remarked:

For low-level FSWs in general, it is difficult to deliver programmes as they are spread out rather than working in one area. It takes time to go from place to place as well as money and as such it [*sic*] not achievable or practical.

Many of them are only contactable via telephone or the Internet. Therefore, it is difficult to estimate the exact numbers operating within Yunnan and there is no way that outreach workers are able to provide services from a particular location.

Additionally, Wang disclosed that there were very few CBOs actually dealing with lower-level sex workers. He states:

> There is a real gap in coverage for those populations and more research needs to be done in these areas in order to find out how best to target these difficult-to-reach low-level populations. The government only supports programmes focusing on the higher-level, easy-access populations.

While there are some drop-in centres that do include lower-level FSWs in their clientele, they more closely resemble offices.

Rather than welcoming spaces where individuals might congregate for support, they are locations where condoms may be collected and where other services (such as rapid testing) can be obtained if desired. Sex workers do not assemble in these locations as they are often afraid the police will have them under surveillance and that they will be arrested when they leave. As a result of this difficulty in accessing FSW populations, there are no simple ways to ensure that education and prevention programmes are reaching the targeted populations with the levels of saturation needed to ensure significant changes in behaviour.

When FSWs are contacted, there are often problems communicating between individuals. Throughout Yunnan, which is home to 25 minority nationality groups (accounting for 33.4 per cent of Yunnan's entire population of 43 million people) and people from neighbouring states that have crossed the border (Lu et al., 2008), language barriers complicate matters as communication with FSWs, and other at-risk groups, in their ethnic language is an enduring problem, due to lack of available translators. For those few in the ethnic minorities who do speak some Mandarin Chinese, there is the possibility that information and understanding may be lost in translation due to a lack of fluency. There may often be a discrepancy in the usage and meaning attributed to the words and concepts being presented. What one party understands may be completely misunderstood by the other, regardless of their ability to use the same words.

This becomes even more of an issue when the concepts being discussed are complex. Explanations concerning prevention methods, educational material and medical concepts revolving around ART regimes are paramount and yet difficult to convey without language fluency. Han Chinese speakers almost exclusively staff the majority of NGOs and CBOs, and while a number of them are able to speak reasonable English, they are generally unable to speak any of the ethnic languages of the region with any fluency. In addition to which, there seemed to be very little information concerning HIV/AIDS available in any of the minority languages. There is little doubt that, in Yunnan, HIV/AIDS outreaches and education and prevention programmes are being hampered by these difficulties in communication.

This is certainly the case in Ruili where there are high numbers of FSWs from Myanmar and rural ethnic areas of Yunnan. Many of these sex workers are young women who have crossed the porous international border between Ruili and Muse. They are poor, uneducated and often as young as 15 years old (Chen, pers. comm., December 2013). There are no real outreaches for these young women and no drop-in centres in the areas where they live and work. Also, there are difficulties in communicating with these FSWs, as the majority of them do not speak Chinese or even Burmese. As a result, because of the vast numbers of minority groups in the border areas near Ruili quite often three or four languages may be represented, making it very difficult for HIV/AIDS prevention programmes to meet their needs linguistically.

This complicates the situation in more than one way as even if they were inclined to seek help (which in general they are not, due to their illegality), they are unable to clearly express their concerns. As such, due to these communication problems; the illegal nature of their profession; and their status as an illegal alien in China, they remain elusive and do not seek the services of medical professionals. They are also reticent in attending outreach services; which makes it difficult for service providers to deliver efficient and worthwhile programmes and services. Due to these difficulties, it is unclear whether these FSWs have any real understanding or even knowledge of HIV/AIDS and the need to use condoms to protect themselves and their clients.

Additionally, there is no clear data on how many FSWs are operating in these areas or the percentage of these FSWs who may be HIV+. One CBO based in Ruili involved in outreach to FSWs also provided some education to the clients of FSWs through the delivery of education programmes to migrant construction workers (which will be discussed in more depth in a later section of this chapter). This CBO also visited villages and provided educational information to women and children before they became involved in sex work, while children of HIV+ individuals were provided with fun programmes and support networks by this CBO.

Zhao (pers. comm., December 2013) oversees these programmes and commented that although their centre operated as an outreach drop-in centre, in reality, very few clients ever came to the premises. Rather, a small number of FSWs act as intermediaries, visiting the centre each evening to collect a large number of condoms, which they then distribute among their peer networks. This was also true of education programmes targeting FSWs. As a result, it was often difficult to ascertain the efficacy of the outreach efforts provided by the CBO. There is no direct empirical evidence being returned about the impact of these services on the levels of increasing HIV/AIDS understanding and awareness, for instance, as is it the peers who do access the services who are relied upon to disseminate the information provided by the CBO. Regardless, the organisation was positive that they were having a tangible, if difficult to measure, impact in addressing some of the higher-risk behaviours of FSWs and their clients.

Unfortunately, there are still high-risk behaviours that the organisation has had little success in influencing, largely because they are steeped in cultural or superstitious reasoning. For example, Zhao commented that one very real issue his organisation faced was the belief that sex workers could not turn away the first client of the day, regardless of concerns they may have about the client. This is due to the belief held by many FSWs that if they declined the first client, then they would have an unsuccessful day/evening of work. Therefore, if the client insisted on not using a condom, the FSWs felt compelled to agree to these terms, despite knowledge of the role of 100 per cent condom use in preventing HIV transmission. This first client has an inordinate amount of power in shaping the sexual interaction and this indicates that it is essential to increase efforts to provide HIV/AIDS programmes to the clients of FSWs. Zhao indicated that there were difficulties in convincing FSWs to use condoms for both commercial and private sexual encounters.

Even when FSWs do adopt a 100 per cent condom use approach to all commercial sexual exchanges, they do not adopt the same approach to their private sexual encounters, thereby increasing their vulnerability to HIV transmission. The absolute necessity of the need for condom use in these private sexual exchanges is clearly demonstrated when one considers that their sexual partners may have multiple sexual encounters with different partners and engage in high-risk behaviours, including intravenous drug use. In addition to this, many FSWs had difficulty understanding that their personal sexual partners may be HIV+ and that they should therefore employ 100 per cent condom usage in their private sexual interactions as well as their commercial sexual exchanges (G. W. Ding et al., 2014).

Some FSWs believe that the use of condoms with their regular partners may create a barrier to intimacy or be viewed as mistrust in their partner (Ulibarri, Roesch, Rangel, Staines, Amaro & Strathdee, 2015). One of the ways that FSWs distinguished between their regular partners and clients was through the use of condoms (Ulibarri et al., 2015), demonstrating that their HIV knowledge concerning how the virus is transmitted remained focused on 'illicit' sex, that is, commercial sexual exchange, rather than all sexual encounters, both commercial and private. Therefore, they pose very serious risks to the HIV status of their partners.

An interview with an FSW advocacy worker and current FSW from Myanmar who was in attendance at the AIDS 2014 conference in Melbourne shed light on the situation. Her anonymity was assured and due to her situation as an advocacy worker and presence at the AIDS 2014 conference (for the specific purpose of providing information concerning FSWs in Myanmar), it was determined that interviewing her posed no fears concerning her safety or vulnerability as a FSW. For the sake of anonymity, a pseudonym, Lily, has been allocated to her. In her interview Lily (pers. comm., July 2014) confirmed that she had worked on the Chinese side of the border as a sex worker. In her role as a FSW advocate she had been given the opportunity to work with many other sex workers both inside Myanmar and along the China/Myanmar border. She suggested that eventually, many of the Myanmar sex workers end up working along the border areas as they feel convinced that there are more opportunities for work there.

When asked about condom usage and whether FSWs were given adequate supplies, Lily responded by recounting an incidence that happened in Myanmar (this is elaborated on in Case study 2.1). She said that there was a problem, particularly in the more remote areas of Myanmar, and that NGO workers exhibited stigmatising attitudes towards FSWs. Lily expressed a great deal of anger at this situation and added that in addition to the attitude of the NGO worker, there were not enough condoms provided to meet the needs of the FSWs in the town.

Lily provided information that suggests that the regular allocation of condoms per FSW for that area was 60 over a three-month period. That allows for 100 per cent condom use for less than one client per day over that time frame. If the FSWs had numerous clients in a month, their supplies would last less than one month. She did report that the situation was better in more urban areas. Anecdotally, then, there seems evidence to suggest that even when condoms are supplied to FSWs, there is an alarming deficit. This does not diminish the need for FSWs to be proactive in securing their own health and undertaking some measure to procure condoms for themselves, but it does reveal a shortfall in current condom supplies administered by HIV/AIDS prevention programmes.

There are also still a number of FSWs who are willing to forgo condom usage when the client offers more money for the transaction. One of the reasons for this is that they still have a poor knowledge or understanding of STIs including HIV (Zhu et al., 2012). One study found that there were a number of significant reasons why FSWs still opted not to use condoms in commercial sexual encounters (Jie, Ciyong, Xueqing, Hui & Lingyao, 2012). First, those who do not use condoms are generally younger, have more customers per day and tend to have lower levels of education. Second, the prevailing climate of the sex venue (or lack of venue) and social support were key determinants. They were also willing to believe that men were safe, based on their word and on their own observations as to whether the client's genitalia appeared normal, their overall cleanliness and appearance, and stereotypes. Lastly, their occupation required them to make money and please the client, therefore if the client did not want to use a condom, and was willing to pay more (some customers pay twice as much), then it was seen as acceptable (Jie et al., 2012).

There is also an emerging HIV/AIDS problem among elderly men in China (those over the age of 50) who are contracting the disease through frequenting low-level FSWs (Wu, pers. comm., November 2013). The men find it difficult to use condoms due to flaccid erections and the FSWs are ill equipped to cope with this. As a result, peer education initiatives are now in progress in order to teach FSWs ways to please their clients without having to use condoms (such as hand jobs and fellatio). They are also teaching FSWs how to use female condoms without the undesirable side effects such as excessive noise during use (Wu, pers. comm., November, 2013). Zhao provided anecdotal evidence to suggest that these initiatives were somewhat successful even though there were still difficulties. When introduced correctly, the female condom could make a positive contribution to condom usage rates for FSWs (Liao et al., 2011). This situation is an ongoing and relatively new phenomenon and, as a result, there is very little conclusive data concerning its success in ensuring 100 per cent condom usage.

Another situation that appears to be emerging in the context of FSWs is the push for FSWs to induce clients to take drugs during sexual encounters (Lily, pers. comm., July 2014). This is specifically the case along the China/Myanmar border areas. In interviewing Lily, she revealed that in sex worker establishments on both the Chinese and Myanmar side of the border, sex workers are compelled to push drugs on their customers. It was revealed that when they fail to do so, they are given a monetary fine by the brothel. When asked what kinds of drugs were being pushed, Lily stated that in general they were using synthetic drugs, such as methamphetamine and amphetamine-type stimulants, such as ecstasy and ketamine. She reported that coerced injection drug use was not likely. The FSWs were also expected to use the drugs along with the customers. This is an alarming trend considering the established research linking drug use with high-risk behaviours (Yao et al., 2012).

Notably, Chen (pers. comm., December 2013) stated that there was very little understanding of the scope of the problem for FSWs in Ruili, and in China in general, due to lack of research in this area. He commented that within the city of Ruili, there were only three CBOs involved in outreach to sex workers. Added to which, the scope of services to FSWs was limited, not only by lack of funding but also due to some of the issues raised above. This is particularly concerning, since the main clientele of FSWs in Ruili are highly mobile long-distance truck drivers.

The impact of long-distance truck drivers on HIV/AIDS epidemics on the Yunnan/Myanmar border confirms the established literature concerning the global impact of long-distance truck drivers in the spread of HIV (Oluwoye, 2007; Zhang, Li, Hong, Zhou, Liu & Stanton, 2013). While there is little data concerning their influence in the HIV epidemic in Yunnan, there is ample evidence linking them to the spread of HIV in other epidemics. Some of the reasons for this include extensive time away from family support networks, frequent encounters with FSWs, drug taking, and low levels of condom use with partners and FSWs (Apostolopoulos, Sönmez & Massengale, 2013; Sunmola, 2005; Zhang et al., 2013). High-risk behaviours, when combined with their ability to introduce HIV long distances into new locations along trucking routes make long-distance truck drivers a serious threat to the spread of HIV. Issues of high mobility; lack of community connection; the need to sleep in their trucks at loading sites; and low incomes contribute to a lack of human security in these cohorts. Their high-risk behaviours have a direct correlation to the situation faced by FSWs and contribute to bridging scenarios for HIV passing into the general population.

PWID

In Yunnan, many of the same problems associated with accessing FSW populations remain true for IDUs. They are very wary of those not already forming a part of their circle of known associates. There is an extremely high level of stigma attached to this cohort of individuals. This is particularly the case when they have tested HIV+. There are few opportunities for employment and those who are employed before ascertaining their HIV status often find themselves unable to work in their previous occupations due to people's rejection of them as HIV+ individuals. In short, they were no longer considered acceptable as members of the general community. Additionally, while many PWID access MMT programmes, there are still a number of those individuals also continuing to use injection drugs such as heroin, meaning their risk factor to HIV transmission remains the same, it does not drop. High rates of drug use seem to be the case in many locations throughout Yunnan. For example, Yuxi, a city renowned for drug trafficking and high usage rates, has some of the highest rates of HIV and STIs in China. From 2005 to 2016, there were 3,092 unique HIV+ diagnoses, of which 326 were newly infected in 2016 (Su et al., 2018).

Having observed a number of micro-financing interviews for families impacted by HIV/AIDS and drug use, it seemed that their stories resonated throughout the community. While they had been previously employed in reputable employment, prior to contracting HIV, after becoming HIV+, they were unable to maintain their positions either through dismissal or, in the case of self-employed individuals, because customers no longer frequented their business. For example, one woman had previously operated a business selling noodles but customers shunned her business upon her HIV+ status becoming public knowledge. For some women, who were responsible for the family income, their only recourse was to turn to sex work. As a result of this, many families visited were living in situations of extreme poverty and facing severe food insecurity.

In another example, a HIV+ PWID had inherited a sizeable home from her deceased parents. While this might have been rented out in other circumstances, she lived there alone (her sister who had also been a PWID had recently died from AIDS-related causes) as no one was prepared to rent a room from her. Her circumstances were dire, as even though she had a prospective source of income, she was unable to access its potential. Rather than being a positive part of her life, owning the house was problematic as she was unable to afford the upkeep and it was deteriorating around her. When we visited her, she was eating one small meal a day and had turned to low-level sex work in order to survive. Her story is representative of all seven interviews that were undertaken with vulnerable families on that day.

In Ruili, another CBO working with PWID had a range of services on offer that extended beyond their main cohort to include FSWs and family members living with PWID. As well as this, they provided HIV blood testing, food, basic medical treatment and essential supplies to homeless PWID who had temporary camps around the city of Ruili. In fact, they commented that 85 per cent of their service outreach was to homeless PWID and their families. They understood the need to deal with individuals holistically, in order to make any real impact in their lives.

For outreach interventions to have a long-term positive impact on the lives of PWID, it is necessary that they have shelter and good nutrition. Addressing these basic needs means that they resist the need for excessive mobility (almost nightly in many cases), thus improving their accessibility and health outcomes. Additionally, the brutal toll on the body of those on ART medications means that good nutrition is essential (Chen, pers. comm., December 2013). Thus, addressing these human security needs allows the optimal cascade of care through continued patient follow-up and increased retention rates for those undertaking ART.

Many of the clients of PWID outreach centres are illegal Myanmar nationals who have crossed the border between Ruili and Muse. Therefore, their outreach programmes for PWID do not distinguish between Chinese and Myanmar nationals. Countless numbers of the PWID receiving services from outreach organisations were suffering from lack of nutrition, illnesses and suppurating sores at needle injection sites on their bodies. As is common with many of the highly mobile PWID and FSWs, they were also loath to seek official help in any form. Organisations in Ruili provide services for each individual regardless of the existing official policy, which states that only Chinese nationals are eligible for services and treatment. Many Chinese officials in Ruili and other parts of China are aware of these activities and supportive of CBOs providing these services to nationals of the surrounding states who are residing in China. While this does not infer that Beijing as a whole or the officers as individuals are supportive of a human security approach, it does provide scope for NGOs and CBOs to implement services that may mitigate some of the human (in)security prevalent among these populations.

These organisations are also involved in Naloxone Hydrochloride (Naloxone) peer programmes that involve training up individuals to be able to administer the drug in cases of overdose. Naloxone works in overdose situations by blocking opioids like heroin and methadone from attaching to the opioid receptors in the brain (Morgan & Jones, 2018). As such, it reverses the overdose symptoms. In China, PWID outreach programmes train peers to provide immediate response to overdoses of heroin by members of their network. Once trained, they are then provided with a number of doses of Naloxone. They commit to being available 24 hours a day, seven days a week. They provide PWID in their network with a mobile phone number that they can call in case of accidental overdose. The peer is then able to attend to the overdose victim by administering Naloxone. This is an essential service, as many PWID will not seek out medical interventions due to fear of arrest. The organisations involved with this outreach estimate that a number of individuals have been successfully revived due to this intervention.

In terms of human security, this is a positive initiative as it lessens stigma (by using peer outreach); strengthens community linkages (by developing relationships within the cohorts); and addresses the fundamental need for these groups to have access to medical services (life-saving medicines in case of overdose). These services are offered, irrespective of nationality or financial considerations. The individual needing the service is the main referent being considered in this bottom-up approach to addressing the health needs of PWID as key populations in HIV/AIDS epidemics.

Migrants

In Yunnan, there are large numbers of migrants. It is both a high destination province and a source province for migrants both from other areas and across international borders. One study in 2012–2016 tested 2,961,530 individuals at China's frontier entrance and exit ports (including land, sea and air). They found a prevalence rate of 0.95 per cent, of which 79.0 per cent were Chinese and the remaining 21.0 per cent were foreigners (Wang, Yang., Zhu, Mo & Tan, 2018). When considering that prevalence rates over 1 per cent constitute a generalised epidemic, this figure is alarming. Of the people tested, 54.4 per cent of the individuals were migrant labour.

While many of these migrants are engaging in legitimate, legal enterprises, many are in China illegally, and engaged in illegal HIV/AIDS high-risk behaviours. FSWs and PWID populations can be considered 'migrant' in their high mobility but they are categorised differently from economic migrants, who are engaged in 'legitimate' employment endeavours. However, the economic migrants in Yunnan often also turn to drug use or become clients of FSWs.

One interviewee delivering outreach programmes to migrant construction and factory workers works in conjunction with organisations, such as the All-China Women's Federation and China's construction authorising body, to present mandatory HIV/AIDS education and prevention programmes. In addition, they provide these groups with free condoms and lubricants. In combination with other travelling businessmen and workers, the floating migrants generally form a large percentage of the clients of FSWs. The groups are extremely important vectors for the expansion of HIV/AIDS in China and thus are a non-traditional security threat.

Zhao (pers. comm., December 2013) remarked that these migrants relocated every three months so it was difficult to ascertain how much of the knowledge gained through these education programmes is acted upon in a long-term manner. However, they are able to receive some immediate feedback concerning the efficacy of these programmes. They administer an end-of-course test that provides a reasonable, if incomplete, picture of levels of migrant workers' understanding. They also monitor numbers of condoms received by these clients. There is also anecdotal evidence from FSWs to suggest that migrant workers who have been through these programmes have increased their rates of condom usage. Conversely, the dearth of empirical evidence does not allow confirmation that the programmes are being delivered in the best possible manner or the long-term behavioural changes that may ensue.

The clients of FSWs, in general, and particularly labour migrants, are an under-researched vector for HIV/AIDS transmission in China. Within these migrant communities, issues of stigma towards individuals with STIs and PLWHA create barriers that prevent migrants from initiating self-protection activities, such as HIV and STI testing and communication with partners concerning positive diagnosis (Mendelsohn, Calzavara, Light, Burchell, Ren & Kang, 2015). Therefore, outreach and education programmes for the current

250 million migrants, whether in the workplace or in drop-in centres, should be increased in order to maximise coverage for these populations. There is still a shortage of such programmes in China. The lack of information available is an unequivocal human security risk as high-risk behaviours continue to threaten both individual security as well as the security of the nation-state.

This is particularly germane in the case of long-distance truck drivers crossing international borders between Myanmar and China, or Vietnam and China, or Laos and China. High levels of boredom, language barriers and a lack of finances make these economic migrants especially vulnerable, as research confirms that they are more likely to engage in high-risk behaviours. Consideration of these truck drivers is exceptionally apropos considering the general ignorance concerning HIV/AIDS predominant in Myanmar.[1]

In Ruili, at any one time, there are thousands of truck drivers from Myanmar. In general, truck drivers crossing the border are required to offload their cargos and reload them onto Chinese trucks for the journey into China. The reverse exchange also operates in the same manner. In this way, foreign truck drivers do not drive in another nation-state. Due to this exchange, truck drivers are often required to wait in border areas for as long as three weeks before their loads are processed. They live in their truck during that time and service industries have set up around these encampments. In general, the truck drivers are poorly educated and have little to no understanding or knowledge of HIV/AIDS. Due to their high levels of boredom, they are prone to seeking diversion with sex workers and other high-risk behaviours. As a result of their low incomes, they are only able to frequent lower hierarchy FSWs who themselves have little understanding of issues surrounding HIV/AIDS. These FSWs operate from hairdressing and massage shopfronts in streets and alleys in the vicinity of the long-distance truck driver encampments.

One recent study found that 5 per cent of long-distance truck drivers from Myanmar had sex with occasional sexual partners, including FSWs. Additionally, 7.1 per cent reported that they did not use condoms during these encounters. A number of them were also found to be PWID (Zhou et al., 2014). When assessing the HIV prevalence of these truck drivers, it was reported to be as high as 3.5–8.8 per cent (Zhou et al., 2014). The study speculates that due to their ability to spread the HIV virus over long distances, they may be implicated in the spread of HIV from Myanmar into China. The tendency for long-distance truck drivers to exacerbate the spread of HIV in regional epidemics and the global pandemic as a whole has been confirmed in other research. Epidemiological results suggest that long-distance truck drivers may also have played a significant role in the expansion of HIV sub-type CRF01_AE from heterosexuals to PWID (Zhou et al., 2014).

An existing truck driver drop-in centre in Ruili provides an important service to long-distance truck drivers from Myanmar and may have significant implications in halting the spread of HIV in the region. Currently, they have a turnover of about 1,000 truck drivers per month. The drop-in centre is located at the hub of one of the main encampment areas for Myanmar truck drivers. They have an onsite manager who is able to speak both Mandarin Chinese and Burmese fluently. His role is to provide assistance to truck drivers seeking services or simply to be available to discuss issues of HIV and simple counselling services.

The centre also provides outreach services for HIV/AIDS education, including condom distribution; referral to medical services for those seeking to become cognisant of their HIV status or who have tested HIV+; and they have a frequent (monthly) schedule of HIV information sessions. They also have HIV information posters on their walls in both Chinese and Burmese. One of the main services they provide is a place for truck drivers to congregate to relieve their boredom through activities as well as being educated about HIV/AIDS.

The centre is set up with chairs and tables, so truck drivers can eat their meals and play games and chat with other drivers there. They also have an area set aside where patrons can watch television and movies. At the time of writing, there was only one drop-in centre of its kind in the whole of Ruili. Considering the global research linking long-distance truck drivers with the expansion of HIV, this is a serious lacuna in Beijing's HIV/AIDS policy. Lack of information and services for long-distance truck drivers increases the non-traditional security threat that they pose in HIV epidemics.

Conclusion

The situation for HIV/AIDS in Yunnan is still one that has yet to be brought under control. HIV rates have continued to expand each year and in no part of the province (or China in general) are infection rates declining. There are many challenges concerning HIV/AIDS that make addressing the disease in Yunnan difficult. The situation for highly mobile and marginalised populations remains precarious. Their elusiveness, fear of stigma and arrest and a generally insufficient number of CBOs and NGOs working with them on the ground mean that there are substantial shortfalls in both coverage and obtainability of programmes.

Additionally, out-of-pocket treatment costs are prohibitive for most PLWHA. While there does appear to be some positive changes in the requirements for migrants to be able to access ART; the financial burden of tests and counselling; travel to and from clinics; and continuing need for stability and regular attendance at government-run hospitals and clinics create issues for those needing to access therapy. Unless Beijing implements further cost-cutting initiatives for these groups, adherence to ART regimes and voluntary testing and treatment will become more complicated as the human (in)security of key populations continues to increase. In each area where human security is lacking, there is a vicious circle. For example, lack of access to health care (through stigma or lack of financial accessibility) leads to poorer health and the inability to find employment. This often leads to social exclusion, depression, stigma, and further high-risk behaviours, leading to poor health. This situation is serious as the epidemic has now become sexually driven due to unsafe sexual practices and therefore has the scope to make debilitating inroads into the general population.

A solution to the spread of HIV/AIDS in FSW populations continues to elude Beijing's efforts. The fact that sexual transmission is known to be the main means of transmission into the general population (and generalised HIV epidemics) indicates this is an area of concern (H. Wang et al., 2018). High-risk behaviours continue and an understanding of HIV/AIDS has failed to encourage FSWs to adapt their behaviours. Cultural belief and a normal desire to treat their non-commercial partners differently from those they deal with as an occupation outweigh their current understandings of the devastating impact that HIV might have on their lives. FSWs are still neglecting to use condoms where commercial partners are willing to walk away or where they are willing to pay extra money. As well as this, they are often disinclined to use condoms with their non-commercial partners.

This situation is one that is mirrored in the case of PWID populations. The situation for PWID in Yunnan is exacerbated by the high availability of cheap drugs and very porous international borders. There are large numbers of homeless PWID living in a type of 'no-man's land' on either side of the international border between China and Myanmar. There are exemplary efforts by existing CBOs who provide NSPs, Naloxone, blood testing and general care and assistance to these highly mobile impoverished PWID. However, these programmes are few and peer workers struggle to meet the demands of the many PWID ostracised by their communities and living in conditions that threaten their human security on a daily basis. Many of them do not have access to employment; access to basic living conditions; or the food and nutritional requirements to survive the instigation and maintenance of ART. Already there is a high rate of drug resistance in this cohort and therefore starting the programme and being unable to continue is worse for them, and for the expanding HIV/AIDS profile as a non-traditional security threat, than not starting at all.

The situation of labour migrants is marginally better than that for FSWs and PWID, due to their ability to find employment. Nonetheless, they are marginalised from the societies that they work in, they move every three months or so and have relatively low incomes. Construction workers are provided with mandatory HIV/AIDS education and this seems an excellent step in the right direction to propagate the knowledge needed to avoid the potential pitfalls of high-risk behaviours. However, there is little empirical evidence to show whether this programme is doing enough for the migrant workers. Although there is anecdotal evidence from FSWs to suggest that higher numbers are using condoms, there needs to be more research into this cohort's role as clients of FSWs.

Like the construction and factory workers, long-distance truck drivers engage in high-risk behaviours. Additionally, having an income does not preclude the possibility of poverty. Low incomes and poor living conditions where services remain unaffordable often mean that high-risk behaviours become acceptable. When this is coupled with boredom and inactivity, then the situation is optimal for the spread of HIV. It is a well-known global phenomenon that HIV/AIDS travels like cargo along trucking routes throughout the world. This is certainly true of Yunnan and the cross-border truck drivers from Myanmar. Thus, the current gaps in Beijing's HIV/AIDS prevention and education programmes directed towards these populations exacerbate HIV/AIDS as a non-traditional security threat.

While there are many excellent programmes in operation in Yunnan, considering the scope of the problem, they are inadequate to address the requirements for prevention and education outreach. The non-traditional threat of HIV/AIDS, due to the current spread of HIV as a sexually driven epidemic, can wreck havoc due to the overwhelming number of people in China. At a grassroots level, individuals experience a lack of human security due to a lack of medical treatment; unemployment; stigma and being ostracised from community support; and a lack of nutritional requirements to optimally sustain ART regimes.

Gaps in current programming mean that the inadequate coverage leaves key populations vulnerable and exposes the general population to the virus through these cohorts. While there are a number of NGOs dealing with issues of HIV/AIDS in urban areas, there are relatively few organisations in rural areas. The current climate in China for NGOs and the recent withdrawal of INGOs have added to the burden of those CBOs and NGOs that are still in operation, creating even more gaps in coverage. Thus, the infrastructure for the operation of INGOs, NGOs and CBOs, which have been found to play an essential role in HIV/AIDS programmes, is shown to be insufficient.

Significantly, considering that the necessary funding to maintain existing programmes is in doubt, there is only a small chance that outreach services will be expanded in the future. With the 2014 allocation of only 5 million yuan for HIV/AIDS programmes for the entire province of Yunnan, it is probable that many of these programmes may even close. Beijing seems to be indicating that its commitment to halting the spread of HIV/AIDS is no longer a high priority. Without an expanded commitment to provide the funding and necessary services, it seems probable that no real change can happen. The previous forward momentum is likely to be wiped out and may result in worst-case scenarios resulting in a full-blown HIV/AIDS epidemic in China. In a synergistic nexus, China's reluctance to embrace HIV/AIDS as a human security threat for its individual citizens may be blinding it to the non-traditional threat it poses to the nation-state.

China's top-down static hierarchy, which may work well in other community health scenarios, is ineffective for HIV/AIDS epidemics where the needs of the individual must be addressed to render effective change. Beijing has made some significant steps in adopting GBP in its HIV/AIDS epidemic. However, a lack of funding and their insistence on dealing with the problem as a public health issue can create a negative environment that is not up to meeting the human security needs of PLWHA. The individual is a poor cousin in the fundamental 'groupthink' of the public health model. The elusive, highly mobile, marginalised and stigmatised individual exists only as a problem to be solved. Added to which, a lack of significant and persistent research and provision of treatment and prevention initiatives hamper efforts to halt the continued spread of HIV throughout China.

Additionally, they must do the following:

- address the current gaps in HIV/AIDS education and prevention access;
- reassess the existing health policies with regards to user-pay services supplementary to the free ART provided in the 'Four Free and One Care' initiative;
- expand research to more clearly understand the impact of long-distance truck drivers and labour migrants in HIV/AIDS epidemics.

Ultimately, there is a significant lack of understanding of the true nature of the epidemic in Yunnan and particularly in the Myanmar/China border areas.

Case study 7.1 Chen's story

This case study documents my meeting with Chen. As much of the conversation with Chen has already been presented in this chapter, this case study provides an informal glimpse into my interactions with him on one particular journey. It provides my first-hand impressions and some of my observations not already included in the text. Thus, unlike the previous case studies highlighting a specific issue, this case study is more of a reflection on the overall situation within China and the frustrations and determination of one man who is doing his best to improve the situation for PLWHA, who are living in conditions of human insecurity. As with all the other case studies the name has been changed to protect the individual and I do not identify where he is located except to say that he works in China somewhere and was willing to travel to meet me in Ruili.

I met Chen soon after my arrival in Yunnan Province. Chen is a modest man and when I met him, he was quiet but very welcoming and gracious. He has an inordinate amount of knowledge about the situation for PLWHA in Yunnan. He is one of the coordinators at an NGO that runs several outreach programmes. He is involved in drop-in centres for PWID, education programmes for migrants, drop-in centres for female sex workers in China and several other social impact programmes. In addition to his role at the NGO, Chen is a medical doctor. He understands the HIV/AIDS epidemic from both sides. He has administered ART and been involved with methadone maintenance programming. He understands how the system works and the unique challenges faced by PLWHA.

Chen invited me to meet him in Ruili to see what was happening in the HIV/AIDS community there. I was staying in Kunming at the time and was excited about going down there as it gave me the opportunity to visit the Dehong region of China, which I didn't know, and observe the current situation in the town that was at the epicentre of the original HIV epidemic in China. I hopped on a plane in Kunming and flew down to the nearest airport to Ruili, the Dehong Mangshi Airport, which is situated almost 4 hours drive from Ruili by taxi. I came out of the airport feeling some trepidation about the road trip; I had travelled in taxis in China many times before and always found them to be forays into the unknown. It seems to take a special kind of person to be a taxi driver in China, they are fearless and I have learned to sit back and distract myself by calculating probabilities. Mostly my calculations are pretty basic and simply result in my repeating a mantra to myself, 'Probably we will make it OK.'

This trip was no different. It had been late afternoon when the plane had landed and by the time I got underway in the taxi, the sun was already dipping in the sky. As the taxi sped along the rough roads, the twists and turns seemed to become more and more fraught with danger. We passed by endless numbers of trucks making the run from Ruili to the interior of China. Chen later told me that these trucks carry loads from Myanmar. Carrying the cargo requires a change of truck and driver at a border post in Ruili, as the Myanmar drivers are not allowed to continue past the truck loading area just inside the Chinese border. The Myanmar trucks pull into the loading area and their loads are transferred onto Chinese trucks with Chinese drivers before they head further into China. Each time we passed a truck, the taxi driver would enthusiastically engage the car horn before swinging out into what seemed like an endless stream of oncoming traffic. In daylight it was disconcerting, in the pitch darkness of a Yunnan night, it was terrifying.

After encountering a massive traffic jam somewhere along the journey, the taxi deposited me at my hotel almost 5 hours later. By this stage the fatigue was extreme and I was grateful to simply stagger into my room and collapse on the bed and sleep. I awoke early the next morning to a message from Chen and I called and arranged to meet him outside the hotel. We were to spend the day touring Ruili and going from one drop-in centre to another. We started our day by visiting a drop-in centre for PWID. It was a small rundown space, little more than a half-sized car garage with a roller door and a few stools and table. When we arrived, two men were staffing it. They were PWID peer workers, who had both been injection drug users. They were on methadone maintenance programmes and had a keen desire to help others who were in the same situation that they had previously found themselves in. We spent a lot of time discussing the situation in Ruili and the border area and then they took me out of town to visit the camp of some drug users who had recently been released from mandatory detention (this is discussed in Case study 6.1)

From there, Chen and I caught a taxi to visit a sex worker drop in centre. They were providing several services and operated an outreach programme for the children of sex workers. The woman running the centre told me that only a few of the sex workers came in for condoms and other services. She said that mostly one person would come and collect supplies for a number of friends. After leaving the drop-in centre, we spent time walking around a run-down area adjacent to the border. This was an area where Myanmar sex workers congregated. Most of the establishments were the typical hairdresser/beauty shops that operate as fronts for brothels in China. Dozens of young girls could be seen lounging in the shop-front windows. Squashed on lounges and perched on low stools scrolling through their mobile phones until the next customer walked in. Chen explained to me that there were few Chinese sex workers in this area as it mostly catered to the Myanmar truck drivers from the loading yard nearby, and older or less wealthy Chinese men who could not afford a Chinese sex worker. He said that the majority of the sex workers in the area were from Myanmar or some of the other Chinese ethnic minorities surrounding Ruili.

We visited the loading yard and spent some time at a truck driver drop-in centre that was located there. It was a bright, clean place that provides a place for drivers to hang out. It offers toilet facilities and there are televisions and tables where individuals can play cards and just talk to each other. It provides sex education and activities to truck drivers. The man running the centre told me that the truck drivers sometimes visited sex workers just because they were away from home and lonely. The drop in centre gave them a sense of community and provided a place where they could interact with others in the same situation. The sex education took the form of videos, brochures and short training programmes. In addition to which they supplied condoms. He said that there was very little understanding about HIV/AIDS among the truck drivers and that the education they provided filled a real need.

From there we stopped at a small café near the border crossing between Muse in Myanmar and Ruili in China. As we ate something and drank lemon sodas, we watched the crowds of people gathered in the small area around the gate that separates the two countries. After a while I noticed a tall, brightly dressed woman caught up in the centre of a group of people. It was immediately obvious to me that she was transgender. I do not know what their conversation was about but to me it seemed that heated words were being exchanged. In the end, she hurried off through the car park and was soon lost from view. Chen commented that it was rare to see a transgender woman in the area, as they are not well regarded by most people. In fact, he told me that in China they are known as ghost people (*ren yao*) because it was almost as if they did not exist. I could only wonder how dehumanising it must be to be forced to live in the shadows; to be vilified for daring to stand in the light of the sun. He told me that the situation for men who have sex with men was very difficult but that it was even more difficult for transgender individuals. Chen then shrugged his shoulders and said that, in China, PLWHA were often not treated well and that many of their needs are not met.

He confided that there is never enough money. They do what they can but it really does not make much impact on the overall situation. A part of the problem that they face is that there are not enough long-term NGOs working on the problem of HIV/AIDS. He said that they are like part-time NGOs. Not that they only work part-time but that they only exist part-time. When funding is available, they are active but when the funding dries up, they no longer operate. He discussed the official HIV/AIDS figures and told me that he did not think it could be possible that they were correct.

Yunnan Province alone diagnoses more than 10,000 new cases of HIV every year. He expressed his frustrations at the lack of support for HIV/AIDS initiatives and said he feared that the situation would continue to grow worse. One of his greatest concerns was that the government did not seem to understand that not addressing the needs of PLWHA exacerbated the problem. I asked him about the human security of PLWHA in China and he felt that they had very little. When I asked him whether he felt that the government had been sufficiently informed, he responded that he had been trying to get it through to them for decades. He stated, 'Why don't you try and tell them? Maybe they will listen to you as a researcher.' He explained that there were very few Chinese HIV/AIDS researchers and that most were foreigners like me.

As shown in Chapter 6, the information that was forthcoming in the conversations with Chen is well supported by the literature. He was very communicative in our conversations and provided me with important insights into the situation for PLWHA in China. I had the opportunity to meet Chen again on a subsequent trip to China and, as documented in this chapter, he was able to elucidate on the changing situation. My overarching observation was that those individuals who are engaged in drop-in centres and working in NGOs related to HIV/AIDS are passionate and dedicated people. They care about those that they are helping and have a real desire to see things improve. They operate at the coalface and deal with difficult situations on a daily basis but their enthusiasm is truly inspirational. Their frustration with the current situation is well matched by their determination to see things change.

Note

1 One of the interview participants (a medical doctor) commented that on a recent trip into Myanmar to meet medical personnel, they were horrified to discover that the doctor they were liaising with *had never heard of HIV/AIDS* [emphasis mine]. Subsequently, upon testing the population of the prison that this doctor was overseeing, they found a HIV prevalence rate exceeding 30 per cent of the population (Chen, pers. comm., December 2013).

References

Apostolopoulos, Y., Sönmez, S. & Massengale, K. (2013). Sexual mixing, drug exchanges, and infection risk among long-haul truck drivers. *Journal of Community Health, 38*(2), 385–391.

Ding, G. W., Hsi, J, H., Liu, H. X., Su, Y. Y., Wang, J. J., Jun, B., ... & Wang, N. (2014). HIV-infected female sex workers high risk behavior and attitude changes in Kaiyuan City, Yunnan Province, China. *Biomedical and Environmental Sciences, 27*(6), 444–452.

Ding, Y., Li, L. & Ji, G. (2011). HIV disclosure in rural China: Predictors and relationship to access to care. *AIDS Care, 23*(9), 1059–1066. doi:10.1080/09540121.2011.554524.

Garcia-Prats, A. J., McMeans, A. R., Ferry, G. D. & Klish, W. J. (2010). Nutrition and HIV/AIDS. *HIV Curriculum, 286,* 4–5.

Gill, B. (2006). China's health care and pension challenges. Testimony before the US-China Security and Economic Review Commission hearing on major internal challenges facing the Chinese Leadership, February 2, Washington, DC. Retrieved from www.uscc.gov/hearings/2006hearings/written_testimonies/06_02_02_bates.pdf

Jie, W., Ciyong, L., Xueqing, D., Hui, W. & Lingyao, H. (2012). A syndemic of psychosocial problems places the MSM (men who have sex with men) population at greater risk of HIV infection. *PloS ONE, 7*(3), e32312.

Li, J., Chongsuvivatwong, V., Assanangkornchai, S., McNeil, E. B. & Cai, L. (2018). Comparison of health system responsiveness between HIV and non-HIV patients at infectious disease clinics in Yunnan, China. *Patient Preference and Adherence, 12,* 1129.

Li, R., Zhao, G., Li, J., McGoogan, J. M., Zhou, C., Zhao, Y., ... & Wu, Z. (2018). HIV screening among patients seeking care at Xuanwu Hospital: A cross-sectional study in Beijing, China, 2011–2016. *PloS ONE, 13*(12), e0208008.

Liao, S., Weeks, M. R., Wang, Y., Li, F., Jiang, J., Li, J., ... & Dunn, J. (2011). Female condom use in the rural sex industry in China: Analysis of users and non-users at post-intervention surveys. *AIDS Care, 23,* 66–74. doi:10.1080/09540121.2011.555742.

Lu, L., Jia, M., Ma, Y., Yang, L., Chen, Z., Ho, D. D., ... & Zhang, L. (2008). The changing face of HIV in China. *Nature, 455*(7213), 609–611.

Mendelsohn, J. B., Calzavara, L., Light, L., Burchell, A. N., Ren, J. & Kang, L. (2015). Design and implementation of a sexual health intervention for migrant construction workers situated in Shanghai, China. *Emerging Themes in Epidemiology, 12*(1), 1.

Morgan, J. & Jones, A. L. (2018). The role of naloxone in the opioid crisis. *Toxicology Communications, 2*(1), 15–18.

Oluwoye, J. (2007). Land transport and HIV vulnerability: A conceptual framework of vulnerability of road users, road and environment. *Research Journal of Medical Sciences, 1*(1), 9–12.

Philbin, M. M. & Zhang, F. (2010). Exploring stakeholder perceptions of facilitators and barriers to accessing methadone maintenance clinics in Yunnan province, China. *AIDS Care, 22*(5), 623–629. doi:10.1080/09540120903311490.

Smith, R. J. (2005). Adherence to antiretroviral HIV drugs: How many doses can you miss before resistance emerges? *Proceedings of the Royal Society B: Biological Sciences, 273*(1586), 617–624.

Su, S., Zhang, L., Cheng, F., Li, S., Li, S., Jing, J., ... & Mao, L. (2018). Association between recreational drug use and sexual practices among people who inject drugs in Southwest China: A cross-sectional study. *BMJ Open, 8*(6), e019730.

Sunmola, A. M. (2005). Sexual practices, barriers to condom use and its consistent use among long-distance truck drivers in Nigeria. *AIDS Care, 17*(2), 208–221.

Ulibarri, M. D., Roesch, S., Rangel, M. G., Staines, H., Amaro, H. & Strathdee, S. A. (2015). 'Amar te Duele' ('Love Hurts'): Sexual relationship power, intimate partner violence, depression symptoms and HIV risk among female sex workers who use drugs and their non-commercial, steady partners in Mexico. *AIDS and Behavior, 19*(1), 9–18.

Wang, B., Liang, Y., Feng, Y., Li, Y., Wang, Y., Zhang, A. M., ... & Xia, X. (2015). Prevalence of human immunodeficiency virus 1 infection in the last decade among entry travelers in Yunnan Province, China. *BMC Public Health, 15*(1), 362.

Wang, H., Yang, Z., Zhu, H., Mo, Q. & Tan, H. (2018). High HIV-1 prevalence and viral diversity among entry-exit populations at frontier ports of China, 2012–2016: A cross-sectional molecular epidemiology study. *Infection, Genetics and Evolution, 65,* 231–237.

WHO (World Health Organization). (2014). *HIV prevention, diagnosis, treatment and care for key populations: Consolidated guidelines.* Geneva, Switzerland: World Health Organization.

Xuan, Q., Liang, S., Qin, W., Yang, S., Zhang, A. M., Zhao, T., ... & Xia, X. (2018). High prevalence of HIV-1 transmitted drug resistance among therapy-naïve Burmese entering travelers at Dehong ports in Yunnan, China. *BMC Infectious Diseases, 18*(1), 211.

Yang, L. H. & Kleinman, A. (2008). 'Face' and the embodiment of stigma in China: The cases of schizophrenia and AIDS. *Social Science & Medicine, 67*(3), 398–408. doi:10.1016/j.socscimed.2008.03.011.

Yao, Y., Yang, F., Chu, J., Siame, G., Lim, H. J., Jin, X., ... & Wang, N. (2012). Associations between drug use and risk behaviours for HIV and sexually transmitted infections among female sex workers in Yunnan, China. *International Journal of STD & AIDS, 23*(10), 698–703.

Zhang, C., Li, X., Hong, Y., Zhou, Y., Liu, W. & Stanton, B. (2013). Unprotected sex with their clients among low-paying female sex workers in southwest China. *AIDS Care, 25*(4), 503–506.

Zhang, F., Hsu, M., Yu, L., Wen, Y. & Pan, J. (2006). Initiation of the national free antiretroviral therapy program in rural China. In J. Kaufman, A. Kleinman & T. Saich

(Eds.), *AIDS and social policy in China* (pp. 96–124). Cambridge, MA: Harvard University Asia Center.

Zhou, Y. H., Liang, Y. B., Pang, W., Qin, W. H., Yao, Z. H., Chen, X., ... & Zheng, Y. T. (2014). Diverse forms of HIV-1 among Burmese long-distance truck drivers imply their contribution to HIV-1 cross-border transmission. *BMC Infectious Diseases, 14*(1), 1.

Zhu, B. Y., Bu, J., Huang, P. Y., Zhou, Z. G., Yin, Y. P., Chen, X. S. & Gan, Q. (2012). Epidemiology of sexually transmitted infections, HIV, and related high-risk behaviors among female sex workers in Guangxi Autonomous Region, China. *Japanese Journal of Infectious Diseases, 65*(1), 75–78.

8   Human insecurity and disease

Remove the firewood from under the pot.

从锅底取出木柴

The securitisation of HIV/AIDS created a framework that attracted attention to the pervasive nature of the HIV/AIDS problem. Globally, nation-states began to take notice of the spread of HIV within their own borders. They also began to note that HIV/AIDS presents a non-traditional threat to security. It is a battle that cannot be fought with an army or in the assemblies of political power. It is an enemy that does not respect the sovereignty of nation-states or seek permission to cross national boundaries. HIV/AIDS must be managed in the global political sphere but the real battle takes place on an individual level. The human being must be the main referent object: the individuals contracting and transmitting the virus. Human security, rather than state security, must be ensured in order to make any lasting impact on the spread of the disease. Globally, research has shown that PLWHA and key populations face human insecurity on a daily basis.

'Freedom from fear', 'freedom from want', and 'freedom to live in dignity' are the overriding principles for human security. Individuals must be able to live their lives free from the fears that stigmatise and marginalise them, free from the wants that often drive them to behaviours that are high in risk, and with the dignity and respect deserved as a human being. Economic, food, health, environmental, personal, community and political insecurity represent the seven areas that influence the behaviours of individuals and the outcomes of political initiatives in HIV/AIDS situations. Individuals are driven to do whatever is necessary to survive and the need to feel secure, find shelter and eat today outweighs the threat of disease that may or may not occur tomorrow. While this book discusses the numerous advantages of ensuring that individuals obtain human security, this chapter examines the negative consequences emanating from a lack of security or insecurity.

Thus, human security and human insecurity are different focal points of the same topic. By concentrating on insecurity, this chapter further highlights the imperative to ensure that key populations' human security is paramount. These insecurities do not exist independently of each other. They are ubiquitous, interconnected and often manifest as a web of interwoven relationships. Food insecurity can be the result of economic insecurity and economic insecurity may be the result of political or community insecurity. Thus, there is no single approach that is effective.

Each area of human insecurity must be addressed in order to make an impact on the whole. Situations of food insecurity cannot be solved when economic insecurity continues. Any measures on that level will simply result in short-term solutions. The individual may eat for a time but unless the underlying cause is addressed, no sustainable change can occur, resulting in a return to previous behaviours. That is not to say that benefits do not arise from short-term interventions that dispel human insecurity. When human insecurity is no longer present, then human security is attained, negating many of the unfavourable outcomes currently exacerbating HIV/AIDS epidemics. However, long-term and sustainable behavioural change leading to the reversal or eradication of HIV/AIDS epidemics cannot occur in situations of continuing human insecurity.

Significantly, different HIV/AIDS epidemics may have different human security threats undermining the intervention efforts and driving high-risk behaviour. Further, one area of insecurity may intensify or cause insecurity in another area in a myriad of ways. For example, in situations of conflict, the HIV/AIDS epidemics may be more driven by political instability, leading to personal insecurity, homelessness, economic insecurity, food insecurity and an inability to access health care or educational programmes. In other situations, economic insecurity may drive the epidemics, leading to labour migration, food insecurity, community insecurity, health and environmental insecurity (Figure 8.1). The insecurities that do seem to be consistent across all global HIV/AIDS epidemics are economic insecurity, food insecurity, health insecurity, personal insecurity and community insecurity. Regardless of why they have occurred (whether through environmental or political means), these insecurities have detrimental impacts on HIV/AIDS epidemics and epidemiology to varying degrees. In order to successfully mitigate these impacts, human insecurity interventions must be generated at a macro level with policy frameworks that actively seek to address the reasons for the insecurity being encountered by individuals at a micro level.

Structural determinants affecting HIV/AIDS epidemics originate from a number of different areas from political and social situations (political and community insecurity); health-related policy (health insecurity); economic factors (economic insecurity and food insecurity); the environment surrounding the individual on a personal, work, community and geographical level (with environmental insecurity leading to community disempowerment or unsafe work environments contributing to community and personal insecurity); and cultural norms leading to stigma (community and personal insecurity) (Shannon et al., 2015). While all seven areas of human insecurity have impacts as structural determinants of HIV/AIDS epidemics, and are considered in this chapter, economic, health and food insecurity have the greatest impact at the health outcome level. As such, this chapter particularly focuses on economic, food and health insecurity and their influences on HIV/AIDS epidemics. As already

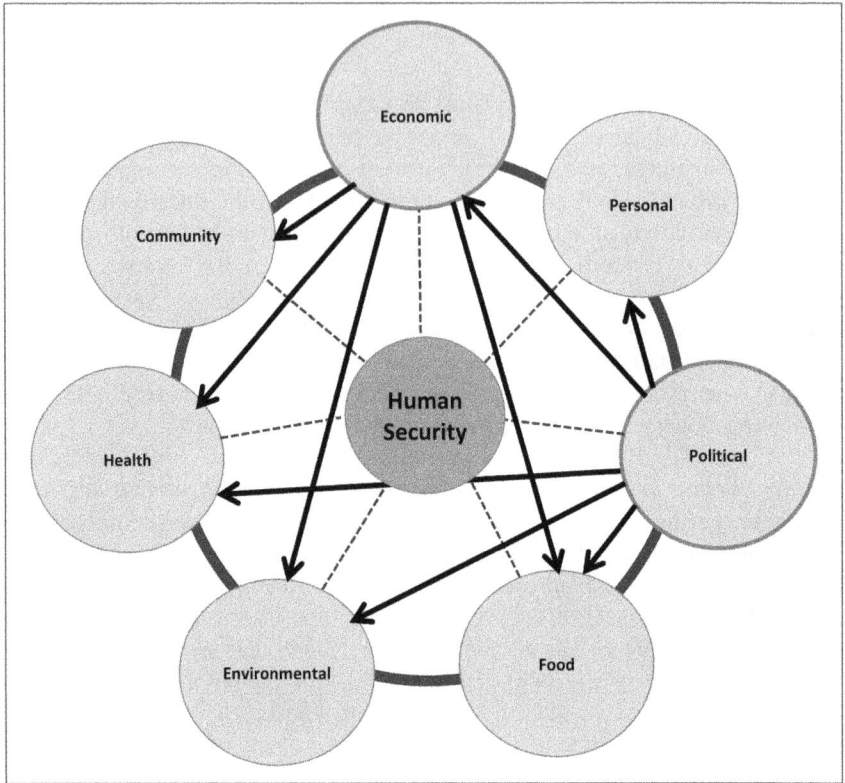

Figure 8.1 Possible interactions between drivers of insecurity.

mentioned, to a large degree, the security threats are concurrent. When there is economic insecurity, there is likely to be food insecurity and health insecurity too.

Economic insecurity in global HIV/AIDS settings

There are a number of different drivers of economic insecurity. Economic insecurity occurs when individuals cannot obtain the financial wherewithal to cover the costs of everyday life. At its basic core it might be defined as a lack of 'an assured basic income – usually from productive and remunerative work, or in the last resort from some publicly financed safety net' (UNDP, 1994, p. 25). Without financial resources, individuals may be unable to gain the education needed to gain basic competencies in order to find work and if they do find employment, they may be unable to afford to obtain the qualifications needed to propel them into higher-income brackets. A lower income or no income at all makes it impossible for individuals to accrue savings, which may be required in times of sickness or unemployment. An individual may not have the necessary economic resources to access the services needed on a daily basis.

Homelessness, poverty and unemployment all constitute economic insecurity. This is particularly problematic in HIV/AIDS epidemics because individuals who are struggling to meet their daily needs are less focused on what might happen in the future than they are about their needs on any given day. Interestingly, economic insecurity has a two-pronged effect in HIV/AIDS epidemics. First, being HIV+ has a detrimental effect on people's ability to obtain economic security, leading to high-risk behaviours that exacerbate HIV transmission. Second, the economic insecurity experienced by PLWHA affects their ability to manage their HIV/AIDS infections, leading to sub-optimal outcomes for ART regimes and often a lack of ability to access medical care.

Influence of HIV/AIDS on economic insecurity

Households affected by HIV/AIDS are likely to experience reduced earning capacities due to unemployment, family members needing to care for HIV+ individuals, and associated costs such as funeral expenses, legal and medical costs (Elbe, 2010). There has been extensive research in Sub-Saharan Africa and the USA that has documented the many ways that HIV/AIDS causes economic insecurity (Conyers, Chiu, Shamburger-Rousseau, Johnson & Misrok, 2015; Salmen et al., 2015). In general, HIV contributes to economic insecurity through the reduced work capacity and productivity of adults. There are also effects due to increased numbers of orphans, which manifests as missed educational opportunities for children as well as their inability to generate an income. Vulnerable women are at risk of losing their income due to ill health and finding themselves in a position where they are negotiating sexual relationships to gain the support of male breadwinners (Ala, 2003; Salmen et al., 2015).

The effects of economic insecurity are far-reaching and comprehensive. In addition to being unable to work for the basic needs of life (such as food), it may result in homelessness (which may also be considered environmental insecurity). The results of HIV/AIDS and homelessness are exacerbated by the conditions that occur as a result of homelessness. In addition to the vulnerability that homelessness produces are the stresses and mental health issues that arise from these conditions. The ongoing ramifications of stress and deteriorating mental health are an exposure to violence and sexual exploitation and drug and alcohol use (Bhunu, 2015). Statistics concerning the correlation between homelessness and HIV indicate that homeless individuals are likely to have infection rates 16 per cent higher than those who have a stable living environment (Bhunu, 2015). PLWHA may be susceptible to losing their home due to the high costs associated with medical care, and figures suggest that at least half of all HIV+ individuals experience homelessness (Aidala, Lee, Abramson, Messeri & Siegler, 2007). In the USA, the figures are between one-third and one-half of all PLWHA experiencing housing instability through unaffordability, placing them in a position of homelessness or imminent homelessness (Bhunu, 2015).

Another result of economic insecurity is high population mobility. Increased numbers of labour migrants are moving from areas of low or no employment to areas where there are greater employment opportunities. The effects of high population mobility include a breakdown in societal structure between those who leave for work and those who stay behind, often resulting in women and children being negatively impacted educationally, and women attempting to address financial lack with subsistence employment (Antman, 2013). This is in addition to the ramifications of labour migration on the individual who is mobile, including increased high-risk behaviours in HIV epidemics.

Economic insecurity has further impacts on other areas of insecurity. Not only does it lead to homelessness, lack of basic needs, and labour migration, it also leads to health insecurity, food insecurity, personal insecurity, community insecurity and environmental insecurity. In HIV/AIDS epidemics, those individuals who are PLWHA, and those who are directly affected by PLWHA (such as partners, children, parents), are often likely to suffer from some degree of economic insecurity. However, in a cyclical, casual sequence, economic insecurity also has an effect on HIV/AIDS epidemics. Thus, economic insecurity is fundamentally entwined with HIV/AIDS epidemics.

Influence of economic insecurity on HIV/AIDS

Economic insecurity is a direct challenge for people undertaking ART regimes. When resources are scarce, they must be used for the most pressing issues, such as food and shelter, resulting in medicine being relegated to an issue to be resolved at a later date. While HIV/AIDS will inevitably result in death without ART, the immediate need to avoid starvation supersedes that future concern. Lack of income and no financial stability inevitably lead to lack of stability and security in other areas. Without the necessary funds, securing a home, food or accessing necessary medication are a challenge that is unable to be met by many people. As a result, health deteriorates and the problems are exacerbated.

Often, even when the drugs themselves are free, the costs of attending clinics, loss of wages, and medical expenses are prohibitive for many (Chen, pers. comm., December 2013). This leads to high rates of attrition from ART programmes and potentially, to increased cases of drug-resistant strains of HIV occurring. For PLWHA, the costs of procuring even 'free' medicines can be unaffordable due to the associated costs, such as loss of income due to time spent away from work while travelling to clinics, transportation costs (Young, Wheeler, McCoy & Weiser, 2014), accommodation costs and supportive medical costs (such as liver function tests) (Chen, pers. comm., December 2013). Considering that HIV/AIDS disproportionally affects the marginalised and poor communities, the need to address economic insecurities may even result in individuals trading or selling ART for food and other resources (Young et al., 2014).

Compounding the problem of the prohibitive costs of health care and medicines, for PLWHA, economic insecurity often leads to transactional sex, including high-risk behaviours, such as not using condoms (women are often unable to successfully negotiate safe sex practices) in order to obtain food or drugs (Conyers et al., 2015; Whittle et al., 2015). Engagement in these unsafe practices further exacerbates HIV/AIDS epidemics through increased transmission of HIV between individuals (Shannon et al., 2015). One of the main drivers of high-risk behaviours during times of economic insecurity is the lack of food security. Food insecurity is such an important component that it is considered to be a separate pillar of human security. Food insecurity adds to the challenges of HIV/AIDS epidemics in that it not only impacts on the transmission of HIV/AIDS through behavioural practices but also impacts the viability and optimisation of ART regimes through a lack of nutritional robustness for individuals.

Food insecurity in global HIV/AIDS settings

Food insecurity occurs when individuals cannot ensure that they can feed themselves. Therefore, manifestations of food insecurity include hunger, malnourishment and famine. Food insecurity occurs when the following conditions are not met:

> [T]hat all people at all times have both physical and economic access to basic food. This requires not just enough food to go around. It necessitates that people have ready access to food – that they have an 'entitlement' to food, by growing it for themselves, by buying it or by taking advantage of a public food distribution system.
>
> (UNDP, 1994, p. 27)

The salient point in the UNDP definition is not only that food is available, but also that individuals have the ability to access that food (Elbe, 2010; UNDP, 1994). Therefore, food insecurity is the limited or inadequate availability of nutritious, safe food or the inability to procure suitable foods in ways that are socially acceptable (Weiser et al., 2011; Whittle et al., 2015, p. 1). In China, for example, food is readily available and yet FSWs, PWID and floating migrants may find it difficult to obtain it. As shown in the case studies, some PLWHA are limited to one meal of rice per day. In one situation an 85-year-old woman who had lost the earning power of three sons to HIV/AIDS-related complications was struggling to survive on the charity of neighbours and less than 50 yuan a month (see Case study 8.1).

Thus, food insecurity occurs when people cannot meet their dietary requirements by accessing enough safe and nutritious food (due to physical, social or economic insufficiencies) to achieve their right as humans to live an active and healthy life (Young et al., 2014). Moreover, while extremely problematic in and of itself, food insecurity inevitably leads to other insecurities. Kalichman et al. (2014) comment: 'Food insecurity was associated with multiple poverty markers, including fewer years of education, greater likelihood of unstable housing, lack of transportation for health care and food/meals and a greater likelihood of receiving food from faith-based services' (p. 1137). Different structural drivers for food insecurity (such as economic insecurity) lead to poverty, lack of education, gender inequality and issues of stigma that alienate individuals from their communities.

Some of the main reasons people in HIV/AIDS settings experience food insecurity include: a lack of economic resources to purchase appropriate amounts of food; and sick family members are unable to work, resulting in lower incomes and care burdens increase (Anema, Vogenthaler, Frongillo, Kadiyala & Weiser, 2009; Bukusuba, Kikafunda & Whitehead, 2007). In addition to which, depression and mental health issues that are directly related to economic insecurity and the stress associated with needing to source food and adequate shelter on a daily basis, may also lead to poor choices and high-risk behaviours (Kang, Delzell, McNamara, Cuffey, Cherian & Matthew, 2015). This point is especially pertinent in HIV/AIDS situations, particularly for key populations who are often already suffering some levels of human insecurity. Food insecurity therefore has wide-ranging impacts for key populations and PLWHA. It directly contributes to the horizontal and vertical transmission of HIV/AIDS and causes continuing problems once the virus has been contracted (Weiser et al., 2011).

In key populations, food insecurity results in the adoption of high-risk behaviours, such as the selling of sex to generate enough money to buy food. For PLWHA, the impacts of food insecurity are increased as it not only leads them into high-risk behaviours but also negatively affects their ability to maintain ART regimes. For some PLWHA suffering from food insecurity, this may appear to constitute legitimate contraindications for optimal health outcomes. Young et al. (2014) state:

> Food insecurity and HIV are 'syndemic': there is a positive biological and social interaction in which one exacerbates the negative health effects of the other. It is increasingly recognized that food insecurity both heightens vulnerability to HIV infection and at the same time exacerbates poor clinical outcomes among PLHIV.
>
> (p. 507)

Among the complications associated with food insecurity in HIV/AIDS settings are:

- incomplete RNA suppression (or viral load suppression);
- declining CD4 counts;
- a lower body mass index;
- increased opportunistic infections and hospitalisations;
- HIV-related mortality (Cox et al., 2016; Ivers et al., 2009; Young et al., 2014).

Thus, for PLWHA, food insecurity is associated with higher morbidity and mortality as well as impaired immunologic and virologic results and ART pharmacokinetics (Benzekri et al., 2015; Cox et al., 2016; Whittle et al., 2015).

Furthermore, the physical side effects of food insecurity may result in decreased ART adherence and high attrition rates due to the inability of PLWHA to cope with the physical side effects of ART (Anema et al., 2009; Chen, pers. comm., December 2013; Cox et al., 2016). Undertaking ART, particularly in the early stages when the body is adapting to the drug cocktail, is difficult without the complications of food insecurity. When taken without food, ART has been known to cause adverse side effects, such as: nausea, vomiting, stomach pains, dizziness, headaches, fainting, sweating, rapid heartbeat and, ultimately, poor adherence (Young et al., 2014).

This is of particular concern in managing the spread and infectiousness of HIV. One of the main reasons for this is that PLWHA are less likely to be taking ART, and if they are taking ART, are less likely to adhere to the regime because they have run out of medications or have to prioritise food over medicine (Kalichman, Hernandez, Cherry, Kalichman, Washington & Grebler, 2014). While this produces a poor outcome for the individual, it also has ramifications for epidemics due to the likelihood of developing drug-resistant strains of HIV and ART failure (Kalichman et al., 2014). Conversely, food security improves treatment outcomes, adherence and the uptake of ART (Claros, de Pee & Bloem, 2014).

Food insecurity is also implicated in high-risk sexual practices (such as unprotected transactional sex), which have a direct correlation with increased acceleration of the virus and increased risk of HIV vertical or horizontal transmission (Aberman, Rawat, Drimie, Claros & Kadiyala 2014; Bukusuba et al., 2007). This may be particularly the case for women who may also engage in intergenerational sex, earlier marriage and abusive relationships (Pascoe et al., 2015). Often transactional sex, undertaken as a method for procuring money or food, is entered into to address severe food shortages and may result in individuals agreeing not to wear condoms out of fear of losing a client or in order to gain extra money (Whittle et al., 2015). The need for food simply outweighs the need to use protection during sex. Significantly, illicit drug-taking environments further disrupt food intake by creating social, economic, physical and policy obstacles that inhibit individuals' access to food (Cox et al., 2016).

Food insecurity and HIV/AIDS are engaged in a cycle of events that increase the severity of each (Anema et al., 2009). The risk factors for food insecurity include: unstable housing, low income, illicit drug use, depression, unemployment and youth (Cox et al., 2016). This cycle is driven by sociodemographic factors (such as homelessness, low income), socioeconomic factors (such as unemployment), behavioral actions (such as illicit drug-taking) and clinical illness (such as depression), which generate increased adverse HIV/AIDS health outcomes, resulting in an inability to acquire food (Cox et al., 2016). Thus, the cycle of insecurity is perpetuated. Addressing this as a human insecurity issue in HIV/AIDS situations is paramount in order to mitigate both the effects that food insecurity has on increased transmission in epidemics and also the impacts that it has on the ability of PLWHA to adhere to ART regimes in TasP health scenarios. The many ways that food insecurity negatively impacts society in general, and global HIV/AIDS epidemics specifically, such as high-risk behaviours resulting in the high attrition rates along the cascade, mean that finding solutions must be considered a primary concern for governments.

While food insecurity may disproportionately affect those who live in poorer areas globally, it also occurs among more affluent urban populations, although this may change as HIV prevalence increases in rural populations (Pascoe et al., 2015). As a part of economic insecurity, food insecurity causes many of the same negative outcomes. Food insecurity has also been linked to lack of education and understanding about HIV/AIDS, flexible attitudes and/or understanding about the HIV/AIDS risk reduction behaviours, and poorer self-sufficiency (Pascoe et al., 2015). While food insecurity is not a direct cause of health insecurity, it does contribute, as individuals are unable or unwilling to use the limited economic resources they have to achieve better health. Ultimately, while death from AIDS might be a future possibility, it loses significance when measured against the very real possibility of imminent starvation.

Health insecurity in HIV/AIDS settings

Human insecurity and health are intrinsically linked because the health of individuals is an essential requirement for human survival and long-term fulfilment (Lo, 2015). No individual should have to endure health insecurity. The WHO Constitution states: 'The enjoyment of the highest attainable standard of health is one of the fundamental rights of every human being, without distinction of race, religion, political belief, economic or social condition' (WHO, 2006, para. 3). It also decrees that health is a 'state of complete physical, mental and social well-being, and not merely the absence of disease or infirmity' (para 2). These two broad statements make it clear that health security should be the right of all people. regardless of their status within the general population. However, in most scenarios. the pursuit of health security remains firmly rooted within public health frameworks.

In order to better define health insecurity, it is useful to first comprehend the historical foundations of health security. Collective health security has existed as a concept since the fourteenth century when quarantine was implemented as a measure to try and stop the spread of the bubonic plague (Heymann, 2015). Additionally, broader concepts of health security concerned with protecting states and individuals from pandemic disease can be further defined as the ability of individuals to access safe and effective health services, technologies and products. as needed. to ensure their own individual health security (Heymann et al., 2015). Furthermore, it incorporates the need to diminish risks to public health by protecting people from environmental and behavioural risk (Quinn, Martins, Cunha, Higuchi, Murph & Bencko, 2014). Health security is therefore fundamental to attaining peace and the security of individuals (Aldis, 2008).

Poor health has a direct correlation to an individual's ability to obtain food, economic security, personal safety, collective security, prevent environmental degradation and achieve political security. Health insecurity has a decisive role in whether individuals, and by extension communities, are able to determine their own course of life and actions in pursuit of personal fulfilment (Nunes, 2014). Therefore, health insecurity threatens the prosperity and the stability of political institutions and societies (Evans, 2010). Therefore, in conditions of disease epidemics, premature loss of life due to an individual's inability to obtain necessary health care represents a great threat (Elbe, 2011a).

Health insecurity occurs when individuals are unable to obtain universal and equitable access to the requisite medications, due to lack of availability or financial constraints preventing their purchase (Yates, Dhillon & Rannan-Eliya, 2015). Protection against the financial risks of medical care can only be achieved through collective and collaborative action by governments both within, and when necessary, external to their own borders (Yates et al., 2015). Arguably, health insecurity is manifest in global infectious disease scenarios when there is no international collaboration or the inclusion of non-state actors and multinational corporations to deliver services (Chiu, Weng, Su, Huang, Chang & Kuo, 2009). Without collective action, it is impossible to prepare for and subsequently reduce the vulnerability of public health from threats that transcend national borders (De Cock, Simone, Davison & Slutsker, 2013).

On the macro level, the threat of naturally emerging and reoccurring infectious disease is just as much a national security dilemma for states as foreign military incursion in terms of mortality, morbidity and economic disruption (Elbe, 2011b). Furthermore, infectious disease has been identified as detrimental to states' abilities to protect themselves militarily from external threats, due to losses of trained individuals in standing and peacekeeping forces. This concept was one of the foundational concerns expressed when pushing for the securitisation of AIDS at the 2000 UN Security Council.

Apart from military concerns in HIV/AIDS epidemics, individuals often endure health insecurity due to sometimes dysfunctional or inefficient health facilities, high costs of medical intervention and preventative services (Nunes, 2014). Certainly, deficiencies in the availability of ART and suboptimal access to sexual health services (including STI testing and contraceptives), safe and sufficient condoms, and HIV testing are major shortfalls in the global efforts to eradicate HIV/AIDS (Shannon et al., 2015). Bearing this in mind, it is essential for nation-states to recognise the insecurity affecting individuals in HIV/AIDS epidemics, not only to halt the spread of the disease but also to ensure that quality of life and personal individual fulfilment are achievable.

On the micro-level, health insecurity is therefore concerned specifically with a lack of power to act and protecting individuals from threats associated with disease. Elbe (2012, p. 321) posits: 'Health security thus takes the provision of security beyond distant theatres and brings it to bear directly on – and indeed inside – the individual body, as the inner biological processes of our bodies become new battlefields of security policy.' The securitisation of AIDS was couched in similar language. The war on AIDS had begun. Once HIV-1 was identified as the enemy in AIDS epidemics, the security focus subtly shifted from humanitarian concerns to war against the virus.

In doing so, the individual only became a consideration within the wider framework of health. Global health models are not concerned with providing services to individuals, rather they are more concerned with ensuring that the health situations of individuals do not affect the broader scope of the population. Thus, the focus becomes preventing the spread of sickness rather than healing the individual. This ignores the idea that healing the individual and providing for their needs actually positively contributes to halting the spread of disease within communities as a whole. Managing the human insecurity needs of key populations and PLWHA by reducing health insecurity will result in lower high-risk behaviours and better optimisation of TasP initiatives. Likewise, the individuals' human insecurity is predicated on their inability to avoid the other six pillars of human insecurity (Elbe, 2010).

Environmental insecurity

Environmental insecurity most often results from the external factors that individuals face. From a macro standpoint, such as that of the globalised society, these include things like conflict, pollution, natural disasters, degradation and drought. These issues tax the financial resources of nation-states and can result in massive losses of income and economic security for individuals. In natural disasters, individuals may lose their homes and jobs. In rural and agrarian-based societies, droughts may lead to a loss of crops and lack of water causing rural industries to decline. Additionally, HIV/AIDS adversely affects commercial and subsistence farming. This is particularly the case for HIV+ subsistence farmers who do not have the financial resources to employ labour and mitigate the impacts of the disease (Ala, 2003).

In addition to resulting in poor living conditions at the point of origin, environmental insecurity often leads to high numbers of labour migrants leaving their home areas and crossing national boundaries and international borders in search of economic security, to avoid environmental insecurity. The effects of labour migration on rates of HIV transmission have been extensively discussed in this book. However, much of the environmental insecurity faced by individuals if also due to everyday environmental factors, such as poor living conditions, unsafe workplaces and conditions of incarceration. This is particularly the case for PLWHA and key populations in HIV/AIDS epidemics.

They are frequently marginalised and stigmatised to such an extent that they live on the edges of society. They are often homeless or suffering from housing instability and economic insecurity, resulting in them becoming mired in poverty and the associated insecurities, leading to poor health outcomes and high-risk behaviours. As a result of poverty, they are likely to encounter unsafe workplace environments, which in the case of FSWs may lead them to sell sex on street corners or off-street through advertisements in newspapers or by phone or text rather than the relative safety of a brothel where there may be safety measures in place (such as client sign-in and removal of violent clients) (Shannon et al., 2015).

In addition to unsafe work environments, FSWs and other key populations are at risk of incarceration due to the criminalisation of sex work and drug usage. Punitive laws and national policies pertaining to sex work in particular may cause environmental insecurity due to the removal of red-light districts, legal restrictions on where FSWs can operate and incarceration (Shannon et al., 2015). These situations have been found to elevate HIV transmissions risks, generate stigma, increase food and economic insecurity, create homelessness due to eviction and economic hardship, and have also been associated with inconsistent condom use. However, the results extend to affect the personal security of individuals in situations of environmental insecurity.

Personal insecurity

Personal insecurity is heightened by the presence of other insecurities. When an individual is homeless or suffering from food insecurity, they are less able to negotiate the spaces they operate within. In HIV/AIDS scenarios, this can often be caused by environmental insecurity and economic insecurity, which leads individuals to undertake sex work or drug usage in areas that are unsafe. In criminalised environments, FSWs are often exposed to violence (including sexual violence) from a host of different people, including clients, police, managers, pimps and other predatory individuals (Shannon et al., 2015). Women, in particular those who are single and homeless, are subject to gender-based violence and are more likely to suffer both domestic violence and sexual abuse (Bhunu, 2015; Taylor, 2016). This type of personal violence is likely to lead to inconsistent use of condoms, both through a lack of power to negotiate their use and client insistence and condom refusal.

The criminalisation of sex work and illicit drug use can create situations of abuse, leading to personal insecurity. Police raids can often lead to displacement, arrests and incarcerations, in addition to the confiscation of condoms and drug-taking paraphernalia, leaving FSWs unable to use barrier protection and PWID having to share needles (Shannon et al., 2015). Not using condoms and lack of needle-sharing practices are well documented as increasing HIV transmission rates and exacerbating HIV/AIDS epidemics. This is in addition to the fear that results from the criminalisation of drug use and sex work, which prevents members of key populations from accessing medical services or ascertaining their HIV status.

Due to homonegativity, MSM and TG populations are very vulnerable to discrimination and mistreatment (Zea et al., 2013). Violence and sexual violence perpetrated against MSMs and TG populations may occur due to stigma and discrimination. Incidental conversations with TG and MSM sex workers at AIDS conference 2014 (pers. comm., July 2014) revealed that they often faced rape, beatings and were forced to perform oral sex both in a community context and in prison. Thus, personal insecurity is directly related to other insecurities such as environmental (poor working conditions and incarceration) and a lack of community support. Without membership of a community, PLWHA and key populations are made more vulnerable to personal insecurity, resulting in violence.

Community insecurity

Strong community support is beneficial to PLWHA as they are more likely to maintain ART regimes and can rely on help from family and friends for the resources needed to access health care, including voluntary testing and ART medicines (Salmen et al., 2015). However, community insecurity means that many PLWHA and key populations are alienated from these potential support networks. The most common outcome of community insecurity in HIV/AIDS settings is stigma. The issue of stigma has been well documented as having extensive detrimental effects in HIV/AIDS epidemics.

In situations of stigma, PLWHA are isolated from family and friends and bear the burden of the disease unaided. In doing so, they may be forced to visit medical practitioners and take ART medications in secret; and make difficult decisions about their health; and navigate challenging economic situations without support or advice (Salmen et al., 2015). Conversely, they may choose not to access medical advice at all and remain ignorant of their HIV seroconversion. This also has implications for MTCT as women may be aware that breastfeeding can result in vertical transmission of HIV but due to both high costs of replacement formulas and cultural norms that dictate breastfeeding, women may continue to breastfeed rather than risk exposure as a PLWHA (Buesseler, Kone, Robinson, Bakor & Senturia, 2014). This situation is one of high stress and anxiety, which further complicates the lives of HIV+ women.

Thus, in addition to dealing with the challenges of HIV/AIDS without assistance or with very little assistance, PLWHA have to cope with increased stress, anxiety and depression which may lead to thoughts of suicide and, in severe cases, attempts at suicide (Sun, Wu, Qu, Lu & Wang, 2014). Stress has also been linked to lower adherence to ART regimes and negative effects on immune functions, which are compromised in HIV/AIDS infections (Mukund & Gopalan, 2015). In China, the stress, anxiety and depression as a result of stigma have led to 40.1 per cent of PLWHA in a research cohort having thoughts of revenge by deliberately infecting other individuals (Sun et al., 2014). Thus, community insecurity has major implications for the treatment and prevention of HIV/AIDS.

Political insecurity

Political insecurity can have a devastating effect on HIV/AIDS rates of transmission and treatment outcomes. Globally, political insecurity leads to high migration, economic insecurity and personal and community insecurity. Political insecurity is a driver of other insecurity. TasP and an efficient cascade require staff that are trained in its administration and a regular and adequate supply of medications. In situations of conflict, hospitals and medical clinics may be forced to shut down, resulting in disruptions to HIV testing and HIV/AIDS treatment due to drug stocks being diminished. Internal political situations may also impact HIV/AIDS epidemics due to lack of political investment. In most countries domestic HIV responses are inadequate to successfully address the epidemics (Ávila, Loncar, Amico & De Lay, 2013).

Unstable political environments also result in economic insecurity due to displacement and lack of economic development (Alesina, Özler, Roubini & Swagel, 1996). Displacement is a major problem globally with individuals being forced to leave their homes and flee the effects of armed conflict, generalised violence or man-made disasters (Zea et al., 2013). The impact of displacement due to political insecurity and its relationship with HIV/AIDS can fuel HIV epidemics due to rape being used as a weapon of war, economic insecurity, personal insecurity, food insecurity and community insecurity. This loss of community may lead to anxiety, stress and mental health issues, resulting in changed behaviours (Friedman et al., 2013; Zea et al., 2013). These changed behaviours may manifest as high-risk sexual practices and drug-taking.

Insecurity in China's HIV/AIDS epidemics

This chapter has revealed that the seven areas of insecurity that need to be addressed within human security frameworks all overlap and one area of insecurity can cause insecurity in another. This is certainly the case for the HIV/AIDS situation in China. The human insecurity of individuals is manifold and, as a result, the HIV/AIDS epidemics are continuing to spread and become generalised. Economic insecurity is extensive in key populations, particularly for PLWHA, and the results of this are manifest in the lack of affordability to access ART and high levels of food insecurity. This is regardless of the 'Four Free and One Care' initiatives. Considering China's adoption of TasP as their primary methodology for dealing with HIV/AIDS, this presents real problems as high attrition rates and lack of ART initiation (due to lack of finances or other issues related to poverty) mean that optimal outcomes are unattainable.

Food insecurity and health insecurity are particular problems causing leakage in the TasP cascade. The high costs of health care create situations of health insecurity as individuals are often unable to use the health services that are available. Additionally, PLWHA may choose not to attend government-run medical services due to fear of stigma and exposure as FSWs or PWID and the negative implications of that for their personal and community security. Many migrants are still unaware that PLWHA are able to access testing and ART outside of their *hukou*. Food insecurity has been shown to cause high attrition rates and poor nutrition may result in being unable to undertake ART at all (Garcia-Prats, McMeans, Ferry & Klish, 2010). Added to which, the pressures of food insecurity may result in CSWs agreeing to forgo condom usage out of fear of losing a client or in order to receive higher payments for services.

The marginalisation and mobility of key populations and PLWHA in China mean that community insecurity is extensive. Issues related to Confucian values and alienation of populations considered inferior or disgusting prevent individuals from obtaining family support, employment and housing. Many PLWHA in China are loath to expose their family members to public censure and therefore choose to remain ignorant of their status or keep it hidden. This causes high levels of stress, anxiety and depression as they navigate medical services and attempt to maintain ART regimes in secrecy. This in turn may lead to other high-risk behaviours such as injection drug use and lack of protected sex.

Having become disconnected from their communities, PLWHA and key populations are often placed in situations of environmental and personal insecurity. They may be forced into work and living environments that are unsafe and which expose them to violence and sexual predation and abuse. This is particularly the case for TG and MSM populations, as increased stigma and homonegativity may lead to personal attacks, rape and other forms of violence. Often FSWs in lower hierarchies face exposure as street-level sex workers without any of the protection that may be available in establishments. They are vulnerable to sexual violence and being coerced into unprotected sex. They are also likely to be less discriminating when choosing clients (or feel unable to refuse clients) in order to address issues of food insecurity.

Finally, the political situation in China means that PLWHA and key populations face political insecurity. HIV/AIDS is a sensitive topic for China and it is often still disinclined to discuss the situation with outsiders. It is viewed as a state problem and entwined within other issues, such as national border protection (in the case of migrants crossing national borders from Myanmar and Vietnam). State-run newspapers report on HIV/AIDs according to party policy and often do not disseminate inclusive information. Government policy means that prevention and education programmes are insufficient to meet the needs of China's HIV/AIDS epidemics. As a result, China's HIV/AIDS epidemics are continuing to expand and have now crossed into the general population and become sexually driven.

Conclusion

The complex nature of HIV/AIDS epidemics and the societal and personal dynamics inherent in the lives of PLWHA and key populations mean that human security frameworks are essential to make an impact on the present epidemics in China and globally. In HIV/AIDS contexts, insecurity results in high-risk behaviours such as unprotected transactional sex in exchange for food or money to buy food, homelessness, depression, stress and anxiety and an inability to obtain the resources necessary to obtain good health. Economic insecurity leads to PLWHA being unable to afford the medicines and tests needed to maintain ART regimes. Additionally, the ancillary costs such as travel, accommodation and subsequent testing are often prohibitive. Lastly, economic insecurity results in poverty and food insecurity. Without sufficient food security, the significant side effects of ART drug cocktails lead to high attrition rates, sub-optimal regime responses and potentially drug-resistant strains of the virus.

This results in increased vertical and horizontal transmission rates of HIV. Without the medical services needed to address HIV/AIDS, PLWHA become less able to work and more of a burden on family and the community. This generates a cyclical effect where health insecurity creates situations of economic insecurity and food insecurity, which further creates health insecurity. All seven areas of insecurity are impacted by each other. Political insecurity may lead to high mobility, lack of health services and medications and high personal insecurity. High mobility and lack of economic security lead to environmental insecurity in the workplace and homes. Communities also become fractured and individuals are left to navigate homelessness, anxiety, fear and stigma unaided. Ultimately, unless the human insecurity of PLWHA is sustainably addressed, the conditions under which HIV/AIDS continues to spread will continue to hamper efforts to address the problem. Case study 8,1 is an example of situations that may occur due to human insecurity.

Case study 8.1 Lijuan's story

Lijuan's story reveals the difficulties that arise for the families of PLWHA. Often research is concerned with key populations and their impacts on HIV epidemics but far less is understood about how families are affected. Human insecurity has a trickle-down effect. When the member of the family that is generally tasked with being the provider can no longer provide, then, inevitably, a climate of insecurity will result. In China, it is the son's role to care for their elderly parents. In Lijuan's case, the elderly parent has been struggling to care for the sons; those who have not already died from HIV/AIDS-related diseases.

It was a cold winter's day when I went to the village where I met Lijuan. I travelled with a group of people, and from Kunming the journey had taken about two hours. The village was large and bustling and, when driving in, we were surrounded by buildings coated with layers of brown dust as they fronted narrow footpaths and roads filled with holes. The village was very old, I was told, and modern buildings had come to overshadow the small, carved wooden buildings of the past. Every now and then I could see them struggling to peer out from behind the concrete monstrosities that blocked them from view.

The village had been notorious during the time of China's opium upsurge, when it had played a significant role as a part of the trafficking network. Its present remained a reflection of its past as it was still well known as a transit point for drugs that originated in the Golden Triangle and travelled to other parts of China. Everyone in the village seemed to be in a hurry; and car horns clamored in cacophony like some kind of movie soundtrack playing in the background as we drove towards the main street and our prearranged meeting with a local PWID peer worker.

We picked him up on a street corner and as we travelled around town, I chatted with him. He told me that he was HIV+ and had been on a methadone maintenance programme for about two years. He explained to me that it had been a struggle but that he now had a young daughter and desperately wanted to make a good life for her. He shook his head and sighed that it was all too easy to obtain drugs in the town and that there were many drug users. The main drug used was heroin as it was relatively cheap and readily available. On that day he guided us to various locations around town to visit families who were in desperate situations. So, I spent the next few hours meeting people and listening to their stories.

Eventually, the peer worker mentioned that there was an old lady living alone who had no one to help her. And so I tagged along with the group and we went to meet her. In order to get to her home, we had to leave the car and walk through the back streets of the village. We walked past those old wooden buildings with long shutters and carved lintels; and I imagined a past time when men and women dressed in brightly coloured traditional costume would sit at the windows and hurry down the alleyways. The present scene was much less evocative of simpler days, as lounging in those same windows and spread out under carved lintels and down side alleys were PWID. They seemed to have no fear of arrest as they injected themselves in full daylight. Or perhaps they had stopped caring and were simply intent on satisfying their body's need for heroin.

We walked past them as we continued our excursion to see an old woman who had seen more bad things than any of us. We crossed alleyways that were narrow and made of cobblestones; their drains were littered with paper, plastic bottles and other detritus. The further we walked, the more rustic the buildings became. Increasingly, they had thick wooden beams forming door lintels and stoops, embedded within mud and concrete walls. They were all small and closely pressed together, forming a densely populated neighbourhood of dwellings. They were a uniform grey colour, so it was sometimes difficult to tell where one building finished and another began. Eventually, the peer worker ran on ahead of us to let Lijuan know that we were coming so that she had time to prepare herself.

As we approached Lijuan's home, she came out to greet us. My first impression of her was deceptive, as I saw a grey-haired, elderly woman, who was short but very rotund. She seemed to be in good health and obviously eating well. As I got closer, I began to notice the discrepancies. I found it difficult to reconcile the thinness of her face with the bulk of her body. She was shivering in the cold and I realised that she was wearing many layers of clothing. They were old and seemed to have been washed to the point of being threadbare. I asked the peer worker why she was wearing so many layers and he replied that she was wearing everything she owned in order to try and stay warm. Her home had no heating and like many others, she never removed her clothing because she had nothing to replace it with while she laundered. It was too cold for her to remain in her underclothes while waiting for washing to dry.

She invited us into her home, which consisted of two small rooms. The interior was very dark even though it was still full daylight outdoors and when my eyes had adjusted, I realised it was because there was just one small window and the walls were covered in soot. The house had no electricity so Lijuan had to use candles when it became too dark to see anything and over time the smoke from their wicks had stained the walls. The only furniture in the room was a couple of short stools, a little table and a dark wood cupboard holding a small gas burner. The room did not have a sink or running water and in place of this there was a small water bucket. The other room was the size of a closet and simply held a sleeping mat and a covered bucket. There was no bathroom and no toilet in the house. The place was so small that with Lijuan and the two men I was travelling with inside, there was no room for me. Instead I sat on the wooden doorframe and leaned in, ready to listen to their conversation.

However, Lijuan would not settle and was bustling around in the tiny space searching the brown cupboard trying to find food to present to us. In Chinese culture, it is unforgivably rude not to provide guests with refreshments and Lijuan was distressed that she did not have something that she felt was worthy to give us. She found a half head of wilted lettuce and along with a brown substance in a glass jar offered it to us with water from the bucket. Not wanting to eat what was obviously the only food she had we thanked her and explained that we had just come from lunch and could not eat anything more. Lijuan seemed content that we were not in need and began to lower herself to the floor, before one of the men quickly stood up and insisted that she take the stool. Having settled down, she grabbed the hem of her jacket, wiped the tears from her eyes and began to tell us her story.

Lijuan told us that she was 85 years old and had been struggling to get by for a long time. Her husband had died many years previously but she had once had three sons and thought that she would be well cared for. In China, it is the son's duty to care for his elderly parents. Unfortunately for Lijuan, her sons had all become heroin users and all three had contracted HIV through shared needles and risky behaviours. She explained that her eldest son had died of an AIDS-related illness a couple of years previously. The middle son was very sick and could not work. Her youngest son had overdosed at one time and was now mentally handicapped.

Lijuan did what she could to care for him but she was old and did not have the means to support him or his older brother. She said that she did not receive any income but that when she could, she would gather flowers and try and sell them at the market. Sometimes the people who lived nearby would give her food and occasionally they would give her a few yuan but most people in the area were also poor so they could not do so all the time. The lettuce and jar of brown paste that Lijuan had offered us was all the food she had. At the time of our visit she had not eaten anything but lettuce for several days and was destitute but she said that there were times when she went without eating at all.

The men I was with asked her how they could help her. They were also not in a position to offer long-term support. She replied that she thought if she could get enough money together, she might be able to start a small business. Perhaps she would make enough to support herself and her sons. The men told her that they would see what they could do and we prepared to depart. As we all stood and gathered just outside the door of her home, I asked one of the men why the government did not give Lijuan any support. He replied that she must have slipped through the cracks because generally the government would give elderly people with no one to care for them a small stipend.

As she stepped outside, Lijuan was still softly weeping and wiping away the tears. Then, as we turned to go one of the men grabbed her hand and pressed a 100 yuan note into her fingers, an amount that would last her a couple of weeks. Lijuan began sobbing loudly and tried to get the words out to thank all of us. As we left, she followed us, clutching at us as she tried to kneel down in the dirt before us and kiss our feet. Dismayed, we begged her, 'Grandmother, please do not kneel in the dirt at our feet.'

Lijuan's story is by no means an isolated one. It highlights the grave insecurity of people who are affected by HIV/AIDS, either indirectly as family members or directly as PLWHA. This chapter has explained in some detail the impact of human insecurity for these marginalised populations. Food insecurity, health insecurity and economic insecurity have all created conditions of deprivation, stress and hardship for Lijuan and her sons. Without being able to access the necessary finances to generate an income, the outlook for Lijuan is very grim.

In many ways the story of Lijuan is the silent backstory; the challenges faced by PLWHA are more likely to be spoken of but the truth is that HIV/AIDS has more victims than those who test positive. Without government policies in place to address the human security needs of the most vulnerable, there is very little that people can do but try and survive as best they can. In situations like this, individuals will sometimes adopt high-risk behaviours, which further expose them to disease, stigmatisation and marginalisation. For others, like Lijuan, their existence is one of abject poverty, relying on the insecure and irregular generosity of others for survival, many of who are themselves struggling.

References

Aberman, N. L., Rawat, R., Drimie, S., Claros, J. M. & Kadiyala, S. (2014). Food security and nutrition interventions in response to the AIDS epidemic: Assessing global action and evidence. *AIDS and Behavior, 18*(5), 554–565. doi:10.1007/s10461-014-0822-z.

Aidala, A. A., Lee, G., Abramson, D. M., Messeri, P. & Siegler, A. (2007). Housing need, housing assistance, and connection to HIV medical care. *AIDS and Behavior, 11*(2), 101–115.

Ala, J. (2003). AIDS as a new security threat. *From Cape to Congo: Southern Africa's evolving security challenges* (pp. 131–158). Boulder, CO: Lynne Rienner.

Aldis, W. (2008). Health security as a public health concept: A critical analysis. *Health Policy and Planning, 23*(6), 369–375. doi:10.1093/heapol/czn030.

Alesina, A., Özler, S., Roubini, N. & Swagel, P. (1996). Political instability and economic growth. *Journal of Economic Growth, 1*(2), 189–211.

Anema, A., Vogenthaler, N., Frongillo, E. A., Kadiyala, S. & Weiser, S. D. (2009). Food insecurity and HIV/AIDS: Current knowledge, gaps, and research priorities. *Current HIV/AIDS Reports, 6*(4), 224–231.

Antman, F. M. (2013). 16 The impact of migration on family left behind. In A. F. Constant & K. F. Zimmermann (Eds.), *International handbook on the economics of migration*. Cheltenham, UK: Edward Elgar.

Ávila, C., Loncar, D., Amico, P. & De Lay, P. (2013). Determinants of government HIV/AIDS financing: A 10-year trend analysis from 125 low-and middle-income countries. *BMC Public Health, 13*(1), 673. doi:10.1186/1471-2458-13-673.

Benzekri, N. A., Sambou, J., Diaw, B., Sall, F., Niang, A., Ba, S., ... & Gottlieb, G. S. (2015). High prevalence of severe food insecurity and malnutrition among HIV-infected adults in Senegal, West Africa. *PloS ONE, 10*(11), e0141819.

Bhunu, C. P. (2015). Assessing the impact of homelessness on HIV/AIDS transmission dynamics. *Cogent Mathematics, 2*(1021602). http://dx.doi.org/10.1080/23311835.2015.1021602.

Buesseler, H. M., Kone, A., Robinson, J., Bakor, A. & Senturia, K. (2014). Breastfeeding: The hidden barrier in Côte d'Ivoire's quest to eliminate mother-to-child transmission of HIV. *Journal of the International AIDS Society, 17*(1).

Bukusuba, J., Kikafunda, J. K. & Whitehead, R. G. (2007). Food security status in households of people living with HIV/AIDS (PLWHA) in a Ugandan urban setting. *British Journal of Nutrition, 98*(01), 211–217.

Chiu, Y. W., Weng, Y. H., Su, Y. Y., Huang, C. Y., Chang, Y. C. & Kuo, K. N. (2009). The nature of international health security. *Asia Pacific Journal of Clinical Nutrition, 18*(4), 679–683.

Claros, J. M., de Pee, S. & Bloem, M. W. (2014). Adherence to HIV and TB care and treatment, the role of food security and nutrition. *AIDS and Behavior, 18*(5), s.459–s.464. doi:10.1007/s10461-014-0870-4.

Conyers, L. M., Chiu, Y. C., Shamburger-Rousseau, A., Johnson, V. & Misrok, M. (2015). Common threads: An integrated HIV prevention and vocational development intervention for African American women living with HIV/AIDS. *Journal of Health Disparities Research and Practice, 7*(2), 118–140.

Cox, J., Hamelin, A. M., McLinden, T., Moodie, E. E., Anema, A., Rollet-Kurhajec, K. C., ... & Canadian Co-infection Cohort Investigators. (2016). Food insecurity in HIV-hepatitis C virus co-infected individuals in Canada: The importance of co-morbidities. *AIDS and Behavior, 20*(2), 1–11. doi:10.1007/s10461-016-1326-9.

De Cock, K. M., Simone, P. M., Davison, V. & Slutsker, L. (2013). The new global health. *Emerging Infectious Diseases, 19*(8), 1192–1197. http://dx.doi.org/10.3201/eid1908.130121.

Elbe, S. (2010). *Security and global health.* Cambridge, UK: Polity.

Elbe, S. (2011a). Pandemics on the radar screen: Health security, infectious disease and the medicalisation of insecurity. *Political Studies, 59*(4), 848–866. doi:10.1111/j.1467-9248.2011.00921.x.

Elbe, S. (2011b). The art of medicine: Should health professionals play the global health security card? *The Lancet, 377*, 220–221. doi:http://dx.doi.org/10.1016/S0140-6736(11)61114-8.

Elbe, S. (2012). Bodies as battlefields: Toward the medicalization of insecurity. *International Political Sociology, 6*(3), 320–322.

Evans, J. (2010). Pandemics and national security. *Global Security Studies, 1*(1), 100–109. Retrieved from http://globalsecuritystudies.com/Evans%20PANDEMICS.pdf

Friedman, S. R., Sandoval, M., Mateu-Gelabert, P., Rossi, D., Gwadz, M., Dombrowski, K., ... & Perlman, D. (2013). Theory, measurement and hard times: Some issues for HIV/AIDS research. *AIDS and Behavior, 17*(6), 1915–1925.

Garcia-Prats, A. J., McMeans, A. R., Ferry, G. D. & Klish, W. J. (2010). Nutrition and HIV/AIDS. *HIV Curriculum, 286*, 4–5.

Heymann, D. L. (2015). The true scope of health security. In D. L. Heymann, L. Chen, K. Takemi, D. P. Fidler, J. W. Tappero, M. J. Thomas, ... & R. P. Rannan-Eliya. Global health security: The wider lessons from the West African Ebola virus disease epidemic. *The Lancet, 385*(9980), 1884–1887.

Heymann, D. L., Chen, L., Takemi, K., Fidler, D. P., Tappero, J. W., Thomas, M. J., ... & Kalache, A. (2015). Global health security: The wider lessons from the West African Ebola virus disease epidemic. *The Lancet, 385*(9980), 1884–1901.

Ivers, L. C., Cullen, K. A., Freedberg, K. A., Block, S., Coates, J., Webb, P. & Mayer, K. H. (2009). HIV/AIDS, undernutrition, and food insecurity. *Clinical Infectious Diseases, 49*(7), 1096–1102.

Kalichman, S. C., Hernandez, D., Cherry, C., Kalichman, M. O., Washington, C. & Grebler, T. (2014). Food insecurity and other poverty indicators among people living with HIV/AIDS: Effects on treatment and health outcomes. *Journal of Community Health, 39*(6), 1133–1139. doi:10.1007/s10900-014-9868-0.

Kang, E., Delzell, D. A., McNamara, P. E., Cuffey, J., Cherian, A. & Matthew, S. (2015). Poverty indicators and mental health functioning among adults living with HIV in Delhi, India. *AIDS Care*, 1–7. doi:10.1080/09540121.2015.1099604.

Lo, C. Y. P. (2015). *HIV/AIDS in China and India: Governing health security.* Basingstoke UK: Palgrave Macmillan.

Mukund, B. & Gopalan, R. T. (2015). Impact of mental wellbeing and quality of life on depression, anxiety and stress among people living with HIV/AIDS (PLWHA). *The International Journal of Indian Psychology, 3*(1), 5–17.

Nunes, J. (2014). Questioning health security: Insecurity and domination in world politics. *Review of International Studies, 40*(05), 939–960. doi:10.1017/S02602105 14000357.

Pascoe, S. J., Langhaug, L. F., Mavhu, W., Hargreaves, J., Jaffar, S., Hayes, R. & Cowan, F. M. (2015). Poverty, food insufficiency and HIV infection and sexual behaviour among young rural Zimbabwean women. *PloS ONE, 10*(1), e0115290.

Quinn, J. M., Martins, N., Cunha, M., Higuchi, M., Murphy, D. & Bencko, V. (2014). Fragile states, infectious disease and health security: The case for Timor-Leste. *Journal of Human Security, 10*(1), 14–31. doi:10.12924/johs2014.10010014.

Salmen, C. R., Hickey, M. D., Fiorella, K. J., Omollo, D., Ouma, G., Zoughbie, D., ... & Geng, E. (2015). 'Wan Kanyakla' (We are together): Community transformations in Kenya following a social network intervention for HIV care. *Social Science & Medicine, 147*, 332–340.

Shannon, K., Strathdee, S. A., Goldenberg, S. M., Duff, P., Mwangi, P., Rusakova, M., ... & Boily, M. C. (2015). Global epidemiology of HIV among female sex workers: Influence of structural determinants. *The Lancet, 385*(9962), 55–71.

Sun, W., Wu, M., Qu, P., Lu, C. & Wang, L. (2014). Psychological well-being of people living with HIV/AIDS under the new epidemic characteristics in China and the risk factors: A population-based study. *International Journal of Infectious Diseases, 28*, 147–152.

Taylor, S. (2016). An overview of the risk for HIV/AIDS among young women in South Africa: Gender-based violence. *World Academy of Science, Engineering and Technology, International Journal of Medical, Health, Biomedical, Bioengineering and Pharmaceutical Engineering, 10*(5), 179–184.

UNDP (United Nations Development Program). (1994). *Human development report 1994.* Oxford: Oxford University Press.

Weiser, S. D., Young, S. L., Cohen, C. R., Kushel, M. B., Tsai, A. C., Tien, P. C., ... & Bangsberg, D. R. (2011). Conceptual framework for understanding the bidirectional links between food insecurity and HIV/AIDS. *The American Journal of Clinical Nutrition, 94*(6), 1729S–1739S.

Whittle, H. J., Palar, K., Napoles, T., Hufstedler, L. L., Ching, I., Hecht, F. M., ... & Weiser, S. D. (2015). Experiences with food insecurity and risky sex among low-income people living with HIV/AIDS in a resource-rich setting. *Journal of the International AIDS Society, 18*(1), 1–6.

WHO (World Health Organization). (2006). *Basic documents.* Forty-fifth edition, Supplement, October. Geneva, Switzerland: WHO. Retrieved from: www.who.int/governance/eb/who_constitution_en.pdf

Yates, R., Dhillon, R. S. & Rannan-Eliya R. P. (2015). Universal health coverage and global health security. In D. L. Heymann, L. Chen, K. Takemi, D. P. Fidler, J. W. Tappero, M. J. Thomas, ... & R. P. Rannan-Eliya. Global health security: the wider lessons from the West African Ebola virus disease epidemic. *The Lancet, 385*(9980), 1897–1901.

Young, S., Wheeler, A. C., McCoy, S. I. & Weiser, S. D. (2014). A review of the role of food insecurity in adherence to care and treatment among adult and pediatric populations living with HIV and AIDS. *AIDS and Behavior, 18*(5), 505–515.

Zea, M. C., Reisen, C. A., Bianchi, F. T., Gonzales, F. A., Betancourt, F., Aguilar, M. & Poppen, P. J. (2013). Armed conflict, homonegativity and forced internal displacement: Implications for HIV among Colombian gay, bisexual and transgender individuals. *Culture, Health & Sexuality, 15*(7), 788–803.

Conclusion

Heading towards the light

An ant may well destroy an entire dam.

千里之堤溃于蚁穴

It seems counterintuitive to treat a disease rather than the individuals living with it and yet that seems to be the case for HIV/AIDS. Conceptually, in many cases, HIV/AIDS appears to be a disease that has individuals rather than a group of individuals that have a disease. The bodies of PLWHA are treated as battlefields in the ongoing war with HIV/AIDS. The referent object appears to be the HIV-1 virus rather than the individuals living with it and the repercussions it exposes them to on a daily basis. Of course, it is essential to understand the challenges presented by the pathogenesis and epidemiology of the disease and continue to seek ways to prevent its continuing spread. However, in the past, there has been a disproportionate focus on addressing the mechanisms for stopping the spread of the HIV virus rather than recognising the human security deficits faced by PLWHA.

Human security frameworks are intended to address the security of individuals and ensure that they are free from fear and want and are able to live life with dignity. This book is particularly concerned with human security and its seven underpinning processes, namely, economic security, health security, food security, community security, environmental security, personal security and political security, and their applicability in global and Chinese HIV/AIDS contexts. Using Yunnan and the three cohorts – FSWs, PWID and floating migrants – provides an excellent case study for understanding both the history of the disease and the main drivers of the present epidemics. When added to the individual case studies at the end of each chapter, a holistic and comprehensive rendering is possible. Human security's theoretical foundations enable an understanding of China's HIV/AIDS situation in the light of GBP, and reveal the manner in which human security can contribute to the mitigation of HIV/AIDS infectiousness.

HIV/AIDS is a non-traditional threat to security, specifically human security. China's lack of engagement with the concept of human security, and resulting lack of political will to address the health needs of individuals rather than the population as a collective, are resulting in programming shortfalls at a grassroots level. Also, in considering the HIV/AIDS epidemic to be an internal problem for the nation-state, Beijing exhibits a lack of transparency concerning the spread of HIV/AIDS within China. In conjunction with the stigma attached to, and experienced by PLWHA, this is an area that is problematic for researchers as it is difficult to obtain correct figures or to engage with large numbers of stakeholders and key populations in China.

The pathogenesis of HIV and the virus's exploitation of the human body are a challenge in China's HIV/AIDS epidemics. The ability to form recombinant strains, its mutability and the manner in which it targets and destroys the very cells needed to keep it from running rampant, mean that it is a formidable threat to populations. This is seen in the epidemiology of the virus throughout China and the new and emerging circulating recombinant forms (CRFs) in key populations. When added to the challenges and increased infectiousness of individuals who have STIs, the problems surrounding HIV/AIDS conflate into an even more difficult problem. Additionally, the virus's biological abilities are facilitated when individuals fail, whether through lack of education or misunderstanding, to recognise the implications of their behavioural choices. High–risk behaviours increase the chances of infection spreading between individuals. Thus, it is essential that programming which educates individuals and addresses high-risk behaviours be promoted.

Identifying current global best practice (GBP) in HIV/AIDS epidemics and Beijing's responses and adoption of GBP, highlights that current shortfalls in China's approaches to HIV/AIDS programming stem, in part, from their disinclination to increase NGO participation in addressing HIV/AIDS epidemics. It is recommended that Beijing should increase its engagement with NGOs and CBOs to meet the increasing needs of PLWHA. This will become even more essential as HIV/AIDS becomes a chronic health problem rather than a disease leading to death. Finally, Beijing needs to increase its adoption and adaptation of GBP. The initiatives outlined in GBP have proven to be adaptable and effective in disparate HIV/AIDS epidemics globally. While they are not one-size-fits-all approaches, they do provide basic operational guidelines. That is not to suggest that Beijing has not adopted any GBP – methadone maintenance therapy (MMT), stigma reduction, condom programmes, syringe and needle programmes and TasP are all in use in China. However, to be effective in continuing situations, they must make further efforts to 'know your epidemic, know your response' and increase the viability of their cascade of care.

Examining the historical perspective of HIV/AIDS in China and the research concerning the situation for FSWs, PWID and floating migrants in Yunnan, as specific choices due to their historical and present role in HIV AIDS epidemics, reveals that China still has some ground to cover in support of PLWHA. The highly porous nature of the international border areas of Yunnan presents one of the challenges faced by Beijing in controlling HIV/AIDS epidemics. The cross-border movement of people, whether through international checkpoints or informally, provides a challenging environment for implementing prevention and education programmes due to language and financial constraints. There is also a high burden of foreign nationals crossing into China who are HIV+ and in need of health care. China has stepped up services to these individuals where possible but there are many more who receive no assistance at all. Due to the shortfalls in programming in the region, there has been relatively little research done on the needs of key populations in Yunnan and, arguably, the true nature of the HIV/AIDS epidemic in these areas has yet to be made manifest. However, what is clear from the research is that the cross-border trade in sex and drugs continues to drive the epidemic in Yunnan.

Human insecurity is a major challenge in addressing HIV/AIDS in key populations in China. Environments of human insecurity exacerbate high-risk behaviours. The seven specific areas of insecurity (economic insecurity, food insecurity, health insecurity, environmental insecurity, personal insecurity, community insecurity and political insecurity) are particularly damaging for HIV/AIDS key populations. Without addressing the human insecurity and attitudes of individuals within key populations, it is debatable whether systematic, long-term change can be possible. Human security is not possible without first eliminating human insecurity. Providing services without ensuring that they can be accessed equitably and sustainably renders them ineffective in the long term.

For example, although Beijing has committed to providing free ART and care for those contracting opportunistic infections, the associated costs can be insurmountable for many. Being provided with free ART but needing to pay for subsequent costs can make the free medication unaffordable, resulting in many of the HIV+ population who are eligible for ART choosing not to take the medication. Additionally, many of the individuals in key populations are living in conditions of poverty. People who are undernourished are often unable to sustain ART regimes due to the extreme side effects associated with lack of basic nutrition. Ultimately, this results in sub-optimal responses to the medications, high rates of attrition from ART programmes and mismanagement of dosage and suspending medications. One of the potential far-reaching problems associated with this insecurity is the possibility that inconsistent medication usage may lead to further drug-resistant strains of HIV.

A requirement pivotal to the 'freedom from want' concept of human security is the right of individuals to access adequate and safe health care. Health security is essential in the management of HIV/AIDS epidemics. The availability of sustainable, long-term health care and quality medication cannot be over-emphasised. In China, this is complicated by high levels of stigma and the need for PLWHA to attend public clinics for the management of their ART programme. The human security threats faced by individuals have a real and compounding effect on policy decisions at governmental levels. Beijing does not endorse human security frameworks in addressing HIV/AIDS epidemics. Available funding for programmes not directly related to TasP initiatives and the longer-term condom and MMT programmes is limited.

While MSM and TG populations were not a focus of this book, it is clear that there is a paucity of literature addressing the subject in China contexts. The illegal and hidden nature of MSM result in their marginalisation and they become extremely difficult to approach. While the term *ghost people* was applied specifically to TG men in China, it is also appropriate as a label for MSM populations, and PLWHA in general. Considering that China's HIV epidemics are now sexually driven, identifying ways to mitigate the HIV/AIDS epidemic in MSM populations is essential.

A second area that needs further research is the pressure placed on sex workers (both male and female) to induce their clients to engage in drug-taking as a part of commercial or transactional sex exchanges. Additionally, the fact that brothel gatekeepers impose fines on sex workers for being unsuccessful in pushing drugs is indicative of the absolute perseverance they are expected to bring to bear in these situations. Indicators are that this is a relatively new phenomenon and thus an area that has yet to be researched in any sustained manner.

Lastly, there is very little information concerning the burden of HIV/AIDS in migrant populations (whether internal or external) in China. This is an area that would benefit from extensive research as migrants make significant contributions to the spread of HIV/AIDS. Moreover, due to their transitory nature, they are more likely to spread the disease to areas that may currently have low infection rates. Rural migrants, contracting HIV while working in urban centres, when returning home during national holidays, must be considered possible disseminators of infection into rural areas that may be relatively isolated from other key populations.

In the final instance, after distilling the problem down, the real stakeholders are individuals. Rather than state security issues having a trickle-down effect on the populations within national borders, the impact of the disease on individuals generates a kind of capillary motion resulting in security issues spreading upward to impact the state. Thus, using the same rationale, the solutions must also be generated from a bottom-up as well as a top-down approach. To reiterate, HIV/AIDS is a disease that affects individuals not states. The repercussion of individuals living with the virus and infecting others is what affects states. The extensive economic pressures faced by nation-states; the loss of life; the required medical infrastructures; the need for extensive education and prevention campaigns; the breakdown of community structures; and the potential negative impacts of disease on military forces and cross-border diplomatic relationships are all causal sequences. Bottom-up approaches that operate in accordance with the human security prerogatives and consultation of individuals in key populations, whether living with HIV/AIDS or not, are needed to enlighten top-down policy.

The theory presented is lived out in the case studies throughout this book. They are the stories of real people; people who matter. They are representative of hundreds of thousands of similar stories, told by people living in China. People who continue to struggle to be heard over the everyday rhetoric of a government who thinks that it is doing enough to address the problem. China is not alone in this; human insecurity is a recurring theme in HIV/AIDS situations globally. Lijuan asks us to remember a grandmother facing insecurity on a daily basis, destitute because she has somehow slipped through the cracks of government policy.

The story of Yong reveals the lack of dignity or success inherent in mandatory incarceration programmes for PWID, and again, the lack of security for those attempting to reintegrate into a society that does not want them. Guoliang informed us about the dire lack of human security faced by PWID who struggle to survive along China's border regions. The stories of Lily, Daiyu and Ming-Hua revealing the devastating effects of stigmatisation and lack of education about HIV/AIDS and the way that it can result in a lack of security leading to high-risk behaviours. While sex work should not carry the weight of judgment or stigma, it is distressing to have to do it when all you want to do is sell noodles. Lastly, the story of Chen who dedicates his life to helping those who need it most; his frustrations at being unable to get anyone to understand that providing people with the basics that they need for survival is good policy. What all these stories tell us is that if the human security needs of individuals are met, then lives can be transformed, and those ghost people who are currently living in the shadows due to the complications of living with HIV/AIDS can head back towards the light.

Index

For Product Safety Concerns and Information please contact our EU
representative GPSR@taylorandfrancis.com
Taylor & Francis Verlag GmbH, Kaufingerstraße 24, 80331 München, Germany